ICSA Book Series in Statistics

More information about this series at http://www.springer.com/series/13402

Zhezhen Jin • Mengling Liu • Xiaolong Luo
Editors

New Developments in Statistical Modeling, Inference and Application

Selected Papers from the 2014 ICSA/KISS Joint Applied Statistics Symposium in Portland, OR

Springer

Editors
Zhezhen Jin
Mailman School of Public Health
Department of Biostatistics
Columbia University
New York, NY, USA

Mengling Liu
Division of Biostatistics
NYU School of Medicine
New York, NY, USA

Xiaolong Luo
Senior Director, Biostatistics
Celgene Corporation
Summit, NJ, USA

ISSN 2199-0980 ISSN 2199-0999 (electronic)
ICSA Book Series in Statistics
ISBN 978-3-319-42570-2 ISBN 978-3-319-42571-9 (eBook)
DOI 10.1007/978-3-319-42571-9

Library of Congress Control Number: 2016952641

Printed on acid-free paper

This Springer imprint is published by Springer Nature
The registered company is Springer International Publishing AG Switzerland

Reviewers

Ming-Hui Chen, Ph.D.
Department of Statistics
University of Connecticut
215 Glenbrook Road, U-4120
Storrs, CT 06269
E-mail: ming-hui.chen@uconn.edu

Peng Chen, Ph.D.
Celgene Corporation
300 Cornell Drive
Berkeley Heights, NJ 07922
E-mail: pechen@celgene.com

Suktae Choi, Ph.D.
Associate Director, Statistics
Biostatistics and Programming
Celgene Corporation
300 Cornell Drive
Berkeley Heights, NJ 07922
Email: suchoi@celgene.com

Ming Hu, Ph.D.
Division of Biostatistics
Department of Population Health
New York University School of Medicine
650 1st Ave, 5th Floor
New York, NY 10016
Email: Ming.hu@nyumc.org

Xiang Huang, Ph.D.
Division of Biostatistics
Department of Population Health

New York University School of Medicine
650 1st Ave, 5th Floor
New York, NY 10016
Email: Xiang.huang@nyumc.org

Jaehee Kim, Ph.D.
Department of Statistics
Duksung Women's University
419 Ssangmun-Dong Tobong-Ku
Seoul, S. Korea
E-mail: jaehee@duksung.ac.kr

Sung Duk Kim, Ph.D.
Biostatistics and Bioinformatics Branch
Division of Intramural Population Health Research
Eunice Kennedy Shriver National Institute of Child Health and Human Development (NICHD)
National Institutes of Health
6100 Executive Blvd Room 7B05A, MSC 7510
Bethesda, MD 20892-7510
E-mail: kims2@mail.nih.gov

Gang Li, Ph.D.
Director, Integrative Health Informatics
RWE Analytics, Janssen R&D
1125 Trenton-Harbourton Road
Titusville, NJ 08560
E-mail: gli@its.jnj.com

Huiling Li, Ph.D.
Celgene Corporation
300 Connell Drive, 7th FL, 7037
Berkeley Heights, NJ 07922
Email: huili@celgene.com

Kejian Liu, Ph.D.
Celgene Corporation
300 Cornell Drive
Berkeley Heights, NJ 07922
E-mail: kliu@celgene.com

Antai Wang, Ph.D.
Department of Mathematical Sciences
New Jersey Institute of Technology
University Heights
Newark, NJ 07102
E-mail: aw224@njit.edu

Jinfeng Xu, Ph.D.
Department of Statistics and Actuarial Science
The University of Hong Kong
Rm 228, Run Run Shaw Building
Pokfulam Road, Hong Kong
Email: xhjf@hku.hk

Xiaonan Xue, Ph.D.
Albert Einstein College of Medicine
Jack and Pearl Resnick Campus
1300 Morris Park Avenue
Belfer Building, Room 1303C
Bronx, NY 10461
E-mail: xiaonan.xue@einstein.yu.edu

Xiaojiang Zhan, Ph.D.
Celgene Corporation
300 Cornell Drive
Berkeley Heights, NJ 07922
E-mail: xzhan@celgene.com

Yichuan Zhao, Ph.D.
Department of Mathematics and Statistics
726, 7th Floor, College of Education Building, 30 Pryor Street
Georgia State University
Atlanta, GA 30303-3083
E-mail: yichuan@gsu.edu

Zhigen Zhao, Ph.D.
Department of Statistics
Temple University
342 Speakman Hall
1801 N. 13th Street
Philadelphia, PA 19122
E-mail: zhaozhg@temple.edu

Preface

The 2014 Joint Applied Statistics Symposium of the International Chinese Statistical Association and the Korean International Statistical Society was successfully held from June 15 to June 18, 2014, at the Marriott Downtown Waterfront Hotel, Portland, Oregon, USA. It was the 23rd annual Applied Statistics Symposium of the ICSA and the first of the KISS. Over 400 participants attended the conference from academia, industry, and government agencies around the world including North America, Asia, and Europe. The conference offered three keynote speeches, seven short courses, 76 scientific sessions, student paper sessions, and social events.

The 11 papers in this volume were selected from the presentations in the conference. They cover new methodology and application for clinical research and information technology, including model development, model checking, and innovative clinical trial design and analysis. All papers have gone through peer-review process of at least two referees and an editor. We believe they provide invaluable addition to the statistical community.

We would like to thank the authors for their contribution and their patience and dedication.

We also would like to thank referees who devoted their valuable time for the excellent reviews.

New York, NY, USA	Zhezhen Jin
New York, NY, USA	Mengling Liu
Summit, NJ, USA	Xiaolong Luo

Contents

Part III Novel Applications and Implementation

Contributors

Shuming Bao China Data Center, University of Michigan, Ann Arbor, MI, USA

Ming-Hui Chen Department of Statistics, University of Connecticut, Storrs, CT, USA

Ying Chen QFR Capital Management, L.P., New York, NY, USA

Lu Cui Data and Statistical Science, AbbVie Inc., North Chicago, IL, USA

XiaoTian Dai Department of Mathematics and Statistics, Utah State University, Logan, UT, USA

Dipak K. Dey Department of Statistics, University of Connecticut, Storrs, CT, USA

Yuexiao Dong Department of Statistics, Temple University, Philadelphia, PA, USA

Elisa V. Gomez Global Statistical Sciences, Eli Lilly and Company, Indianapolis, IN, USA

Xin He Department of Epidemiology and Biostatistics, University of Maryland, College Park, MD, USA

Xianzheng Huang Department of Statistics, University of South Carolina, Columbia, SC, USA

Xiyun Jiao Statistics Section, Imperial College, London, UK

Rita C. Kuo Joint Genome Institute, Lawrence Berkeley National Laboratory, Walnut Creek, CA, USA

Yang Li Department of Mathematics and Statistics, University of North Carolina at Charlotte, Charlotte, NC, USA

Rong Liu Department of Mathematics and Statistics, University of Toledo, Toledo, OH, USA

Jyoti N. Rayamajhi Global Statistical Sciences, Eli Lilly and Company, Indianapolis, IN, USA

Hikmatali Shariff Astrophysics Group, Imperial College, London, UK

Bing She China Data Center, University of Michigan, Ann Arbor, MI, USA

Miao Shui China Data Center, University of Michigan, Ann Arbor, MI, USA

Jianguo Sun Department of Statistics, University of Missouri, Columbia, MO, USA

Ning Sun IBM Research Center, Beijing, China

Ramachandran Suresh Global Biometric Sciences, Bristol-Myers Squibb, Plainsboro, NJ, USA

Jürgen Symanzik Department of Mathematics and Statistics, Utah State University, Logan, UT, USA

Roberto Trotta Astrophysics Group, Imperial College, London, UK

David A. van Dyk Statistics Section, Imperial College, London, UK

Deli Wang Global Pharmaceutical Research and Development, AbbVie Inc., North Chicago, IL, USA

Haiying Wang Department of Mathematics and Statistics, University of New Hampshire, Durham, NH, USA

Ming-Dauh Wang Global Statistical Sciences, Eli Lilly and Company, Indianapolis, IN, USA

Xia Wang Department of Mathematical Sciences, University of Cincinnati, Cincinnati, OH, USA

Dominique A. Williams Global Statistical Sciences, Eli Lilly and Company, Indianapolis, IN, USA

Haipeng Xing Department of Applied Mathematics and Statistics, State University of New York, Stony Brook, NY, USA

Bo Yang Biometrics, Global Medicines Development & Affairs, Vertex Pharmaceutical, Boston, MA, USA

Ruji Yao Merck Research laboratory, Merck & Co., Inc., Kenilworth, NJ, USA

Zhou Yu East China Normal University, Shanghai, China

Guoyi Zhang Department of Mathematics and Statistics, University of New Mexico, Albuquerque, NM, USA

Lanju Zhang Data and Statistical Science, AbbVie Inc., North Chicago, IL, USA

Yijie Zhou Data and Statistical Science, AbbVie Inc., North Chicago, IL, USA

Part I
Theoretical Development in Statistical Modeling

Dual Model Misspecification in Generalized Linear Models with Error in Variables

Xianzheng Huang

Abstract We study maximum likelihood estimation of regression parameters in generalized linear models for a binary response with error-prone covariates when the distribution of the error-prone covariate or the link function is misspecified. We revisit the remeasurement method proposed by Huang et al. (Biometrika 93:53–64, 2006) for detecting latent-variable model misspecification and examine its operating characteristics in the presence of link misspecification. Furthermore, we propose a new diagnostic method for assessing assumptions on the link function. Combining these two methods yields informative diagnostic procedures that can identify which model assumption is violated and also reveal the direction in which the true latent-variable distribution or the true link function deviates from the assumed one.

1 Introduction

Since the seminal paper of Nelder and Wedderburn (1972), the class of generalized linear models (GLM) has received wide acceptance in a host of applications (McCullagh and Nelder, 1989). Studies in these applications often involve covariates that cannot be measured precisely or directly. For example, in the Framingham Heart Study (Kannel et al., 1986), a logistic regression model was used to relate the indicator for the presence of coronary heart disease with covariates such as one's smoking status, body mass index, age, serum cholesterol level, and long-term systolic blood pressure (SBP). Among these covariates, measures of one's serum cholesterol level were imprecise, and the actual observed blood pressure of a subject is merely a noisy surrogate of the long-term SBP, which cannot be measured directly. Taking the structural model point of view to account for measurement error as opposed to the functional model point of view (Carroll et al., 2006, Sect. 2.1), one needs to assume a model for the latent true covariates in order to derive the observed data likelihood function. Together the latent-covariate model, the model that relates the true covariates with their noisy surrogates, and the GLM as the conditional model of the response given the true covariates, one has the complete specification

X. Huang (✉)
Department of Statistics, University of South Carolina, Columbia, SC 29208, USA
e-mail: huang@stat.sc.edu

Z. Jin et al. (eds.), *New Developments in Statistical Modeling, Inference and Application*, ICSA Book Series in Statistics, DOI 10.1007/978-3-319-42571-9_1

of a structural measurement error model for the observed data. From that point on, one can draw parametric inference on the regression parameters straightforwardly.

Like most model-based inference, the validity of inference derived from the structure measurement error model relies on the assumed latent-variable model as well as the posited GLM. In the measurement error community there is a general concern about imposing models for unobserved covariates, as one can easily make inappropriate assumptions on unobservable covariates that often lead to misleading inference (Huang et al., 2006). The widely entertained GLMs for a binary response often assume one of the popular links such as logistic, probit, and complementary log-log. The choice of these popular links is mostly encouraged by ease of interpretation, the familiarity among practitioners, and its convenient implementation using standard statistical software. However, for one particular application, a link function outside of this popular suite of links may be able to capture the underlying association between the response and covariates more accurately. Li and Duan (1989) studied the properties of regression analysis under a misspecified link function in general regression settings. Czado and Santner (1992) focused on the effects of link misspecification on regression analysis based on GLMs for a binary response. Without considering measurement error in covariates, these authors provided theoretical and empirical evidence of the adverse effects of a misspecified link in GLM on likelihood-based inference. They showed that the maximum likelihood estimators (MLE) of regression coefficients obtained under an inappropriate link can be biased and inefficient.

In this article, we address both sources of model misspecification and propose diagnostic procedures to assess these model assumptions. There are only a handful of diagnostic methods available for testing either one of these assumptions (e.g., Brown, 1982; Huang et al., 2009; Pregibon, 1980; Stukel, 1988), and most existing tests for GLM, with or without error-prone covariates, are omnibus tests designed for testing overall goodness-of-fit (GOF) rather than assessing specific assumptions of a hierarchical model (e.g., Fowlkes, 1987; Hosmer and Lemeshow, 1989; Le Cessie and van Houwelingen, 1991; Ma et al., 2011; Tsiatis, 1980). To the best of our knowledge, there is no existing work that address the dual misspecification considered in our study. Huang et al. (2006) proposed the so-called remeasurement method, referred to as RM henceforth, to detect latent-variable model misspecification in structural measurement error models. This method also has successes in testing latent-variable model assumptions in the bigger class of joint models (Huang et al., 2009), and was later improved to adapt to more challenging data structures (Huang, 2009). To detect link misspecification without involving error-prone covariates, Pregibon (1980) proposed a test derived from linearizing the discrepancy between the assumed link and the true link. His test was developed under the assumption that the assumed link and the true link belong to the same family, which can be a stringent assumption. Moreover, his test fails easily if the local linear expansion of the true link about the assumed link is a poor approximation of the true link. For logistic regression models in the absence of measurement error, Hosmer et al. (1997) compared nine GOF tests for three types of model misspecification, including link misspecification, and found none of these tests have satisfactory power to detect link misspecification.

Inspired by the rationale behind RM, we propose a new diagnostic method initially aiming to detect link misspecification, called the reclassification method, or RC for short. This new method is described in Sect. 2, where we first define generic notations in a structural measurement error model, followed by a brief review of RM. Both RM and RC are motivated by theoretical findings on the effects of either type of misspecification on MLEs. For illustration purposes, we focus on one particular assumed structural measurement error model for the majority of the study and formulate a class of true flexible models. Under such formulation we present properties of the MLEs in the presence of one or both sources of misspecification in Sect. 3. In Sect. 4 we report finite-sample simulation studies to illustrate the performance of the proposed diagnostic procedures. Two real-life data examples are used to demonstrate the implementation of these methods in Sect. 5. Finally, discussions on our findings and follow-up research directions ensue in Sect. 6.

2 Models and Two Diagnostic Methods

2.1 Models

Denote by Y_i the binary response of subject i, for $i = 1, \ldots, n$, and the true distribution of Y_i conditioning on covariates X_i is specified by a GLM,

$$P(Y_i = 1|X_i; \beta) = H(\beta_0 + \beta_1^t X_i), \quad (1)$$

where $\beta = (\beta_0, \beta_1^t)^t$ is the vector of regression coefficients, and $H(s)$ is the inverse link function, assumed to be a nondecreasing and differentiable function of s. For a succinct exposition, we assume a scalar error-prone covariate X_i in the sequel, and the observed covariate, W_i, relates to X_i via a classical measurement error model (Carroll et al., 2006, Sect. 1.2), for $i = 1, \ldots, n$,

$$W_i = X_i + U_i, \quad (2)$$

where $U_i \sim N(0, \sigma_u^2)$ is the nondifferential measurement error (Carroll et al., 2006, Sect. 2.5). Estimation of σ_u^2 is straightforward when replicate measures of each X_i ($i = 1, \ldots, n$) are available (Carroll et al., 2006, Eq. (4.3)). For notational simplicity, σ_u^2 is assumed known in the majority of this article. Lastly, suppose that $\{X_i\}_{i=1}^n$ is a random sample from a distribution specified by the probability density function (pdf) $f_X^{(t)}(x; \tau)$, indexed by parameters τ. The three component models, (1), (2), and $f_X^{(t)}(x; \tau)$, constitute the structural measurement error model, based on which one has the correct likelihood function of the observed data for subject i, (Y_i, W_i), given by $f_{Y,W}^{(t)}(Y_i, W_i; \Omega^{(t)}, \sigma_u^2) = \int \{H(\beta_0 + \beta_1 x)\}^{Y_i} \{1 - H(\beta_0 + \beta_1 x)\}^{1-Y_i} \sigma_u^{-1} \phi\{(W_i - x)/\sigma_u\} f_X^{(t)}(x; \tau) dx$, where $\phi(s)$ is the pdf of the standard normal distribution, and $\Omega^{(t)} = (\beta^t, \tau^t)^t$ is the vector of all unknown parameters under the correct model specification.

Suppose that one assumes the link function to be $J(s)$, which may differ from $H(s)$ in (1), and one posits a model for X_i with pdf give by $f_X(x;\eta)$, indexed by parameters η. Then one has the assumed likelihood function of the observed data for subject i, denoted by $f_{Y,W}(Y_i, W_i; \Omega, \sigma_u^2)$, similarly derived as above, where $\Omega = (\beta^t, \eta^t)^t$ is the p-dimensional vector of all unknown parameters under the assumed model.

2.2 Remeasurement Method and Reclassification Method

It was shown in Huang et al. (2006) that, when the model for the true covariate, that is, the X-model, is misspecified, the MLE of β is usually inconsistent with bias depending on the measurement error variance. By exploiting this dependence, they proposed further contaminating $\{W_i\}_{i=1}^n$ to generate $W_{b,i}^* = W_i + \sqrt{\lambda}\sigma_u Z_{b,i}$, for $b = 1, \ldots, B$, $i = 1, \ldots, n$, where λ is a user-specified positive constant and $Z_{b,i}$'s are independent pseudo errors from $N(0, 1)$. Note that the measurement error variance associated with $\{W_{b,i}^*, b = 1, \ldots, B\}_{i=1}^n$ is equal to $(1 + \lambda)\sigma_u^2$. They then constructed a test statistic based on the difference between the MLE of β, $\hat{\beta}$, computed using the raw data, $\{(Y_i, W_i)\}_{i=1}^n$, and the counterpart MLE, $\hat{\beta}_r$, obtained from the remeasured data, $\{(Y_i, W_i^*)\}_{i=1}^n$, where $W_i^* = (W_{1,i}^*, \ldots, W_{B,i}^*)$, for $i = 1, \ldots, n$. Take β_1 as an example, the test statistic associated with β_1 is defined by $T_{\beta_1} = (\hat{\beta}_1 - \hat{\beta}_{1r})/\hat{v}_{\beta_1}$, where $\hat{v}_{\beta_1}$ is an estimator of the standard error of $\hat{\beta}_1 - \hat{\beta}_{1r}$. Each so-constructed test statistic for a parameter in Ω follows a Student's t distribution with $n - p$ degrees of freedom asymptotically under the null hypothesis that the two MLEs being compared converge to the same limit as $n \to \infty$. If the value of a test statistic deviates significantly from zero, one finds evidence that the assumed latent-variable model is inappropriate. Derivations of the standard error estimator and the proof of the null distribution, omitted here, are given in Huang et al. (2006).

It is assumed in this existing work that all aspects of the structural measurement error model are correctly specified except for the X-model. But one may legitimately question the adequacy of the assumed link in the GLM. And if the link is indeed misspecified, one may wonder if RM can also detect the link misspecification and how its ability to reveal latent-variable model misspecification is affected by this additional misspecification. As an important step in RM, pseudo measurement error are added to the observed covariates $\{W_i\}_{i=1}^n$ to produce the remeasured data. A natural extension of this idea is to add measurement error to the responses $\{Y_i\}_{i=1}^n$. For binary data, measurement error lead to misclassified binary responses. Parallel with adding noise to W to detect latent-variable model misspecification, we propose to detect link misspecification by adding noise to Y, producing the so-called reclassified data. Now one may think of $\hat{\beta}_r$ as the MLE of β obtained from the reclassified data. If $\hat{\beta}$ is biased due to link misspecification, then $\hat{\beta}_r$ is usually also biased. If the bias of $\hat{\beta}_r$ depends on some parameter in the user-specified reclassification model according to which the reclassified data are created, then $\hat{\beta}_r$ can differ noticeably from $\hat{\beta}$. Such difference can serve as evidence of link misspecification. And test statistics like those constructed in RM can be used to quantify the significance of the difference. We refer to this strategy as the reclassification method, or, RC for short.

Under regularity conditions, the MLE of β follows a normal distribution asymptotically, despite the source of model misspecification (White, 1982) and the type of measurement error. Because both RM and RC rely on the discrepancy between the MLEs of β before and after pseudo measurement error are added (to W or Y), one important clue to answering the question, "Does RM/RC work?", is the means of these asymptotic normal distributions associated with the MLEs from data with measurement error (in X or Y) in the presence of different model misspecification. The next section is devoted to studying these asymptotic quantities, i.e., the limiting MLEs of β.

3 Limiting Maximum Likelihood Estimators

3.1 *Estimating Equations*

Denote by β_m and β_c the limiting MLEs of β associated with the raw data and the reclassified data, respectively, as $n \to \infty$. By the theory of maximum likelihood estimation in the presence of model misspecification (White, 1982), β_m and β_c uniquely satisfy the following score equations respectively,

$$E_{\mathrm{W}}\left[E_{\mathrm{Y|W}}\left\{(\partial/\partial\beta)f_{\mathrm{Y,W}}(Y_i, W_i; \Omega, \sigma_u^2)|_{\beta=\beta_m}\right\}\right] = 0, \tag{3}$$

$$E_{\mathrm{W}}\left[E_{\mathrm{Y^*|W}}\left\{(\partial/\partial\beta)f_{\mathrm{Y^*,W}}(Y_i^*, W_i; \Omega, \sigma_u^2)|_{\beta=\beta_c}\right\}\right] = 0, \tag{4}$$

where $f_{\mathrm{Y^*,W}}(Y_i^*, W_i; \Omega, \sigma_u^2)$ is the likelihood of the reclassified data for subject i, (Y_i^*, W_i), and the subscripts attached to "E" signify that the expectations are defined with respect to the relevant true model.

In order to focus on inference for β, we treat the parameters in the assumed X-model, η, as known constants in (3) and (4). Although in practice one has to estimate η along with β, this seemingly unrealistic treatment of η does not make the follow-up theoretical findings less practically valuable if η can be estimated consistently (in some sense). Consistent estimation of η in the presence of model misspecification is often possible in many scenarios. For example, when both the assumed and the true X-models can be fully parameterized via some moments (included in η) up to a finite order, the interpretation of η remains meaningful even if the assumed X-model differs from the true model, and hence one can still conceptualize the "true" value of η, which are simply the moments of the true X-distribution. Moreover, such η usually can be consistently estimated, say, using the method of moments based on $\{W_i\}_{i=1}^n$, even in the presence of dual misspecification.

In general, the above estimating equations cannot be solved explicitly, thus closed form expressions of their solutions, β_m and β_c, are usually unattainable. Without sacrificing too much the generality of the theoretical investigation, we next formulate the assumed model and true models that make these limiting MLEs more transparent.

3.2 Assumed and True Models

For tractability, we fix the assumed structural measurement error model at the probit-normal model, which is one of the favorite toy examples entertained in the measurement error literature. In this model, one posits a probit link in the primary model (1) and assumes $X \sim N(\mu_x, \sigma_x^2)$. As for the true model, we formulate a class of the so-called mixture-probit-normal models, which contains the probit-normal model as a special member. In this class of true models, the link function $H(s)$ is the cdf of a two-component mixture normal, referred to as the mixture probit. With a mixture probit link, the primary model is a GLM given by

$$P(Y_i = 1|X_i; \beta) = \alpha\Phi\left(\frac{\beta_0 + \beta_1 X_i - \mu_1}{\sigma_1}\right) + (1-\alpha)\Phi\left(\frac{\beta_0 + \beta_1 X_i - \mu_2}{\sigma_2}\right), \quad (5)$$

where $\alpha \in [0, 1]$, μ_k and $\sigma_k > 0$ $(k = 1, 2)$ are chosen such that the corresponding mixture normal, $\alpha N(\mu_1, \sigma_1^2) + (1-\alpha)N(\mu_2, \sigma_2^2)$, is of zero mean and unit variance. The true X-model in this class is a mixture normal.

To achieve explicit likelihood for the reclassified data without being overly restrictive in the creation of reclassified data, we consider reclassification models of the form $P(Y_i^* = Y_i|W_i) = \pi_i$, for $i = 1, \ldots, n$, according to which the reclassified responses, $\{Y_i^*\}_{i=1}^n$, are generated. Combining the assumed raw-data likelihood, $f_{Y,W}(Y_i, W_i; \Omega, \sigma_u^2)$, and the reclassification model yields the likelihood of (Y_i^*, W_i) under the probit-normal model, $f_{Y^*,W}(Y_i^*, W_i; \Omega, \sigma_u^2)$.

Under the formulated assumed and true models, all needed ingredients for deriving the score equations in (3) and (4) become available in closed form. These ingredients include the true mean of Y_i and Y_i^* given W_i, the assumed-model likelihood for the raw data, $f_{Y,W}(Y_i, W_i; \Omega, \sigma_u^2)$, and that for the reclassified data, $f_{Y^*,W}(Y_i^*, W_i; \Omega, \sigma_u^2)$, the true-model likelihood for both types of data, $f_{Y,W}^{(t)}(Y_i, W_i; \Omega^{(t)}, \sigma_u^2)$ and $f_{Y^*,W}^{(t)}(Y_i^*, W_i; \Omega^{(t)}, \sigma_u^2)$. The explicit expressions of these quantities are provided in Appendix 1. Some interesting findings regarding β_m and β_c are presented next, in which we only consider cases where $\beta_1 \neq 0$. The special case with $\beta_1 = 0$ is discussed in Appendix 2, where the expressions of β_m and β_c are derived. This is a rare case where (3) and (4) can be solved explicitly, and also a rare case where the MLE of β_1 is consistent despite the type of model misspecification. When $\beta_1 \neq 0$, although (3) and (4) cannot be solved explicitly, we are able to make use the aforementioned intermediate results in Appendix 1 to study the limiting MLEs.

3.3 Limiting MLEs from Data with Measurement Error Only in X

Fixing the assumed model at the probit-normal model, we consider combinations of five true links and five true X-distributions in the formulation of the true model. The five true links are, (L0) probit link, and four mixture probit links with the following parameter configurations: (L1) $\alpha = 0.3$, $\mu_1 = 0.3$, $\sigma_1 = 0.1$; (L2) $\alpha = 0.3$, $\mu_1 = -0.3$, $\sigma_1 = 0.1$; (L3) $\alpha = 0.7$, $\mu_1 = 0.5$, $\sigma_1 = 0.2$; (L4) $\alpha = 0.7$, $\mu_1 = -0.5$, $\sigma_1 = 0.2$. The upper panels of Fig. 1 depict these five links. For two link functions, $H_1(s)$ and $H_2(s)$, we say that $H_1(s)$ and $H_2(s)$ are symmetric of each other if $H_1(s) = 1 - H_2(-s)$. Among the four mixture probit links, (L1) and (L2) are symmetric of each other, and (L3) and (L4) are symmetric of each other, with the latter two links deviating from probit more than the former two. The five true X-distributions are, (D0) $N(0, 1)$, and four mixture normals with mean zero and variance one formulated by varying the mixing proportion ζ, skewness ξ, and excessive kurtosis κ as follows: (D1) $\zeta = 0.3$, $\xi = -1$, $\kappa = 2$; (D2) $\zeta = 0.3$, $\xi = 1$, $\kappa = 2$; (D3) $\zeta = 0.1$, $\xi = -1.5$, $\kappa = 2$; (D4) $\zeta = 0.1$, $\xi = 1.5$, $\kappa = 2$. The lower panels of Fig. 1 show the pdf's of these five distributions. Among the four mixture normal distributions, (D1) and (D2) are symmetric of each other, and (D3) and (D4) are symmetric of each other, with the latter pair deviating from normal further than the former pair. In the true GLM in (5), we set $\beta_0 = 0$ and $\beta_1 = 1$. For ease of presentation, we use "$\curlywedge$" to connect a true X-model with a true link to refer to a true model specification. For example, (D1)$\curlywedge$(L3) refers to the true model with X following a distribution specified by (D1) and the link configured according to (L3).

Under each of the above true model specifications, we numerically solve (3) for β_m. Figure 2 presents β_m under different true models as σ_u^2 increases from 0 to 1. This range of σ_u^2 yields a reliability ratio ω that drops from 1 to 0.5, where $\omega = \sigma_x^2/(\sigma_x^2 + \sigma_u^2)$. The top panels of Fig. 2, where the true X-model coincides with the assumed, show that β_m only changes slightly as σ_u^2 increases in the presence of link misspecification. This suggests that, unless information in both the raw data and the remeasured data are rich enough to allow detection of the weak dependence of β_m on σ_u^2, RM will have low power to detect link misspecification despite the amount of bias in β_m due to link misspecification. When the true X-model deviates from normal (see the middle and the bottom panels of Fig. 2), although the dependence of β_{1m} on σ_u^2 is stronger than before, β_{1m} changes noticeably mainly over a narrow range of σ_u^2. This phenomenon for cases with dual misspecification indicates that, although RM has been shown to be effective in diagnosing latent-variable model misspecification, its power in this regard can be substantially compromised by the coexistence of link misspecification.

Besides Fig. 2, we show analytically in Appendix 3 that, under certain conditions, β_{1m} is unchanged by a symmetric flip of either the true X-distribution or the true link, and only β_{0m} is affected. This property is stated next, with empirical justification relegated to Appendix 5.

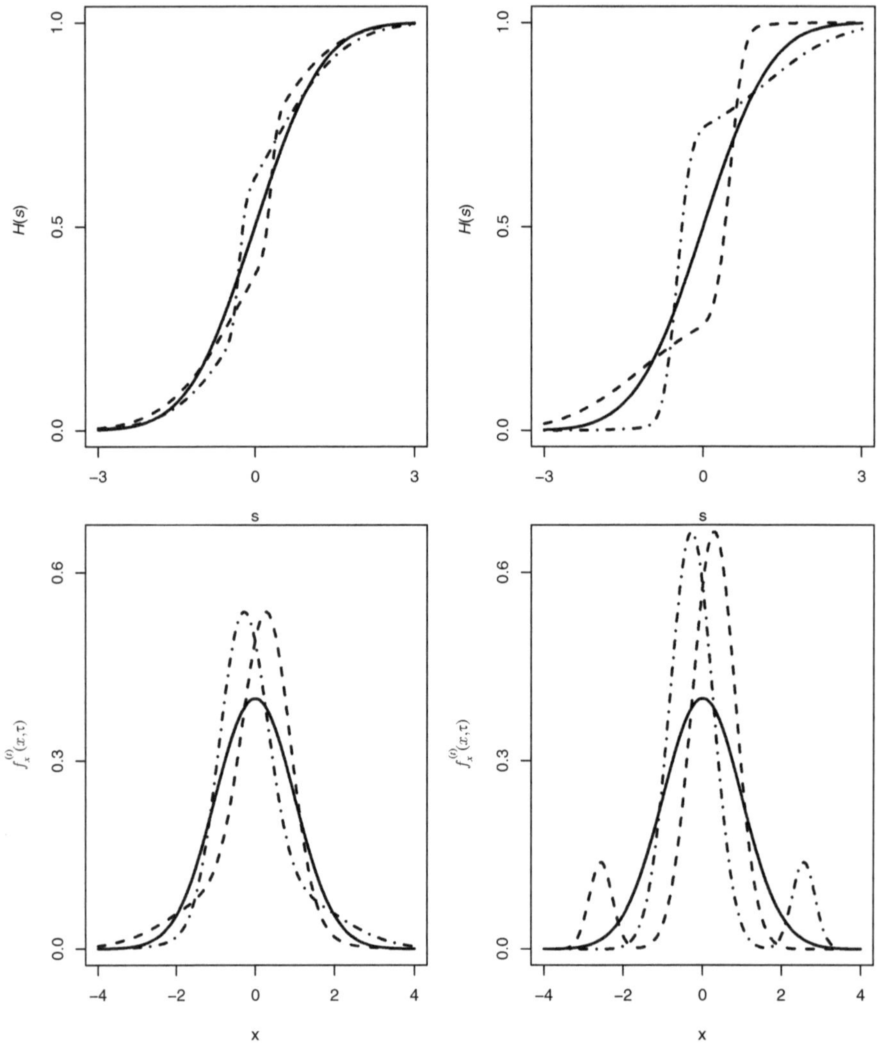

Fig. 1 *Upper panels* give four mixture probit links formulated in Sect. 3.3, where the *upper left panel* gives link (L1) (*dashed line*) and link (L2) (*dot-dashed line*), and the *upper right panel* gives link (L3) (*dashed line*) and link (L4) (*dot-dashed line*). *Solid lines* are the probit link. *Lower panels* show four mixture normal density functions formulated in Sect. 3.3, where the *lower left panel* gives distributions (D1) (*dashed line*) and (D2) (*dot-dashed line*), and the *lower right panel* gives distributions (D3) (*dashed line*) and (D4) (*dot-dashed line*). *Solid lines* are the density function of $N(0,\ 1)$

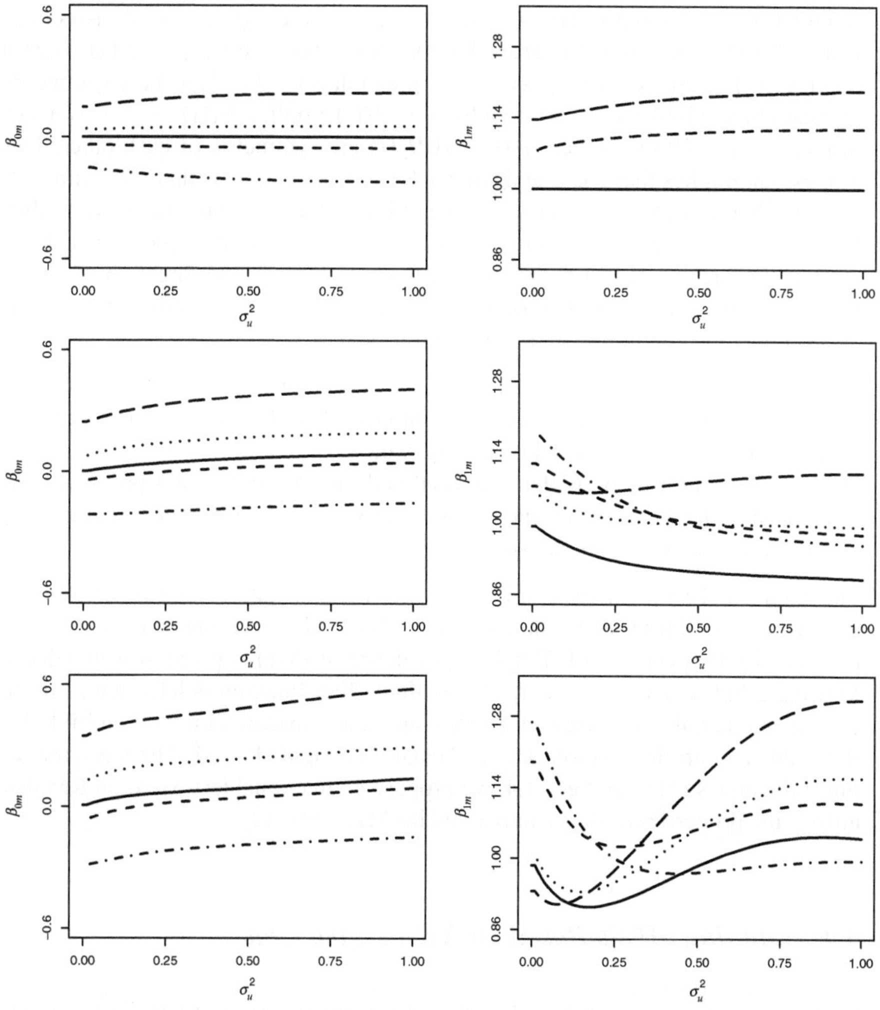

Fig. 2 Plots of β_{0m} (*left column*) and β_{1m} (*right column*) versus σ_u^2 when fixing the true X-model at $N(0, 1)$ (*top row*), (D1) (*middle row*), and (D3) (*bottom row*), respectively, then varying the true link among the five links: probit (*solid lines*), (L1) (*short dashed lines*), (L2) (*dotted lines*), (L3) (*dot-dashed lines*), and (L4) (*long dashed lines*)

Proposition 3.1. *Let $f_1(x)$ and $f_2(x)$ be two pdf's specifying two true X-distributions that are symmetric of each other, and let $H_1(s)$ and $H_2(s)$ be two true links that are symmetric of each other. Denote by $\beta_m^{(jk)}$ the limiting MLE of β based on data with measurement error only in X when the true model is $f_j(x) \curlywedge H_k(s)$, for $j, k = 1, 2$. If $E(X) = \beta_0 = 0$, then $\beta_{0m}^{(11)} = -\beta_{0m}^{(22)}$ and $\beta_{1m}^{(11)} = \beta_{1m}^{(22)}$.*

Note that Proposition 3.1 includes two special cases: one is when $H_1(s) \neq H_2(s)$ and $f_1(x) = f_2(x) = f(x)$, where $f(x)$ is a pdf symmetric around zero; the other is when $f_1(x) \neq f_2(x)$ and $H_1(s) = H_2(s) = H(s)$, where $H(s)$ is the cdf associated with a distribution symmetric around zero. This is because $f_1(x) = f_2(x) = f(x)$ implies $f_1(x) = f_2(-x)$, since $f(x) = f(-x)$, and thus $f_1(x)$ and $f_2(x)$ are symmetric of each other. Similarly, $H_1(s) = H_2(s) = H(s)$ implies $H_1(s) = 1 - H_2(-s)$, as $H(s) = 1 - H(-s)$, hence $H_1(s)$ and $H_2(s)$ are symmetric of each other. This proposition implies that β_{0m} can distinguish two true X-models that are symmetric of each other, and can also tell apart two true links that are symmetric of each other. For the purpose of model diagnosis, one can exploit this and other properties of β_{0m} to obtain a directional test based on RM that can identify the direction of model misspecification. This potential of RM is supported by the following observations of β_{0m} under the conditions stated in Proposition 3.1:

(M1) Despite the skewness of the true link, when the true X-model is not normal, β_{0m} is increasing in σ_u^2 when the true X-model is left-skewed, and it is decreasing in σ_u^2 when the true X-model is right-skewed.

(M2) When the true X-model is normal and the true link is not probit, β_{0m} is increasing in σ_u^2 when the true link is right-skewed, and it is decreasing in σ_u^2 when the true link is left-skewed.

The middle and bottom panels of Fig. 2, which are associated with two left-skewed true X-models, illustrate the first half of (M1), and the second half of (M1) is indicated by Proposition 3.1. Empirical evidence of (M1) is given in Appendix 5. Viewing a link function as a cdf, we say that a link function is left-skewed if the corresponding pdf is left-skewed. Among the four considered mixture probit links, (L1) and (L3) are left-skewed and (L2) and (L4) right-skewed. The top panel of Fig. 2 illustrates (M2). In Sect. 4.4, we propose a directional test based on RM that utilizes the properties of β_{0m} summarized in (M1) and (M2).

3.4 Limiting MLEs Based on Reclassified Data

Under the same configurations for the assumed/true models as in Sect. 3.3, we solve (4) numerically for β_c based on reclassified data generated according to the reclassification model $P(Y_i^* = Y_i|W_i) = \Phi(W_i + \gamma)$, for $i = 1, \ldots, n$, where γ is a constant. Figure 3 presents β_c when $\gamma = 0$, which shows stronger dependence on σ_u^2 compared to Fig. 2, especially for β_{0c}. This implies that, if one applies RM to the reclassified data, T_{β_0} can be much more significant than the counterpart test statistic from RM only (without adding noise to Y).

Viewing β_c as a function of γ and thinking of β_c as $\beta_c(\gamma)$ symbolically, Fig. 4 presents $\beta_c(-2) - \beta_c(0)$ as σ_u^2 varies. This figure reveals that the changes in β_c as γ changes can be substantial when σ_u^2 is small. This phenomenon suggests that RC alone (without adding further noise to W) can have good power to detect X-model misspecification or link misspecification, and the power is higher when the error contamination in X is milder. If the X-model is correctly specified, both β_{0c} and β_{1c} can change substantially as γ varies when σ_u^2 is fixed at a lower level,

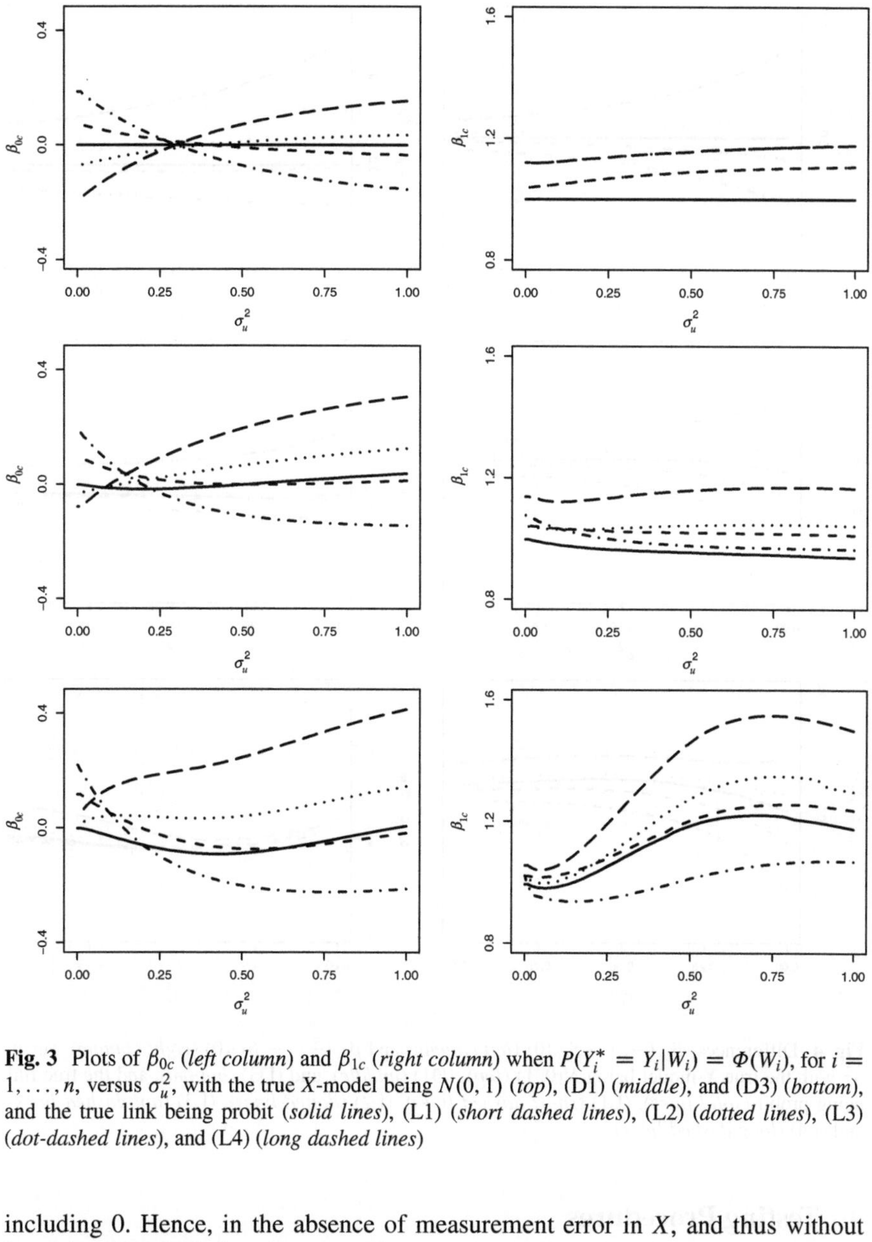

Fig. 3 Plots of β_{0c} (*left column*) and β_{1c} (*right column*) when $P(Y_i^* = Y_i|W_i) = \Phi(W_i)$, for $i = 1, \ldots, n$, versus σ_u^2, with the true X-model being $N(0, 1)$ (*top*), (D1) (*middle*), and (D3) (*bottom*), and the true link being probit (*solid lines*), (L1) (*short dashed lines*), (L2) (*dotted lines*), (L3) (*dot-dashed lines*), and (L4) (*long dashed lines*)

including 0. Hence, in the absence of measurement error in X, and thus without involving RM, RC alone is expected to possess some power to detect moderate to severe link misspecification.

In Appendix 4, we show that, if the reclassification model is $P(Y_i^* = Y_i|W_i) = \pi(W_i)$, where $\pi(t)$ is an even function or when $\pi(t)$ satisfies $\pi(-t) = 1-\pi(t)$, then β_c has the same property of β_m under the same conditions stated in Proposition 3.1. Empirical justification of this finding are given in Appendix 5.

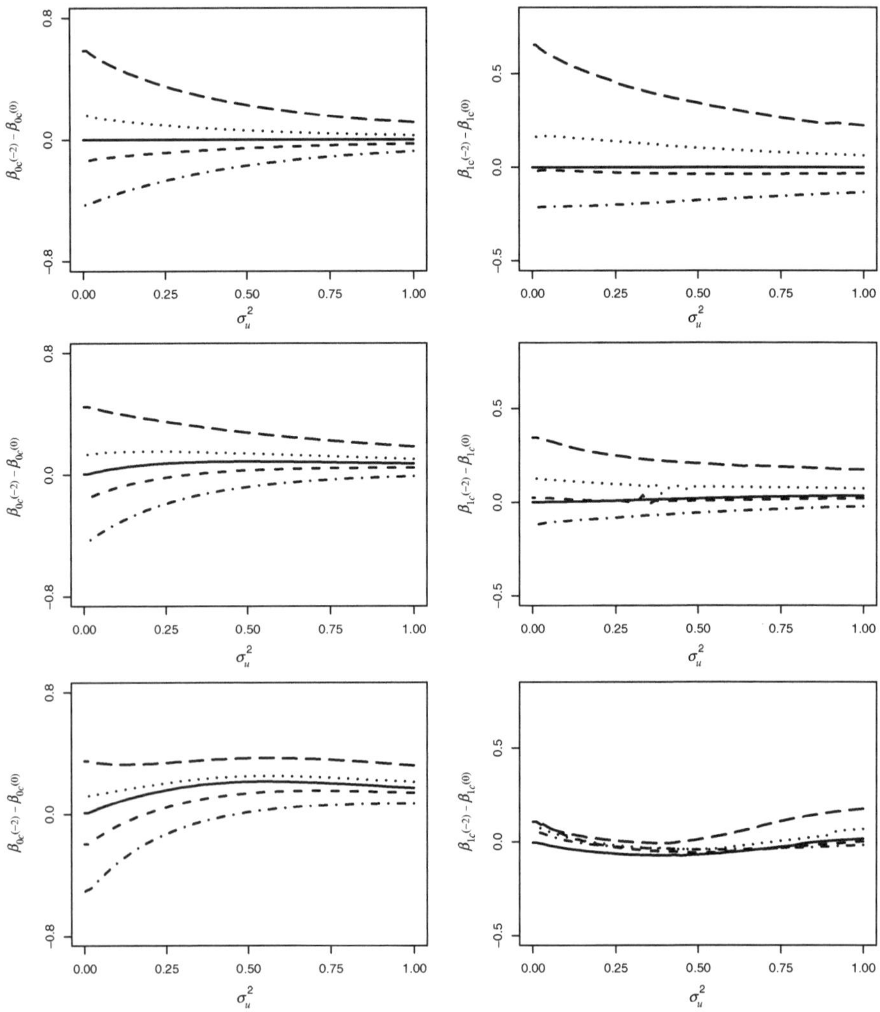

Fig. 4 Differences, $\beta_{0c}(-2) - \beta_{0c}(0)$ (*left column*) and $\beta_{1c}(-2) - \beta_{1c}(0)$ (*right column*), versus σ_u^2 with the true X-model being $N(0, 1)$ (*top*), (D1) (*middle*), and (D3) (*bottom*), and the true link being probit (*solid lines*), (L1) (*short dashed lines*), (L2) (*dotted lines*), (L3) (*dot-dashed lines*), and (L4) (*long dashed lines*)

4 Testing Procedures

The investigation in Sect. 3 on the limiting MLEs of β based on data with measurement error in X or Y in the presence of X-model misspecification or link misspecification are helpful for understanding the operating characteristics of the test statistics, T_{β_0} and T_{β_1}. When the true model is not in the class of mixture-probit-normal models, and the assumed model is probit-normal, the phenomena described in Sects. 3.3 and 3.4 that motivate the upcoming testing strategies are still observed in extensive simulations we carried out. Some of these simulation studies are presented in the upcoming subsections.

Similar comments apply to scenarios where the assumed model is the logit-normal model. This point is practically less relevant because, although one cannot choose a true model in reality, one can choose an assumed model and use it as a reference model for the purpose of exploring features of the unknown true model. Hence, with well-grounded and effective testing procedures developed with a probit-normal assumed model, using this particular assumed model serves the purpose of diagnosing model misspecification well enough. Regardless, for completeness, we present some simulation results in Appendix 5 where the assumed model is a logit-normal model. In this section, we keep the assumed model as probit-normal to first study via simulation the operating characteristics of the aforementioned test statistics resulting from three diagnostic methods: first, RM; second, RC; third, a hybrid method that combines RM and RC. Then we propose more informative testing procedures that can disentangle two sources of misspecification and point at the direction of misspecification.

4.1 Simulation Design

Fixing the sample size n at 500, we create the raw data, $\{(Y_i, W_i)\}_{i=1}^n$, from different true models resulting from varying three factors in the simulation experiments. The first factor is the true X-model, taking five levels (D0)–(D4) as defined in Sect. 3.3. The second factor is the true link function, for which we consider seven true links, (L0)–(L4), i.e., the probit and mixture-probit links formulated in Sect. 3.3, and two generalized logit links (Stukel, 1988), referred to as (L5) and (L6). These two generalized logit links are symmetric of each other, with (L5) left-skewed and (L6) right-skewed, as depicted in Fig. 5. The third factor is the value of σ_u^2 used to generate $\{W_i\}_{i=1}^n$ according to (2), with four values leading to reliability ratio ω ranging from 0.7 to 1 at increments of 0.1. Under each simulation setting, 1000 Monte Carlo (MC) replicates are generated. After each replicate is generated, assuming a probit-normal model, we compute T_{β_0} and T_{β_1} associated with the aforementioned three diagnostic methods.

When implementing RM, $\hat{\beta}_r$ is the MLE from the remeasured data $\{(Y_i, W_i^*)\}_{i=1}^n$, where $W_i^* = (W_{1,i}^*, \ldots, W_{B,i}^*)$, in which $W_{b,i}^* = W_i + \sigma_u Z_{b,i}$, with $Z_{b,i} \sim N(0, 1)$ independent across $b = 1, \ldots, B$, $i = 1, \ldots, n$, and $B = 100$. When carrying out RC, $\hat{\beta}_r$ is the estimate computed from the reclassified data, $\{(Y_i^*, W_i)\}_{i=1}^n$, where the reclassified responses, $Y_i^* = (Y_{1,i}^*, \ldots, Y_{B,i}^*)$, for $i = 1, \ldots, n$, are generated according to $P(Y_{b,i}^* = Y_i|W_i) = \Phi(W_i)$. When employing the hybrid method, we first generate $\{W_{b,i}^*, b = 1, \ldots, B\}_{i=1}^n$ as in RM above, then the reclassified responses are generated according to $P(Y_{b,i}^* = Y_i|W_{b,i}^*) = \Phi(W_{b,i}^*)$; finally one obtains $\hat{\beta}_r$ based on the hybrid data that have measurement error in both X and Y, $\{(Y_{b,i}^*, W_{b,i}^*),$

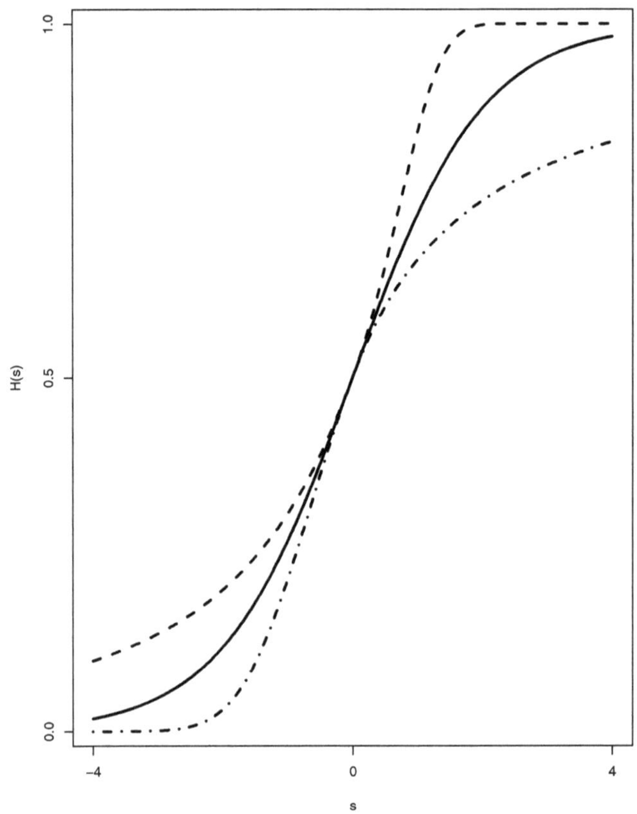

Fig. 5 Two generalized logit links, (L5) (*dashed line*) and (L6) (*dot-dashed line*), in comparison with the logit link (*solid line*)

$b = 1, \ldots, B\}_{i=1}^{n}$. Using a significance level of 0.05, we monitor how often the value of a test statistic turns out significant, leading to rejection of a null hypothesis, which states that two MLEs being compared in the test statistic have the same limit as $n \to \infty$.

4.2 Simulation Results

Table 1 presents the rejection rate of each test statistic under each simulation setting across 1000 MC replicates for a representative subset of all considered true-model configurations. This subset of true models includes five models belonging to the class of mixture-probit-normal models, (D3)⋏(L0), (D0)⋏(L3), (D3)⋏(L3), (D4)⋏(L3), and (D3)⋏(L4); and four models in the class of generalized-logit-normal models, (D0)⋏(L5), (D3)⋏(L5), (D4)⋏(L5), and (D3)⋏(L6). Among these nine

Table 1 Rejection rates across 1000 Monte Carlo replicates of each test statistic under each testing procedure considered in Sect. 4 at different levels of reliability ratio ω when the assumed model is probit-normal

		$\omega = 0.7$			$\omega = 0.8$			$\omega = 0.9$			$\omega = 1$		
True model		RM	RC	HB	RM	RC	HB	RM	RC	HB	RM	RC	HB
(D3)⋏(L0)	T_{β_0}	0.99	0.53	0.85	1.00	0.40	0.75	1.00	0.23	0.38	0	0.09	0.09
	T_{β_1}	0.47	0.51	0.39	0.81	0.52	0.41	0.93	0.34	0.23	0	0.07	0.07
(D0)⋏(L3)	T_{β_0}	0.18	0.75	0.72	0.31	0.92	0.92	0.48	0.98	0.99	0	1.00	1.00
	T_{β_1}	0.04	0.08	0.06	0.05	0.09	0.08	0.08	0.08	0.09	0	0.06	0.06
(D3)⋏(L3)	T_{β_0}	0.82	0.09	0.08	0.88	0.44	0.16	0.76	0.80	0.90	0	0.70	0.70
	T_{β_1}	0.58	0.09	0.05	0.67	0.11	0.16	0.59	0.36	0.62	0	0.63	0.63
(D4)⋏(L3)	T_{β_0}	1.00	0.89	0.97	1.00	0.89	0.96	1.00	0.96	0.96	0	1.00	1.00
	T_{β_1}	0.03	0.53	0.66	0.10	0.74	0.83	0.45	0.81	0.84	0	0.80	0.80
(D3)⋏(L4)	T_{β_0}	1.00	0.85	0.97	1.00	0.89	0.96	1.00	0.95	0.96	0	1.00	1.00
	T_{β_1}	0.03	0.55	0.69	0.11	0.74	0.82	0.45	0.82	0.83	0	0.74	0.74
(D0)⋏(L5)	T_{β_0}	0.08	0.36	0.36	0.13	0.54	0.53	0.18	0.73	0.73	0	0.91	0.91
	T_{β_1}	0.03	0.06	0.06	0.04	0.07	0.06	0.05	0.08	0.09	0	0.06	0.06
(D3)⋏(L5)	T_{β_0}	0.41	0.05	0.21	0.57	0.09	0.06	0.61	0.35	0.17	0	0.89	0.89
	T_{β_1}	0.05	0.08	0.16	0.06	0.06	0.10	0.06	0.05	0.05	0	0.10	0.10
(D4)⋏(L5)	T_{β_0}	0.95	0.86	0.98	1.00	0.89	0.99	1.00	0.89	0.97	0	0.80	0.80
	T_{β_1}	0.54	0.70	0.63	0.87	0.78	0.79	0.96	0.75	0.75	0	0.50	0.50
(D3)⋏(L6)	T_{β_0}	0.90	0.85	0.99	0.99	0.87	0.99	1.00	0.83	0.95	0	0.69	0.69
	T_{β_1}	0.46	0.67	0.65	0.73	0.72	0.77	0.89	0.65	0.71	0	0.45	0.45

true-models configurations, (D3)⋏(L0) represents the scenario where only the X-model is misspecified, (D0)⋏(L3) and (D0)⋏(L5) represent the case where only the link is misspecified, and the remaining six configurations represent cases with dual misspecification. Albeit not included in Table 1, we observe rejection rates for all tests well controlled at around 0.05 when the true model is (D0)⋏(L0), that is, when there is no model misspecification. Some noteworthy observations regarding RM and RC from the simulation are summarized in the following three remarks.

Remark 1. When $\sigma_u^2 = 0$, that is, the covariate is measured without error ($\omega = 1$), RM can detect neither source of misspecification. This is due to the definition of the remeasured data, $W_{b,i}^* = W_i + \sqrt{\lambda}\sigma_u Z_{b,i}$, resulting in the remeasured data identical to the raw data when $\sigma_u^2 = 0$. In contrast, when $\sigma_u^2 = 0$, RC has impressive power to detect link misspecification, whether or not the X-model is also misspecified.

Remark 2. When $\sigma_u^2 \neq 0$, the power of RM to detect X-model misspecification surpasses that of RC if this is the only source of misspecification; but when only the link is misspecified, the test based on T_{β_0} from RC is the clear winner in detecting link misspecification, whose power increases as σ_u^2 decreases.

Remark 3. Although RM is designed for detecting X-model misspecification, and RC is proposed aiming at detecting link misspecification, each of them can be influenced in nontrivial ways by the other source of misspecification. Take RM as an example. When only the X-model is misspecified, such as case (D3)⅄(L0) in Table 1, RM is expectedly effective in picking up this type of misspecification. But its power is mostly weakened by the additional link misspecification as in case (D3)⅄(L3). Note that, when the true model is (D3)⅄(L3), the directions of the two misspecification are the same in the sense that the true X-model is left-skewed and so is the true link. This tampering effect on the power of RM due to the added link misspecification is not observed for T_{β_0} when the dual misspecification are of opposite directions, such as in cases (D3)⅄(L4) and (D3)⅄(L6). Similar nontrivial patterns are observed for RC when X-model misspecification is added on top of link misspecification. In summary, whether or not the added misspecification compromises the power of a method to detect the type of misspecification it is originally designed for depends on how the two types of misspecification interact.

Although the empirical power associated with T_{β_1} from RM lingers around 0.60 in the case (D3)⅄(L3) when $\omega = 0.7, 0.8$, and 0.9, it drops to around 0.33 and 0.22 when $\omega = 0.6$ and 0.55 (not included in Table 1), respectively. This abrupt drop in power can be explained by the large-sample phenomenon in Sect. 3.3 depicted in Fig. 2. It is pointed out there that, in the presence of dual model misspecification, as in case (D3)⅄(L3), β_{1m} changes noticeably mainly over a narrow (lower) range of σ_u^2. For this case in particular, as shown in the lower right panel of Fig. 2 (with the dot-dashed line referring to case (D3)⅄(L3)), β_{1m} stays nearly flat soon after σ_u^2 passes 0.25 (i.e., soon after ω drops below 0.8). The (nearly) flat region of σ_u^2 or ω is where T_{β_1} from RM exhibits low power.

Finally, the hybrid method is the same as RC when $\sigma_u^2 = 0$. And, according to Table 1, when $\sigma_u^2 \neq 0$, the hybrid method performs similarly as RC when only the link is misspecified. In other cases, the power of the hybrid method mostly lies between that of RM and RC. We recommend use the hybrid method with caution due to the amount of information loss when creating the hybrid data.

4.3 Sequential Tests

Although we caution use of the hybrid method in practice, sequentially using test results from RM and those from RC can help to disentangle two types of misspecification. We now illustrate some sequential testing procedures when the covariate is measured with error. To distinguish the test statistics from two methods, denote by $T_\theta^{(m)}$ and $T_\theta^{(c)}$ the test statistics associated with RM and RC, respectively, where θ denotes a generic parameter. Suppose one implements RM, with only W-data further contaminated, and then implements RC, with only Y-data contaminated (and the W-data left as originally observed). Implementing these two methods sequentially yields four test statistics of interest, $T^{(m)}_{\beta_0}$, $T^{(m)}_{\beta_1}$, $T^{(c)}_{\beta_0}$, and $T^{(c)}_{\beta_1}$. In light of the operating characteristics of these test statistics revealed in Sect. 4.2, we consider the following three sequential testing strategies.

First, if $T^{(m)}_{\beta_0}$ is highly significant and $T^{(c)}_{\beta_0}$ is insignificant, one may interpret this as evidence that the X-model is misspecified and the assumed link may be adequate for the observed data. For instance, when the true model is (D3)⋏(L0), using this testing criterion, one concludes "only the X-model is misspecified" 55, 70, and 84 % of the time when $\omega = 0.7, 0.8, 0.9$, respectively, based on the simulation results in Sect. 4.2. When summarizing the preceding rejection rates, we apply the Bonferroni correction for multiple testing and use a significance level of $0.025(= 0.05/2)$ now that two test statistics are used simultaneously.

Second, if $T^{(m)}_{\beta_1}$ turns out insignificant whereas $T^{(c)}_{\beta_0}$ is highly significant, one may view this as indication that the assumed X-model may be appropriate but the assumed link is inadequate. Revisiting the simulation results in Sect. 4.2, when the true model is (D0)⋏(L3), using this sequential testing strategy, one concludes "only the link is misspecified" 67, 86, and 94 % of the time when $\omega = 0.7, 0.8, 0.9$, respectively.

Third, having observed promising power from the above two sequential tests, one would hope that having both $T^{(m)}_{\beta_0}$ and $T^{(c)}_{\beta_0}$ significant can be interpreted as an indication of dual misspecification. Unfortunately, due to the complicated interaction between the two misspecification described in Remark 3 in Sect. 4.2, this criterion is a reliable indicator of dual misspecification only when two misspecification are of opposite directions. For example, when the true model is (D4)⋏(L3), the criterion of both $T^{(m)}_{\beta_0}$ and $T^{(c)}_{\beta_0}$ being significant is met 79, 85, and 93 % of the time across 1000 MC replicates when $\omega = 0.7, 0.8, 0.9$, respectively. Similar high power is also observed when the true model is (D3)⋏(L4), (D4)⋏(L5), or (D3)⋏(L6). However, if the true model is (D3)⋏(L3), the rejection rates according to this same criterion drop to 1, 13, and 29 % when $\omega = 0.7, 0.8, 0.9$, respectively.

Despite the complication arising from dual misspecification, empirical evidence from the above three sequential tests give much encouragement to use the combination of two tests from two diagnostic methods, such as $T^{(m)}_{\beta_0}$ (or $T^{(m)}_{\beta_1}$) and $T^{(c)}_{\beta_0}$, in order to learn more from the data regarding the two model assumptions.

4.4 Directional Tests

The properties of β_{0m} described in (M1)–(M2) in Sect. 3.3 suggest that the sign of $T^{(m)}_{\beta_0}$ can indicate in which direction the true X-model deviates from normal or the true link function deviates from probit (or logit). More specifically, if there is strong evidence against a normal X-distribution, then, despite what the true link is, a significantly negative (positive) $T^{(m)}_{\beta_0}$ implies that the true X-distribution is left-skewed (right-skewed). This is supported by (M1). On the other hand, suppose one has evidence to suggest that the assumed normal X-model is likely appropriate, but

Table 2 Rejection rates associated with a one-sided test based on $T^{(m)}_{\beta_0}$ at significance level 0.05 under different true model configurations defined in Sect. 3.3 at different levels of reliability ratio ω

	(D0)⋏(L1)	(D0)⋏(L3)	(D0)⋏(L4)	(D0)⋏(L5)	
ω	[R]	[R]	[L]	[R]	
0.7	0.09	0.29	0.26	0.15	
0.8	0.10	0.45	0.42	0.22	
0.9	0.13	0.62	0.60	0.27	
	(D1)⋏(L0)	(D3)⋏(L0)	(D4)⋏(L0)	(D1)⋏(L1)	(D2)⋏(L1)
ω	[L]	[L]	[R]	[L]	[R]
0.7	0.87	1.00	1.00	0.83	0.93
0.8	0.98	1.00	1.00	0.95	1.00
0.9	1.00	1.00	1.00	0.99	1.00
	(D3)⋏(L3)	(D3)⋏(L5)	(D3)⋏(L6)	(D4)⋏(L3)	(D4)⋏(L5)
ω	[L]	[L]	[L]	[R]	[R]
0.7	0.95	0.62	0.96	1.00	0.98
0.8	0.98	0.78	1.00	1.00	1.00
0.9	0.96	0.83	1.00	1.00	1.00

Codes beneath the true model codes, [L] and [R], indicate left-sided and right-sided tests, respectively

suspects that the assumed probit link may be inadequate, then one further gains evidence to support a right-skewed link if $T^{(m)}_{\beta_0} < 0$, and left-skewed otherwise. This is justified by (M2).

As empirical evidence, Table 2 presents the rejection rates (at significance level 0.05) from the same simulation study described in Sect. 4.1 but associated with a one-sided test based on $T^{(m)}_{\beta_0}$, assuming one knows a priori the right side of the test (as we do in simulations). The high rejection rates for the cases with X-model misspecification tabulated in Table 2 indicate that, if one is mostly interested in the skewness of the true X-distribution, the sign of $T^{(m)}_{\beta_0}$ is indeed an effective indicator of the direction of skewness, regardless whether or not (and how) the link function is misspecified. In the absence of X-model misspecification, $T^{(m)}_{\beta_0}$ requires milder error contamination in X in order to more effectively reveal the direction of skewness of the true link.

5 Application to Real Data Examples

We now apply the above testing procedures to two data examples, beginning with a data set from the Framingham Heart Study briefly described in Sect. 1.

5.1 Framingham Heart Study

The data considered in this example consist of information on 1615 subjects, who were followed for the development of coronary heart disease over six examination periods. Denote by Y_i the binary indicator of the first evidence of coronary heart disease for subject i within an 8-year follow-up period from the second examination period, for $i = 1, \ldots, 1615$. At each of the second and third examination periods, each subject's SBP was measured twice. We first center all observed SBP measures from the second examination. Then, for subject $i(= 1, \ldots, 1615)$, we compute the average of the two (centered) SBP measures divided by 100 from the second examination, and use it as W_i, the error-contaminated version of the unobservable (centered) long-term SBP, X_i. Using the two replicate measures in the second exam and applying Eq. (4.3) in Carroll et al. (2006) gives an estimated ω for the so-defined W as around 0.92. Assuming a probit-normal structural measurement error model for the observed data $\{(Y_i, W_i)\}_{i=1}^{1615}$, we apply RM with $\lambda = 1$ and $B = 100$. The resulting test statistics are $T^{(m)}_{\beta_0} \approx 2.349$ (0.019) and $T^{(m)}_{\beta_1} \approx -2.387$ (0.017), with the corresponding p-values in parentheses. These test results yield significant evidence that the normality assumption on X is inadequate. This finding is not new (see, e.g., Huang, 2009; Huang et al., 2006). What is new here is that, because now $T^{(m)}_{\beta_0}$ is significantly positive (at significance level 0.05), using the directional test described in Sect. 4.4, we also find evidence that the true X-distribution is right-skewed. This new finding (from a model diagnostics standpoint) agrees with the kernel density estimate for X in Wang and Wang (2011, Fig. 5), who applied the deconvoluting kernel density estimation (Stefanski and Carroll, 1990) to estimate the density of X based on W-data.

We also apply the RC method using the reclassification model, $P(Y_i^* = Y_i|W_i) = \Phi(W_i)$, for $i = 1, \ldots, 1615$, to generate the reclassified data. The resultant test statistics are $T^{(c)}_{\beta_0} \approx -1.474$ (0.141) and $T^{(c)}_{\beta_1} \approx 1.474$ (0.141), with the associated p-values in parentheses. Based on these we conclude that the current data do not give sufficient evidence to imply that the probit link is inappropriate for this application. To this end, we are comfortable with the probit link in the GLM and lean toward a right-skewed distribution for X as opposed to normal.

5.2 Beetle Mortality

Pregibon (1980) studied the association between mortality of adult beetles and exposure to gaseous carbon disulfide. Using his test for link specification, he found strong evidence to support an asymmetric link as opposed to the logit link. The data include logarithm of dosages of carbon disulfide exposure for a total of 481 adult beetles, and the status (being killed or surviving) of each beetle after 5 h exposure. Let Y_i denote the indicator of being killed after exposure to carbon disulfide for the ith beetle, and denote by X_i the standardized (via centering and scaling) logarithm of dosage this beetle was exposed to, for $i = 1, \ldots, 481$. Here, the covariate of interest, log(dosage), is free of measurement error, making assumptions on X-model irrelevant to estimating β. Hence, we first focus on using RC to assess the adequacy of a probit GLM relating Y and X. The reclassification model used for this purpose is $P(Y_i^* = Y_i|X_i) = 0.2$, for $i = 1, \ldots, 481$. The values of the test statistics of interest are, with the corresponding p-values in parentheses, $T_{\beta_0}^{(c)} \approx 3.184$ (0.002) and $T_{\beta_1}^{(c)} = 0.241$ (0.810). This round of test provides strong evidence that the assumed probit link may be inappropriate.

Log transformation is a popular transformation used by data analysts in biology and medicine to alleviate departure from normality of data. We are now curious about what RM can tell us about the normality assumption on the covariate, log(dosage), in this study. To make RM applicable, we create noisy surrogate covariate data, $\{W_i\}_{i=1}^{481}$, according to (2) with an estimated ω to be 0.8. Using the new data, $\{(Y_i, W_i)\}_{i=1}^{481}$, treating them as the "raw" observed data, and assuming a probit-normal model, we implement RM, RC, and the hybrid method, successively. When carrying out RM, the remeasured data, $\{W_{b,i}^*, b = 1, \ldots, 100\}_{i=1}^{481}$, are generated according to $W_{b,i}^* = W_i + \sigma_u Z_{b,i}$ with $Z_{b,i} \sim N(0, 1)$, for $b = 1, \ldots, 100$, $i = 1, \ldots, 481$. For RC and the hybrid method, the reclassified responses are generated according to $P(Y_{b,i}^* = Y_i|W_i) = 0.2$ and $P(Y_{b,i}^* = Y_i|W_{b,i}^*) = 0.2$, respectively, for $b = 1, \ldots, 100$, $i = 1, \ldots, 481$. The resultant test statistics are listed below, with p-values in parentheses. From RM, $T_{\beta_0}^{(m)} \approx -0.618$ (0.537) and $T_{\beta_1}^{(m)} \approx -1.724$ (0.085); from RC, $T_{\beta_0}^{(c)} \approx 2.904$ (0.004) and $T_{\beta_1}^{(c)} \approx 0.090$ (0.929); and finally, from the hybrid method, $T_{\beta_0} \approx 2.903$ (0.004) and $T_{\beta_1} \approx 0.086$ (0.932). The pattern of these three sets of tests is mostly consistent with what is observed in Sect. 4.2 when only the link is misspecified. Following the sequential testing strategy proposed in Sect. 4.3, with the insignificant $T_{\beta_1}^{(m)}$ and the highly significant $T_{\beta_0}^{(c)}$ (at significance level 0.025), one can also conclude that the current data only provide strong evidence against the assumed link but not the normality assumption on log(dosage). In addition, using the directional test described in Sect. 4.4, although insignificant, the negative sign of $T_{\beta_0}^{(m)}$ may be an indication that the true link is right-skewed.

For illustration purposes, we drop the log transformation on the dosage levels in the raw data and view the standardized dosage as the true covariate X. Then we repeat the same data generation procedure to create the (hypothetical) error-contaminated observed data, $\{(Y_i, W_i)\}_{i=1}^{481}$, based on which we further generate the remeasure data and the reclassified data as above, and implement RM, RC, and the hybrid method. The test statistics are: from RM, $T_{\beta_0}^{(m)} \approx -1.192$ (0.234) and $T_{\beta_1}^{(m)} \approx -4.067$ (0.000); from RC, $T_{\beta_0}^{(c)} \approx 1.938$ (0.053) and $T_{\beta_1}^{(c)} \approx -1.320$ (0.188); from the hybrid method, $T_{\beta_0} \approx 1.253$ (0.211) and $T_{\beta_1} \approx -0.843$ (0.400). Now the test based on $T_{\beta_1}^{(m)}$ from RM indicates that the assumed normality on "dosage" is highly suspicious. The nearly significant $T_{\beta_0}^{(c)}$ (at significance level 0.05) from RC may also suggest the probit link questionable, although the evidence is weaker than the previous round of testing from RC when log(dosage) is the true covariate. This seems to suggest that the power of RC to detect link misspecification is somewhat compromised by the coexistence of an inappropriate assumed X-model. Finally, using the directional test proposed in Sect. 4.4, the fact that $T_{\beta_0}^{(m)} < 0$, although insignificant, may be evidence that the true distribution of dosage is left-skewed.

6 Discussion

In this study we tackle the challenging problem of model diagnostics for GLM with error-prone covariates, where there are two potential sources of model misspecification. Motivated by the rationale behind the remeasurement method (RM) designed for assessing latent-variable model assumptions, we propose the reclassification method (RC) mainly for detecting a misspecified link in GLM. We carry out rigorous theoretical investigation to study the properties of MLEs for the regression coefficients in GLM when only the link is misspecified, and also when both the assumed link and the assumed latent-variable distribution differ from the truth. These estimators include MLEs resulting from data with measurement error only in the covariate, and also MLEs based on data with measurement error in the binary response. These properties of the estimators justify use of RM and RC for assessing different model assumptions, and further motivate more informative sequential/directional tests that can reveal how the true link or true latent-variable model deviates from the assumed one.

Although starting from Sect. 3.2 we focus on the (mixture-)probit-normal model as the assumed/true models, the theoretical findings in Sects. 3.3 and 3.4 have broader implications beyond this formulation. For example, when the assumed link is logit and/or the true link belongs to the class of generalized logit links, plenty empirical evidence (partly given in Sect. 4 and Appendix 5) suggest that most properties of β_m and β_c stated in Sects. 3.3 and 3.4 are still observed. Hence, the assumed/true models formulated in Sect. 3.2 help us make great strides toward understanding the asymptotic properties of MLEs in the presence of model misspecification, and the findings under this formulation provide answers to more general questions like "What happen to the MLE when one assumes a symmetric (not necessarily normal/probit) X-model/link whereas the true X-model/link is asymmetric?". Because of the generality of their implications, similar operating characteristics of the proposed testing procedures described in Sect. 4.2 also carry over to cases outside of the (mixture-)probit-normal formulation, as evidenced in Table 1 and Appendix 5.

When multiple model assumptions are in question simultaneously, a potential obstacle for model diagnostics, and for inference in general, is non-identifiability. For example, in the framework of generalized linear mixed models (GLMM), it is only meaningful to test a posited model for the random effects when one assumes that the model for the response given the random effects is correct because these two models cannot be identified/validated simultaneously (Alonso et al., 2010; Verbeke and Molenberghs, 2010). In the context of our study, although the true covariate X in the primary model is a latent variable like random effects in GLMM, the existence of an observed surrogate W, which relates to X via a known model, clears the obstacle of non-identifiability encountered in GLMM, and thus it is possible to assess the assumed primary model and the assumed latent-variable model simultaneously. Concrete evidence of such identifiability is partly given by Proposition 3.1.

In the actual implementation of RC, one open question relates to the choice of reclassification model. In this work, we choose this model mostly for ease of deriving the reclassified-data likelihood and also try to avoid too much information loss in the reclassified responses. An interesting follow-up research topic is to find some optimal ways of creating reclassified data to maximize the power of RC. This direction of research will require involvement of the asymptotic variance of the MLE of β, a quantity yet to be studied besides the asymptotic means which we focus on in this article. Other practical concerns worth addressing in the future research are incorporation of multivariate error-prone covariates and relaxing the normality assumption on the measurement error.

Appendix 1: Likelihood and Score Functions Referenced in Sect. 3.2

Likelihood and Score Functions Under the Assumed Model

If one posits a probit link in the primary model and assumes $X \sim N(\mu_x, \sigma_x^2)$, the observed-data likelihood for subject i is

$$f_{Y,W}(Y_i, W_i; \Omega, \sigma_u^2) = e_i[\Phi\{h_i(\beta)\}]^{Y_i}[\Phi\{-h_i(\beta)\}]^{1-Y_i}, \quad \text{for } i = 1, \ldots, n, \tag{6}$$

where $\Phi(\cdot)$ is the cumulative distribution function (cdf) of $N(0, 1)$, and

$$e_i = \frac{1}{\sqrt{\sigma_u^2 + \sigma_x^2}}\phi\left(\frac{W_i - \mu_x}{\sqrt{\sigma_u^2 + \sigma_x^2}}\right), \tag{7}$$

$$h_i(\beta) = \left(\beta_0 + \beta_1\frac{\sigma_x^2 W_i + \sigma_u^2\mu_x}{\sigma_u^2 + \sigma_x^2}\right)\left(1 + \frac{\beta_1^2\sigma_u^2\sigma_x^2}{\sigma_u^2 + \sigma_x^2}\right)^{-1/2}. \tag{8}$$

If the reclassification model is

$$P(Y_i^* = Y_i|W_i) = \pi_i, \text{for } i = 1, \ldots, n, \tag{9}$$

the likelihood of the ith reclassified data, (Y_i^*, W_i), under the assumed model is

$$f_{Y^*,W}(Y_i^*, W_i; \Omega, \sigma_u^2) = e_i[\pi_i \Phi\{h_i(\beta)\} + (1-\pi_i)\Phi\{-h_i(\beta)\}]^{Y_i^*} \times [(1-\pi_i)\Phi\{h_i(\beta)\} + \pi_i \Phi\{-h_i(\beta)\}]^{1-Y_i^*}. \quad (10)$$

Differentiating the logarithm of (6) with respect to β yields the normal scores associated with β based on the raw data with measurement error only in X; and, similarly, differentiating the logarithm of (10) with respect to β gives the counterpart normal scores for the reclassified data with measurement error in both X and Y. These two sets of scores are respectively

$$\psi_m(\beta; Y_i, W_i) = h_i'(\beta)\phi\{h_i(\beta)\}\Phi^{-1}\{-h_i(\beta)\}\left[\frac{Y_i}{\Phi\{h_i(\beta)\}} - 1\right], \quad (11)$$

$$\psi_c(\beta; Y_i^*, W_i) = h_i'(\beta)\phi\{h_i(\beta)\}\Phi^{-1}\{-h_i(\beta)\}d_i^{-1}(\beta) \times \left[\frac{Y_i^*(2\pi_i - 1)\Phi\{-h_i(\beta)\}}{1 - d_i(\beta)} + 1 - d_i(\beta) - \pi_i\right], \quad (12)$$

where

$$d_i(\beta) = (1-\pi_i)\Phi\{h_i(\beta)\} + \pi_i\Phi\{-h_i(\beta)\}, \quad (13)$$

and $h_i'(\beta) = (\partial/\partial\beta)h_i(\beta)$ consists of the following two elements,

$$\frac{\partial h_i(\beta)}{\partial\beta_0} = \left(1 + \frac{\beta_1^2\sigma_u^2\sigma_x^2}{\sigma_u^2 + \sigma_x^2}\right)^{-1/2},$$

$$\frac{\partial h_i(\beta)}{\partial\beta_1} = \frac{(\sigma_x^2 W_i + \sigma_u^2\mu_x)\{(\partial/\partial\beta_0)h_i(\beta)\}^{-1} - \beta_1\sigma_u^2\sigma_x^2 h_i(\beta)}{\sigma_u^2 + \sigma_x^2 + \beta_1^2\sigma_u^2\sigma_x^2}.$$

A close inspection of the scores in (11) and (12) reveals some values of π_i that one should avoid when specifying the reclassification model in (9). First, note that the score function in (12) is identically zero if $\pi_i = 0.5$ for all $i = 1, \ldots, n$. Consequently, β is non-estimable from the reclassified data generated according to $P(Y_i^* = Y_i|W_i) = 0.5$ for all $i = 1, \ldots, n$. This is not surprising as, with all π_i's equal to 0.5, $\{Y_i^*\}_{i=1}^n$ virtually contains no information of the true responses. Second, the two sets of scores are equal when $\pi_i = 0$ for $i = 1, \ldots, n$, or, $\pi_i = 1$ for $i = 1, \ldots, n$. This is also expected as this is the case where $\{Y_i^*\}_{i=1}^n$ literally contains the same information as $\{Y_i\}_{i=1}^n$, and hence MLEs of β from these two data sets are identical, whether or not the assumed model is correct. Therefore, for the purpose of model diagnosis, we avoid setting π_i in (9) identically as 0.5, or 0, or 1, for all $i = 1, \ldots, n$.

Score Estimating Equations

Under regularity conditions, the limiting MLE of β based on the raw data and that based on the reclassified data as $n \to \infty$, β_m and β_c, uniquely satisfy the following score equations respectively,

$$E_{\mathrm{Y,W}}\left\{\psi_m(\beta_m; Y_i, W_i)\right\} = 0, \tag{14}$$

$$E_{\mathrm{Y^*,W}}\left\{\psi_c(\beta_c; Y_i^*, W_i)\right\} = 0, \tag{15}$$

where the subscripts attached to $E\{\cdot\}$ signify that the expectations are defined with respect to the relevant true model.

Using iterated expectations, one can show that (14) boils down the following set of two equations,

$$E_{\mathrm{W}}\left[\phi\{h_i(\beta_m)\}\frac{p_i - \Phi\{h_i(\beta_m)\}}{\Phi\{h_i(\beta_m)\}\Phi\{-h_i(\beta_m)\}}\right] = 0, \tag{16}$$

$$E_{\mathrm{W}}\left[W_i\phi\{h_i(\beta_m)\}\frac{p_i - \Phi\{h_i(\beta_m)\}}{\Phi\{h_i(\beta_m)\}\Phi\{-h_i(\beta_m)\}}\right] = 0, \tag{17}$$

where p_i is the mean of Y_i given W_i under the true model, that is, $p_i = P^{(t)}(Y_i = 1|W_i)$ evaluated at β (the true parameter value), for $i = 1, \ldots, n$. Similarly, one can deduce that (15) is equivalent to the following system of equations,

$$E_{\mathrm{W}}\left[\phi\{h_i(\beta_c)\}\frac{(1-2\pi_i)\{1-d_i(\beta_c)-q_i\}}{d_i(\beta_c)\{1-d_i(\beta_c)\}}\right] = 0, \tag{18}$$

$$E_{\mathrm{W}}\left[W_i\phi\{h_i(\beta_c)\}\frac{(1-2\pi_i)\{1-d_i(\beta_c)-q_i\}}{d_i(\beta_c)\{1-d_i(\beta_c)\}}\right] = 0, \tag{19}$$

where q_i is the mean of Y_i^* given W_i under the true model, that is,

$$q_i = P^{(t)}(Y_i^* = 1|W_i) = \pi_i p_i + (1-\pi_i)(1-p_i), \quad \text{for } i = 1, \ldots, n. \tag{20}$$

Likelihood Function Under the True Model

Under the mixture-probit-normal model specified in Sect. 3.2, the likelihood of (Y_i, W_i) is

$$f^{(t)}_{\mathrm{Y,W}}(Y_i, W_i; \Omega^{(t)}, \sigma_u^2) = \rho e_{1i} p_{1i}^{Y_i}(1-p_{1i})^{1-Y_i} + (1-\rho)e_{2i}p_{2i}^{Y_i}(1-p_{2i})^{1-Y_i},$$

where, for $\ell = 1, 2$,

$$e_{\ell i} = \frac{1}{\sqrt{\sigma_u^2 + \sigma_{x\ell}^2}} \phi \left(\frac{W_i - \mu_{x\ell}}{\sqrt{\sigma_u^2 + \sigma_{x\ell}^2}} \right),$$

$$p_{\ell i} = \alpha \Phi(h_{\ell 1i}) + (1 - \alpha) \Phi(h_{\ell 2i}),$$

$$h_{\ell ki} = \left(\beta_0 - \mu_k + \beta_1 \frac{\sigma_{x\ell}^2 W_i + \sigma_u^2 \mu_{x\ell}}{\sigma_u^2 + \sigma_{x\ell}^2} \right) \left(\sigma_k^2 + \frac{\beta_1^2 \sigma_u^2 \sigma_{x\ell}^2}{\sigma_u^2 + \sigma_{x\ell}^2} \right)^{-1/2}, \quad \text{for } k = 1, 2.$$

It follows that, as the true mean of Y_i given W_i,

$$p_i = P^{(t)}(Y_i = 1 | W_i) = \frac{\rho e_{1i} p_{1i} + (1 - \rho) e_{2i} p_{2i}}{\rho e_{1i} + (1 - \rho) e_{2i}}, \quad \text{for } i = 1, \ldots, n. \tag{21}$$

Evaluating (20) at this p_i, one obtains the true mean of Y_i^* given W_i, that is, $q_i = P^{(t)}(Y_i^* = 1 | W_i)$, and further deduces that the true-model likelihood of the reclassified data (Y_i^*, W_i) is, for $i = 1, \ldots, n$,

$$f_{Y^*, W}^{(t)}(Y_i^*, W_i; \Omega^{(t)}, \sigma_u^2) = \{\rho e_{1i} + (1 - \rho) e_{2i}\} q_i^{Y_i^*} (1 - q_i)^{1 - Y_i^*}.$$

Appendix 2: Limiting Maximum Likelihood Estimators When $\boldsymbol{\beta}_1 = 0$

When $\beta_1 = 0$, the limiting MLEs of β are given in the following proposition.

Proposition 1. *Suppose that the true primary model is a GLM with a mixture probit link and $\beta_1 = 0$. Under the assumed probit-normal model, $\beta_c = \beta_m = (\beta_{0m}, 0)^t$, where*

$$\beta_{0m} = \Phi^{-1} \left\{ \alpha \Phi \left(\frac{\beta_0 - \mu_1}{\sigma_1} \right) + (1 - \alpha) \Phi \left(\frac{\beta_0 - \mu_2}{\sigma_2} \right) \right\}. \tag{22}$$

The proof is given next, which does not depend on the true X-model or the reclassification model. Proposition 1 indicates that, if $\beta_1 = 0$, β_m does not depend on σ_u^2, suggesting that RM cannot detect either misspecification. Also, β_c does not depend on π_i, which defeats the purpose of creating reclassified data, hence RC does not help in model diagnosis either. This implication should not raise much concern because, after all, now $\beta_{1m} = \beta_{1c} = \beta_1 (= 0)$, suggesting that MLEs of β_1 remain consistent despite model misspecification.

Proof. By the uniqueness of the solution to (14), it suffices to check if $\beta_m = (\beta_{0m}, 0)^t$ solves (16)–(17), where β_{0m} is given in (22).

Because $\beta_1 = 0$,

$$\begin{aligned}
p_i &= P^{(t)}(Y_i = 1|W_i) \\
&= \frac{f^{(t)}(Y_i = 1, W_i; \Omega^{(t)}, \sigma_u^2)}{f_{\mathrm{W}}^{(t)}(W_i; \tau, \sigma_u^2)} \\
&= \frac{\int P^{(t)}(Y_i = 1|x; \beta) f_{\mathrm{W|X}}^{(t)}(W_i|x; \sigma_u^2) f_{\mathrm{X}}^{(t)}(x; \tau) dx}{f_{\mathrm{W}}^{(t)}(W_i; \tau, \sigma_u^2)} \\
&\quad [\text{Notethat } P^{(t)}(Y_i = 1|x; \beta) \text{ isfreeof } x \text{ when } \beta_1 = 0.] \\
&= \frac{P^{(t)}(Y_i = 1|x; \beta) f_{\mathrm{W}}^{(t)}(W_i; \tau, \sigma_u^2)}{f_{\mathrm{W}}^{(t)}(W_i; \tau, \sigma_u^2)} \\
&= \alpha \Phi \left(\frac{\beta_0 - \mu_1}{\sigma_1} \right) + (1 - \alpha) \Phi \left(\frac{\beta_0 - \mu_2}{\sigma_2} \right). \qquad (23)
\end{aligned}$$

Suppose one assumes for now that $\beta_{1m} = 0$, then by, (8), $h_i(\beta_m) = \beta_{0m}$. With both $h_i(\beta_m)$ and p_i in (23) free of W_i, (16) reduces to $p_i - \Phi\{h_i(\beta_m)\} = 0$, or, $\Phi(\beta_{0m}) = p_i$. Therefore, $\beta_{0m} = \Phi^{-1}(p_i)$, which proves (22). And with $p_i - \Phi\{h_i(\beta_m)\} = 0$, (17) holds automatically. This completes proving the result regarding β_m.

Next we show that β_m established above also solves (18)–(19), that is, $\beta_c = \beta_m$. Suppose $\beta_{1c} = 0$, then $h_i(\beta_c) = \beta_{0c}$, and $d_i(\beta_c) = (1 - \pi_i)\Phi(\beta_{0c}) + \pi_i\Phi(-\beta_{0c})$. Note that, inside (18), with $q_i = \pi_i p_i + (1-\pi_i)(1-p_i)$ and $d_i(\beta_c) = (1-\pi_i)\Phi(\beta_{0c}) + \pi_i\Phi(-\beta_{0c})$, one has $1 - d_i(\beta_c) - q_i = (1 - 2\pi_i)\{p_i - \Phi(\beta_{0c})\}$. Therefore, if $\beta_{0c} = \Phi^{-1}(p_i)$, then $1 - d_i(\beta_c) - q_i = 0$ and (18) holds for all π_i. Furthermore, $1 - d_i(\beta_c) - q_i = 0$ immediately makes (19) hold. This shows that $\beta_c = \beta_m$.

This completes the proof for Proposition 1. □

Appendix 3: Proof of Proposition 3.1

The following four results are crucial for proving Proposition 3.1. For clarity, we incorporate the dependence of $h_i(\beta)$ in (8) on W_i by re-expressing this function as $h(\beta_0, \beta_1, w)$, with the subscript i suppressed.

- (R1) If $\mu_x = 0$, then $h(-\beta_{0m}, \beta_{1m}, -w) = -h(\beta_{0m}, \beta_{1m}, w)$.
- (R2) If $\mu_x = 0$, then $\phi\{h(-\beta_{0m}, \beta_{1m}, -w)\} = C\phi\{h(\beta_{0m}, \beta_{1m}, w)\}$, where C does not depend on w.
- (R3) If $f_1(x) = f_2(-x)$ and $f_{\mathrm{U}}(u) = f_{\mathrm{U}}(-u)$, then $f_{\mathrm{W}}^{(1)}(w) = f_{\mathrm{W}}^{(2)}(-w)$, where $f_{\mathrm{U}}(u)$ is the pdf of the measurement error U, $f_{\mathrm{W}}^{(1)}(w)$ and $f_{\mathrm{W}}^{(2)}(w)$ are the pdf of W when the pdf of X is $f_1(x)$ and $f_2(x)$, respectively.

- (R4) If $f_1(x) = f_2(-x)$, $f_U(u) = f_U(-u)$, $H_1(s) = 1 - H_2(-s)$, $\mu_x = 0$, and $\beta_0 = 0$, then $p^{(22)}(-w) = 1 - p^{(11)}(w)$, where $p^{(jk)}(w)$ denotes the conditional mean of Y_i given $W_i = w$ under the true model $f_j(x) \curlywedge H_k(s)$, for $j, k = 1, 2$.

The first two results, (R1) and (R2), follow directly from the definition of $h_i(\beta)$ in (8); (R3) can be easily proved by using the convolution formula based on the error model given in Eq. (2) in the main article. The proof for (R4) is given next.

Proof. By the definition of $p^{(jk)}(w)$, one has, with $\beta_0 = 0$,

$$p^{(11)}(w) = P^{(t)}(Y_i = 1|W_i = w) = \int_{-\infty}^{\infty} H_1(\beta_1 x) f_U(w-x) f_1(x) dx / f_W^{(1)}(w).$$

Similarly, $p^{(22)}(-w)$ is equal to

$$\begin{aligned}
&\int_{-\infty}^{\infty} H_2(\beta_1 x) f_U(-w-x) f_2(x) dx / f_W^{(2)}(-w)\\
&= \int_{-\infty}^{\infty} \{1 - H_1(-\beta_1 x)\} f_U(-w-x) f_1(-x) dx / f_W^{(1)}(w), \text{by(R3)},\\
&= \int_{-\infty}^{\infty} f_U(-w-x) f_1(-x) dx / f_W^{(1)}(w) - \int_{-\infty}^{\infty} H_1(-\beta_1 x) f_U(-w-x) f_1(-x) dx / f_W^{(1)}(w)\\
&= \int_{-\infty}^{\infty} f_U(-w+s) f_1(s) ds / f_W^{(1)}(w) - \int_{-\infty}^{\infty} H_1(\beta_1 s) f_U(-w+s) f_1(s) ds / f_W^{(1)}(w)\\
&= \int_{-\infty}^{\infty} f_U(w-s) f_1(s) ds / f_W^{(1)}(w) - \int_{-\infty}^{\infty} H_1(\beta_1 s) f_U(w-s) f_1(s) ds / f_W^{(1)}(w)\\
&= 1 - p^{(11)}(w).
\end{aligned}$$

This completes the proof of (R4).

Now we are ready to show Proposition 3.1. In essence, we will show that, if (β_{0m}, β_{1m}) solves (16)–(17) when the true model is $f_1(x) \curlywedge H_1(s)$, then $(-\beta_{0m}, \beta_{1m})$ solves (16)–(17) when the true model is $f_2(x) \curlywedge H_2(s)$. More specifically, evaluating (16) and (17) at its solution under the true model $f_1(x) \curlywedge H_1(s)$, we will show that the following two equations,

$$\int_{-\infty}^{\infty} \phi\{h(\beta_{0m}, \beta_{1m}, w)\} \frac{p^{(11)}(w) - \Phi\{h(\beta_{0m}, \beta_{1m}, w)\}}{\Phi\{h(\beta_{0m}, \beta_{1m}, w)\}\Phi\{-h(\beta_{0m}, \beta_{1m}, w)\}} f_W^{(1)}(w) dw = 0, \tag{24}$$

$$\int_{-\infty}^{\infty} w\phi\{h(\beta_{0m}, \beta_{1m}, w)\} \frac{p^{(11)}(w) - \Phi\{h(\beta_{0m}, \beta_{1m}, w)\}}{\Phi\{h(\beta_{0m}, \beta_{1m}, w)\}\Phi\{-h(\beta_{0m}, \beta_{1m}, w)\}} f_W^{(1)}(w) dw = 0, \tag{25}$$

imply the following two identities,

$$\int_{-\infty}^{\infty} \phi\{h(-\beta_{0m},\beta_{1m},w)\} \frac{p^{(22)}(w) - \Phi\{h(-\beta_{0m},\beta_{1m},w)\}}{\Phi\{h(-\beta_{0m},\beta_{1m},w)\}\,\Phi\{-h(-\beta_{0m},\beta_{1m},w)\}} \times f_{\mathrm{W}}^{(2)}(w)dw = 0, \tag{26}$$

$$\int_{-\infty}^{\infty} w\phi\{h(-\beta_{0m},\beta_{1m},w)\} \frac{p^{(22)}(w) - \Phi\{h(-\beta_{0m},\beta_{1m},w)\}}{\Phi\{h(-\beta_{0m},\beta_{1m},w)\}\,\Phi\{-h(-\beta_{0m},\beta_{1m},w)\}} \times f_{\mathrm{W}}^{(2)}(w)dw = 0. \tag{27}$$

Take (27) as an example, the left-hand side of it is equal to, by (R1)–(R4) and $\Phi(-t) = 1 - \Phi(t)$,

$$\begin{aligned}
&\int_{-\infty}^{\infty} (-v)\phi\{h(-\beta_{0m},\beta_{1m},-v)\} \frac{p^{(22)}(-v) - \Phi\{h(-\beta_{0m},\beta_{1m},-v)\}}{\Phi\{h(-\beta_{0m},\beta_{1m},-v)\}\,\Phi\{-h(-\beta_{0m},\beta_{1m},-v)\}} \\
&\times f_{\mathrm{W}}^{(2)}(-v)dv \\
&= -C\int_{-\infty}^{\infty} v\phi\{h(\beta_{0m},\beta_{1m},v)\} \frac{1 - p^{(11)}(v) - \Phi\{-h(\beta_{0m},\beta_{1m},v)\}}{\Phi\{-h(\beta_{0m},\beta_{1m},v)\}\,\Phi\{h(\beta_{0m},\beta_{1m},v)\}} f_{\mathrm{W}}^{(1)}(v)dv \\
&= -C\int_{-\infty}^{\infty} v\phi\{h(\beta_{0m},\beta_{1m},v)\} \frac{1 - p^{(11)}(v) - 1 + \Phi\{h(\beta_{0m},\beta_{1m},v)\}}{\Phi\{h(\beta_{0m},\beta_{1m},v)\}\,\Phi\{-h(\beta_{0m},\beta_{1m},v)\}} f_{\mathrm{W}}^{(1)}(v)dv \\
&= C\int_{-\infty}^{\infty} v\phi\{h(\beta_{0m},\beta_{1m},v)\} \frac{p^{(11)}(v) - \Phi\{h(\beta_{0m},\beta_{1m},v)\}}{\Phi\{h(\beta_{0m},\beta_{1m},v)\}\,\Phi\{-h(\beta_{0m},\beta_{1m},v)\}} f_{\mathrm{W}}^{(1)}(v)dv \\
&= 0, \text{according to (25).}
\end{aligned}$$

Following similar derivations, one can show that the left-hand side of (26) is equal to

$$-C\int_{-\infty}^{\infty} \phi\{h(\beta_{0m},\beta_{1m},v)\} \frac{p^{(11)}(v) - \Phi\{h(\beta_{0m},\beta_{1m},v)\}}{\Phi\{h(\beta_{0m},\beta_{1m},v)\}\,\Phi\{-h(\beta_{0m},\beta_{1m},v)\}} f_{\mathrm{W}}^{(1)}(v)dv,$$

which is also equal to 0 according to (24). Therefore, $\beta_{0m}^{(11)} = -\beta_{0m}^{(22)}$ and $\beta_{1m}^{(11)} = \beta_{1m}^{(22)}$. This completes the proof of Proposition 3.1.

Appendix 4: A Counterpart Proposition of Proposition 3.1 for $\boldsymbol{\beta}_c$

Proposition 2. *Let $f_1(x)$ and $f_2(x)$ be two pdf's specifying two true X-distributions that are symmetric of each other, and let $H_1(s)$ and $H_2(s)$ be two true links that are symmetric of each other. Denote by $\beta_c^{(jk)}$ the limiting MLE of β based on reclassified* *data generated according to* $P(Y_i^* = Y_i|W_i) = \pi(W_i)$ *when the true model is* $f_j(x) \curlywedge H_k(s)$, *for* $j, k = 1, 2$. *If* $\mu_x = \beta_0 = 0$ *and* $\pi(t)$ *is an even function or* $\pi(t)$ *satisfies* $\pi(-t) = 1 - \pi(t)$, *then* $\beta_{0c}^{(11)} = -\beta_{0c}^{(22)}$ *and* $\beta_{1c}^{(11)} = \beta_{1c}^{(22)}$.

We will elaborate the proof when $\pi(t)$ is an even function in this Appendix. The following two lemmas are needed in the proof, one lemma concerning $d_i(\beta)$ defined in (13), and the other relates to q_i defined in (20). To elaborate the dependence of $d_i(\beta)$ on W_i in (13), we re-express this function as $d(\beta_0, \beta_1, w)$, with the subscript i suppressed.

Lemma 1. *If* $\mu_x = 0$ *and* $\pi(t)$ *is an even function, then* $d(-\beta_{0c}, \beta_{1c}, -w) = 1 - d(\beta_{0c}, \beta_{1c}, w)$.

Proof. By (13),

$$
\begin{aligned}
& d(-\beta_{0c}, \beta_{1c}, -w) \\
&= \{1 - \pi(-w)\}\, \Phi\{h(-\beta_{0c}, \beta_{1c}, -w)\} + \pi(-w)\Phi\{-h(-\beta_{0c}, \beta_{1c}, -w)\} \\
&= \{1 - \pi(w)\}\, \Phi\{-h(\beta_{0c}, \beta_{1c}, w)\} + \pi(w)\Phi\{h(\beta_{0c}, \beta_{1c}, w)\} \\
&\qquad [\text{Nextuse(R1)andthefactthat}\pi(t) = \pi(-t).] \\
&= \{1 - \pi(w)\}\,[1 - \Phi\{h(\beta_{0c}, \beta_{1c}, w)\}] + \pi(w)\,[1 - \Phi\{-h(\beta_{0c}, \beta_{1c}, w)\}] \\
&= 1 - d(\beta_{0c}, \beta_{1c}, w).
\end{aligned}
$$

This completes the proof of Lemma 1. □

Lemma 2. *If* $f_1(x) = f_2(-x)$, $f_U(u) = f_U(-u)$, $H_1(s) = 1 - H_2(-s)$, $\mu_x = 0$, $\beta_0 = 0$, *and* $\pi(t)$ *is an even function, then* $q^{(22)}(-w) = 1 - q^{(11)}(w)$, *where* $q^{(jk)}(w)$ *denotes the conditional mean of* Y_i^* *given* $W_i = w$ *under the true model* $f_j(x) \curlywedge H_k(s)$, *for* $j, k = 1, 2$.

Proof. By (20),

$$
\begin{aligned}
& q^{(22)}(-w) \\
&= \{1 - \pi(-w)\}\left\{1 - p^{(22)}(-w)\right\} + \pi(-w)p^{(22)}(-w) \\
&= \{1 - \pi(w)\}\, p^{(11)}(w) + \pi(w)\left\{1 - p^{(11)}(w)\right\}, \text{by(R4)and } \pi(-t) = \pi(t), \\
&= 1 - q^{(11)}(w).
\end{aligned}
$$

This completes the proof of Lemma 2. Following similar derivations, one can show that $q^{(12)}(-w) = 1 - q^{(21)}(w)$.

If, instead of being an even function, $\pi(t)$ satisfies $\pi(-t) = 1 - \pi(t)$, then the conclusion in Lemma 1 becomes $d(-\beta_{0c}, \beta_{1c}, -w) = d(\beta_{0c}, \beta_{1c}, w)$, and the conclusion in Lemma 2 changes to $q^{(22)}(-w) = q^{(11)}(w)$.

Now we are ready to show that, if (β_{0c}, β_{1c}) solves (18)–(19) under the true model $f_1(x) \curlywedge H_1(s)$, then $(-\beta_{0c}, \beta_{1c})$ solves (18)–(19) under the true model

$f_2(x) \curlywedge H_2(s)$. Given that (β_{0c}, β_{1c}) solves (18) and (19) under the true model $f_1(x) \curlywedge H_1(s)$, one has, by elaborating (18) and (19),

$$\int_{-\infty}^{\infty} \frac{\phi\{h(\beta_{0c}, \beta_{1c}, w)\}}{d(\beta_{0c}, \beta_{1c}, w)\{1-d(\beta_{0c}, \beta_{1c}, w)\}}\{1-2\pi(w)\}$$
$$\left\{1-q^{(11)}(w)-d(\beta_{0c}, \beta_{1c}, w)\right\} f_{\mathrm{W}}^{(1)}(w)dw = 0, \tag{28}$$
$$\int_{-\infty}^{\infty} w \frac{\phi\{h(\beta_{0c}, \beta_{1c}, w)\}}{d(\beta_{0c}, \beta_{1c}, w)\{1-d(\beta_{0c}, \beta_{1c}, w)\}}\{1-2\pi(w)\}$$
$$\left\{1-q^{(11)}(w)-d(\beta_{0c}, \beta_{1c}, w)\right\} f_{\mathrm{W}}^{(1)}(w)dw = 0. \tag{29}$$

Now we check if $(-\beta_{0c}, \beta_{1c})$ solves (18)–(19) under the true model $f_2(x) \curlywedge H_2(s)$. Plugging $(-\beta_{0c}, \beta_{1c})$ in (18) gives, where we set $v = -w$ in the first equality,

$$\int_{-\infty}^{\infty} \frac{\phi\{h(-\beta_{0c}, \beta_{1c}, w)\}}{d(-\beta_{0c}, \beta_{1c}, w)\{1-d(-\beta_{0c}, \beta_{1c}, w)\}}\{1-2\pi(w)\}$$
$$\left\{1-q^{(22)}(w)-d(-\beta_{0c}, \beta_{1c}, w)\right\} f_{\mathrm{W}}^{(2)}(w)dw$$
$$= \int_{-\infty}^{\infty} \frac{\phi\{h(-\beta_{0c}, \beta_{1c}, -v)\}}{d(-\beta_{0c}, \beta_{1c}, -v)\{1-d(-\beta_{0c}, \beta_{1c}, -v)\}}\{1-2\pi(-v)\}$$
$$\left\{1-q^{(22)}(-v)-d(-\beta_{0c}, \beta_{1c}, -v)\right\} f_{\mathrm{W}}^{(2)}(-v)dv$$
$$[\mathrm{Next use (R1)--(R3), Lemmas\ 1, 2, and}\ \pi(t) = \pi(-t).]$$
$$= \int_{-\infty}^{\infty} \frac{C\phi\{h(\beta_{0c}, \beta_{1c}, v)\}}{\{1-d(\beta_{0c}, \beta_{1c}, v)\}d(\beta_{0c}, \beta_{1c}, v)}\{1-2\pi(v)\}$$
$$\left\{-1+q^{(11)}(v)+d(\beta_{0c}, \beta_{1c}, v)\right\} f_{\mathrm{W}}^{(1)}(v)dv$$
$$= -C\int_{-\infty}^{\infty} \frac{\phi\{h(\beta_{0c}, \beta_{1c}, v)\}}{d(\beta_{0c}, \beta_{1c}, v)\{1-d(\beta_{0c}, \beta_{1c}, v)\}}\{1-2\pi(v)\}$$
$$\left\{1-q^{(11)}(v)-d(\beta_{0c}, \beta_{1c}, v)\right\} f_{\mathrm{W}}^{(1)}(v)dv$$
$$= 0, \text{by (28)}.$$

Similarly, one can show that (29) implies

$$\int_{-\infty}^{\infty} w \frac{\phi\{h(-\beta_{0c}, \beta_{1c}, w)\}}{d(-\beta_{0c}, \beta_{1c}, w)\{1-d(-\beta_{0c}, \beta_{1c}, w)\}}\{1-2\pi(w)\}$$
$$\left\{1-q^{(22)}(w)-d(-\beta_{0c}, \beta_{1c}, w)\right\} f_{\mathrm{W}}^{(2)}(w)dw = 0.$$

Hence, $(-\beta_{0c}, \beta_{1c})$ does solve (18)–(19) under the true model $f_2(x) \curlywedge H_2(s)$. In other words, $\beta_{0c}^{(11)} = -\beta_{0c}^{(22)}$ and $\beta_{1c}^{(11)} = \beta_{1c}^{(22)}$. Following parallel arguments as above one can show that $\beta_{0c}^{(12)} = -\beta_{0c}^{(21)}$ and $\beta_{1c}^{(12)} = \beta_{1c}^{(21)}$. This completes the proof of Proposition 2. □

Appendix 5: Additional Simulation Results from Sect. 4

When the assumed model is not probit-normal or the true model is not in the class of mixture-probit-normal, analytic exploration, as elaborated in Appendices 1–4 leading to the properties of the limiting MLEs of β, β_m and β_c, become infeasible. To provide empirical justification of these results, such as those summarized in Proposition 3.1 and (M1) in Sect. 3.3, under and outside this assumed/true-model configuration, Table 3 presents Monte Carlo averages of $\hat{\beta}_m$ and $\hat{\beta}_c$ obtained under some simulation settings considered or mentioned in Sect. 4. When computing $\hat{\beta}_c$, we consider two forms of $\pi(t)$ in the reclassification model $P(Y^*_{b,i} = Y_i|W_i) = \pi(W_i)$. One is used in Sect. 4, i.e., $P(Y^*_{b,i} = Y_i|W_i) = \Phi(W_i)$, and the other is $P(Y^*_{b,i} = Y_i|W_i) = 0.2$. The former $\pi(t)$ satisfies the condition that $\pi(-t) = 1 - \pi(t)$, and the latter is an even function, providing two examples satisfying the condition regarding $\pi(t)$ under Proposition 2.

Table 4 provides rejection rates across 1000 Monte Carlo replicates when data are generated from four true models in the class of generalized-logit-normal and the assumed model is logit-normal. Overall the operating characteristics of all considered tests are very similar to those when the assumed model is probit-normal

Table 3 Averages of maximum likelihood estimates of β across 1000 Monte Carlo replicates under different true models

Assumed model	True model	ω	$\hat{\beta}_{0m}$	$\hat{\beta}_{1m}$	$\hat{\beta}^{(1)}_{0c}$	$\hat{\beta}^{(1)}_{1c}$	$\hat{\beta}^{(2)}_{0c}$	$\hat{\beta}^{(2)}_{1c}$
Probit-normal	(D3)⋏(L4)	0.7	0.431	0.874	0.210	0.980	0.490	0.903
	(D4)⋏(L3)		−0.428	0.874	−0.207	0.983	−0.488	0.905
	(D3)⋏(L4)	0.8	0.409	0.881	0.168	1.001	0.467	0.892
	(D4)⋏(L3)		−0.407	0.881	−0.164	1.001	−0.465	0.894
	(D3)⋏(L4)	0.9	0.381	0.903	0.117	1.023	0.436	0.909
	(D4)⋏(L3)		−0.380	0.902	−0.114	1.022	−0.434	0.910
Probit-normal	(D3)⋏(L6)	0.7	−0.050	0.585	−0.228	0.671	−0.032	0.540
	(D4)⋏(L5)		0.045	0.635	0.226	0.730	0.022	0.585
	(D3)⋏(L6)	0.8	−0.059	0.599	−0.249	0.693	−0.037	0.547
	(D4)⋏(L5)		0.056	0.653	0.249	0.757	0.029	0.594
	(D3)⋏(L6)	0.9	−0.070	0.621	−0.257	0.711	−0.046	0.563
	(D4)⋏(L5)		0.071	0.682	0.262	0.783	0.041	0.617
Logit-normal	(D3)⋏(L6)	0.7	−0.073	0.951	−0.379	1.116	−0.042	0.881
	(D4)⋏(L5)		0.069	1.030	0.380	1.223	0.034	0.950
	(D3)⋏(L6)	0.8	−0.087	0.973	−0.421	1.160	−0.051	0.890
	(D4)⋏(L5)		0.086	1.061	0.427	1.277	0.046	0.966
	(D3)⋏(L6)	0.9	−0.108	1.009	−0.452	1.205	−0.067	0.916
	(D4)⋏(L5)		0.109	1.111	0.464	1.337	0.068	1.007

Monte Carlo standard errors associated with the averages are in the range between 0.002 and 0.005. Results under $\hat{\beta}^{(1)}_c$ are for the case when $P(Y^*_{b,i} = Y_i|W_i) = \Phi(W_i)$. Results under $\hat{\beta}^{(2)}_c$ are for the case when $P(Y^*_{b,i} = Y_i|W_i) = 0.2$

Table 4 Rejection rates across 1000 Monte Carlo replicates of each test statistic under each testing procedure considered in Sect. 4 at different levels of reliability ratio ω when the assumed model is logit-normal

		$\omega = 0.7$			$\omega = 0.8$			$\omega = 0.9$			$\omega = 1$		
True model		RM	RC	HB	RM	RC	HB	RM	RC	HB	RM	RC	HB
(D0)⅄(L5)	T_{β_0}	0.03	0.37	0.40	0.03	0.57	0.58	0.04	0.76	0.76	0	0.92	0.92
	T_{β_1}	0.04	0.06	0.07	0.04	0.06	0.08	0.04	0.09	0.10	0	0.10	0.10
(D3)⅄(L5)	T_{β_0}	0.67	0.05	0.18	0.89	0.09	0.06	0.95	0.32	0.18	0	0.87	0.87
	T_{β_1}	0.04	0.08	0.14	0.08	0.06	0.08	0.13	0.04	0.04	0	0.12	0.12
(D4)⅄(L5)	T_{β_0}	0.81	0.87	0.98	0.98	0.90	0.98	1.00	0.91	0.97	0	0.90	0.90
	T_{β_1}	0.36	0.78	0.75	0.67	0.85	0.87	0.91	0.87	0.88	0	0.74	0.74
(D3)⅄(L6)	T_{β_0}	0.73	0.86	0.99	0.94	0.89	0.98	1.00	0.87	0.95	0	0.80	0.80
	T_{β_1}	0.29	0.68	0.73	0.56	0.77	0.84	0.82	0.75	0.80	0	0.62	0.62

"HB" refers to the hybrid method

(see the lower half of Table 1). Indeed, from a practical point of view when it comes to model diagnosis, it should not matter whether one assumes probit-normal or logit-normal. If one concludes existence of model misspecification under one assumed model, certainly one should not believe in the other assumed model. If one concludes lack of sufficient evidence of model misspecification under one assumed model, the other assumed model is clearly equally plausible. After all, the logit link and the probit link are virtually indistinguishable in most inference contexts (Chambers and Cox, 1967).

References

Alonso, A., Litière, S., & Laenen, A. (2010). A note on the indeterminacy of the random-effects distribution in hierarchical models. *The American Statistician, 64*, 318–324.

Brown, C. C. (1982). On a goodness-of-fit test for the logistic model based on score statistics. *Communications in Statistics, 11*, 1087–1105.

Carroll, R. J., Ruppert, D., Stefanski, L. A., & Crainiceanu, C. M. (2006). *Measurement error in non-linear models: A modern perspective* (2nd ed.). Boca Raton: Chapman & Hall/CRC.

Chambers, E., & Cox, D. (1967). Discrimination between alternative binary response models. *Biometrika, 67*, 250–251.

Czado, C., & Santner, T. J. (1992). The effect of link misspecification on binary regression inference. *Journal of Statistical Planning and Inference, 33*, 213–231.

Fowlkes, E. B. (1987). Some diagnostics for binary regression via smoothing. *Biometrika, 74*, 503–515.

Hosmer, D. W., Hosmer, T., Le Cessie, S., & Lemeshow, S. (1997). A comparison of goodness-of-fit tests for the logistic regression model. *Statistics in Medicine, 16*, 965–980.

Hosmer, D. W., & Lemeshow, S. (1989). *Applied logistic regression*. New York: Wiley.

Huang, X. (2009). An improved test of latent-variable model misspecification in structural measurement error models for group testing data. *Statistics in Medicine, 28*, 3316–3327.

Huang, X., Stefanski, L. A, & Davidian, M. (2006). Latent-model robustness in structural measurement error models. *Biometrika, 93*, 53–64.

Huang, X., Stefanski, L. A., & Davidian, M. (2009). Latent-model robustness in joint modeling for a primary endpoint and a longitudinal process. *Biometrics*, *65*, 719–727.

Kannel, W. B., Neaton, J. D., Wentworth, D., Thomas, H. E., Stamler, J., Hulley, S. B., et al. (1986). Overall and coronary heart disease mortality rates in relation to major risk factors in 325,348 men screened for MRFIT. *American Heart Journal*, *112*, 825–836.

Le Cessie, S., & van Houwelingen, J. C. (1991). A goodness-of-fit test for binary data based on smoothing residuals. *Biometrics*, *47*, 1267–1282.

Li, K., & Duan N. (1989). Regression analysis under link violation. *The Annals of Statistics*, *17*, 1009–1052.

Ma, Y., Hart, J. D., Janicki, R., & Carroll, R. J. (2011). Local and omnibus goodness-of-fit tests in classical measurement error models. *Journal of the Royal Statistical Society: Series B*, *73*, 81–98.

McCullagh, P., & Nelder, J. A. (1989). *Generalized linear models* (2nd ed.). Boca Raton: Chapman & Hall/CRC.

Nelder, J. A., & Wedderburn, R. W. M. (1972). Generalized linear models. *Journal of the Royal Statistical Society: Series A 135*, 370–384.

Pregibon, D. (1980). Goodness of link tests for generalized linear models. *Journal of the Royal Statistical Society: Series C 29*, 15–24.

Stefanski, L. A., & Carroll, R. J. (1990). Deconvoluting kernel density estimators. *Statistics*, *21*, 169–184.

Stukel, T. A. (1988). Generalized logistic models. *Journal of American Statistical Association*, *83*, 426–431.

Tsiatis, A. A. (1980). A note on a goodness-of-fit test for logistic regression model. *Biometrika*, *67*, 250–251.

Verbeke, G., & Molenberghs, G. (2010). Arbitrariness of models for augmented and coarse data, with emphasis on incomplete-data and random-effects models. *Statistical Modelling*, *10*, 391–419.

Wang, X., & Wang, B. (2011). Deconvolution estimation in measurement error models: The R package decon. *Journal of Statistical Software*, *39*, 1–24.

White, H. (1982). Maximum likelihood estimation of misspecified models. *Econometrica*, *50*, 1–25.

Joint Analysis of Longitudinal Data and Informative Observation Times with Time-Dependent Random Effects

Yang Li, Xin He, Haiying Wang, and Jianguo Sun

Abstract Longitudinal data occur in many fields such as the medical follow-up studies that involve repeated measurements. For their analysis, most existing approaches assume that the observation or follow-up times are independent of the response process either completely or given some covariates. In practice, it is apparent that this may not be true. We present a joint analysis approach that allows the possible mutual correlations that can be characterized by time-dependent random effects. Estimating equations are developed for the parameter estimation and the resulting estimators are shown to be consistent and asymptotically normal.

1 Introduction

Longitudinal data occur in many fields such as the medical follow-up studies that involve repeated measurements. In these situations, study subjects are generally observed only at discrete times. Therefore, for the analysis of longitudinal data, two processes need to be considered: one is the response process, which is usually of the primary interest but not continuously observable; the other one is the observation process, which is nuisance but gives rise to the discrete times when the responses are observed.

Y. Li (✉)
Department of Mathematics and Statistics, University of North Carolina at Charlotte, Charlotte, NC, USA
e-mail: Y.Li@uncc.edu

X. He
Department of Epidemiology and Biostatistics, University of Maryland, College Park, MD, USA
e-mail: xinhe@umd.edu

H. Wang
Department of Mathematics and Statistics, University of New Hampshire, Durham, NH, USA
e-mail: HaiYing.Wang@unh.edu

J. Sun
Department of Statistics, University of Missouri, Columbia, MO, USA
e-mail: sunj@missouri.edu

Z. Jin et al. (eds.), *New Developments in Statistical Modeling, Inference and Application*, ICSA Book Series in Statistics, DOI 10.1007/978-3-319-42571-9_2

An extensive literature exists for the analysis of longitudinal data. Sun and Kalbfleisch (1995) and Wellner and Zhang (2000) investigated nonparametric estimation of the mean function when the response process is a counting process. Cheng and Wei (2000), Sun and Wei (2000), Zhang (2002) and Wellner and Zhang (2007) developed some semiparametric approaches for regression analysis under the proportional means models. However, with respect to the observation process, most existing approaches assume that the observation times are independent of the underlying response process either completely or given some covariates. For the analysis with a correlated observation process, there is limited work and most of them assume independent censoring or require some restrictive conditions such as the Poisson assumption or specified correlation structure for dependence (He et al. 2009; Huang et al. 2006; Kim et al. 2012; Li et al. 2013; Sun et al. 2007; Zhao and Tong 2011; Zhao et al. 2013; Zhou et al. 2013).

In many situations, however, the response process, the observation and censoring times may be mutually correlated. In addition, such correlations may be time-dependent. For instance, both the observation times and longitudinal responses may depend on the stage of disease progression. Their correlation may change over time and so are their correlations with the follow-up times. He et al. (2009) considered such correlations in shared frailty models. However, their method requires the assumptions that the underlying random effect is normally distributed and the observation process is a nonhomogeneous Poisson process. Also all correlations between the three processes are assumed to be fixed over time. Zhao et al. (2013) proposed a robust estimation procedure and relaxed the Poisson assumption required in He et al. (2009). However, the follow-up times are assumed to be independent from covariates, responses and observation times; and the possible correlations between responses and observation times are time-independent. More recently, Sun et al. (2012) presented a joint model with time-dependent correlations between the response process, the observation times and a terminal event, where the random effect associated with the terminal event is fixed over time and follow a specified distribution. In practice, however, such conditions may not hold or be difficult to check when informative censoring involves.

We consider regression analysis of longitudinal data when the underlying response process, the observation and censoring times are mutually correlated and none of the correlations is restricted by specified forms or distributions. A general estimation approach is proposed. The remainder of this chapter is organized as follows: In Sect. 2, we introduce the notation and present the model. Section 3 presents the estimation procedure and establishes the asymptotic properties of the resulting estimators. In Sect. 4, a simulation study is performed to evaluate the finite sample properties of the proposed estimators. Some concluding remarks are given in Sect. 5.

2 Notation and Models

Consider a longitudinal study in which the response process of interest is observed only at some discrete sampling time points. For each subject i, $i = 1, \cdots, n$, let $N_i(t)$ be the observation process, which gives the cumulative number of observation times up to time t. In practice, one observes $\widetilde{N}_i(t) = N_i(t \wedge C_i)$ where $a \wedge b = min(a, b)$ and C_i denotes the censoring or follow-up time. Let $Y_i(t)$ denote the response process, which gives the response of interest at time t but is observed only at m_i discrete observation times $\{T_{i,1}, \cdots, T_{i,m_i}\}$ when $\widetilde{N}_i(t)$ has jumps. Suppose that there exists a p-dimensional vector of covariates denoted by $\mathbf{Z}_i$, which will be assumed to be time-independent.

In the following, we model the correlation between $Y_i(t)$, $N_i(t)$ and C_i through an unobserved random vector $\mathbf{b}_i(t) = (b_{1i}(t), b_{2i}(t), b_{3i}(t))'$, which could be time-dependent. Define $\mathscr{B}_{it} = \{\mathbf{b}_i(s), s \leq t\}$. It will be assumed that the $\mathbf{b}_i(t)$'s are independent and identically distributed, $\mathscr{B}_{it}$ is independent of $\mathbf{Z}_i$, and given $\mathbf{Z}_i$ and $\mathscr{B}_{it}$, C_i, $N_i(t)$ and $Y_i(t)$ are mutually independent. To be specific, the mean function of $Y_i(t)$ is assumed to follow the proportional means model

$$E\{Y_i(t)|\mathbf{Z}_i, \mathbf{b}_i(t)\} = \Lambda_0(t) \exp\{\beta'\mathbf{Z}_i + b_{1i}(t)\}, \tag{1}$$

where $\Lambda_0(t)$ is an unknown baseline mean function and β denotes a vector of p-dimensional regression coefficients. When $b_{1i}(t) = 0$ meaning that $Y_i(t)$ is independent of both $N_i(t)$ of C_i, model (1) has been considered extensively by Cheng and Wei (2000), Sun and Wei (2000), Zhang (2002) and Hu et al. (2003) among others. When $b_{1i}(t)$ is time-independent, model (1) is equivalent to model (3) considered in Zhao et al. (2013). In general, $b_{1i}(t)$ is unknown and may follow an arbitrary distribution.

The observation process $N_i(t)$ follows the proportional rates model

$$E\{dN_i(t)|\mathbf{Z}_i, \mathbf{b}_i(t)\} = \exp\{\gamma'\mathbf{Z}_i + b_{2i}(t)\}d\mu_0(t)\,, \tag{2}$$

where γ is a vector of unknown parameters and $d\mu_0(t)$ is an unknown baseline rate function. For the $C_i's$, motivated by the additive hazards models that have been commonly used in survival analysis (Kalbfleisch and Prentice 2002; Lin and Ying 2001; Zhang et al. 2005), we consider the additive hazards model. That is, the hazard $\lambda_i(t|\mathbf{Z}_i, \mathbf{b}_i(t))$ of C_i, defined as the rate of observing C_i at time t provided that C_i is no larger than t, is given by

$$\lambda_i(t|\mathbf{Z}_i, \mathbf{b}_i(t)) = \lambda_0(t) + \xi'\mathbf{Z}_i + b_{3i}(t)\,. \tag{3}$$

Here $\lambda_0(t)$ is an unknown baseline hazard function and ξ denotes the effect of covariates on the hazard function of $C_i's$. Note that instead of model (3), one may consider the proportional hazards model. As pointed out by Lin et al. (1998) and others, the additive model (3) can be more plausible than the proportional hazards model in many applications. Related applications and model-checking techniques of model (3) can be found in Yuen and Burke (1997), Kim and Lee (1998), Ghosh (2003) and Gandy and Jensen (2005) among others.

In the above, models (1)–(3) can be viewed as natural generalizations of some existing and commonly used models. In fact, when any of the $b_{ki}(t)$'s ($k = 1, 2, 3$) is zero or independent from other $b_{ji}(t)$'s ($j = 1, 2, 3$ and $j \neq k$), the corresponding process is independent from the others. Therefore, the proposed joint model also applies to special cases when either the observation or censoring times are noninformative. In general, since the form or distribution of $\mathbf{b}_i(t)$ is arbitrary and completely unspecified, the joint model described above is quite flexible compared to many existing procedures.

Note that in models (1)–(3), for simplicity, we have assumed that the set of covariates that may affect $Y_i(t)$, $N_i(t)$ and C_i is the same. In practice, it is apparent that this may not be the case and actually the estimation procedure proposed below still applies as long as one replaces $\mathbf{Z}_i$ by appropriate covariates. As an alternative, one can define a single and big covariate vector by combining all different covariates together. In the following, we will focus on estimation of regression parameters β along with γ and ξ. For this, it is easy to see that the use of the existing procedures that assume independence could give biased or even misleading results.

3 Estimation Procedure

In this section, we will present an inference procedure for estimation of β which is usually of the primary interest. For this, first note that the counting process $\widetilde{N}_i(t) = N_i(t \wedge C_i)$ jumps by one at time t if and only if $C_i \geq t$ and $dN_i(t) = 1$. Also we have

$$
\begin{aligned}
E\{d\widetilde{N}_i(t)|\mathbf{Z}_i\} &= E\{I(t \leq C_i)dN_i(t)|\mathbf{Z}_i\} \\
&= E\left[E\{I(t \leq C_i)dN_i(t)|\mathbf{Z}_i, \mathscr{B}_{it}\}\middle|\mathbf{Z}_i\right] \\
&= E\left[E\{I(t \leq C_i)|\mathbf{Z}_i, \mathscr{B}_{it}\}E\{dN_i(t)|\mathbf{Z}_i, \mathscr{B}_{it}\}\middle|\mathbf{Z}_i\right] \\
&= E\left[exp\{-\Lambda_0^*(t) - B_i(t) - \xi'\mathbf{Z}_i^*(t)\}\exp\{\gamma'\mathbf{Z}_i + b_{2i}(t)\}d\mu_0(t)\middle|\mathbf{Z}_i\right] \\
&= \exp\{\gamma'\mathbf{Z}_i - \xi'\mathbf{Z}_i^*(t)\}d\Lambda_1^*(t), \qquad (4)
\end{aligned}
$$

where

$$
\Lambda_0^*(t) = \int_0^t \lambda_0(s)ds, \quad B_i(t) = \int_0^t b_{3i}(s)ds, \quad \mathbf{Z}_i^*(t) = \int_0^t \mathbf{Z}_i ds
$$

and

$$
d\Lambda_1^*(t) = \exp\{-\Lambda_0^*(t)\}E[exp\{b_{2i}(t) - B_i(t)\}]d\mu_0(t).
$$

Define

$$dM_i^*(t;\eta) = d\widetilde{N}_i(t) - e^{\eta'\mathbf{X}_i(t)} d\Lambda_1^*(t)$$

and $dM_i^*(t) = dM_i^*(t;\eta_0)$, where $\eta = (\gamma, \quad \xi)'$, $\mathbf{X}_i(t) = (\mathbf{Z}_i, \quad -\mathbf{Z}_i^*(t))'$ and η_0 denotes the true value of η. It can be shown that $M_i^*(t)$ is a mean-zero stochastic process. It follows that the estimators of η and $d\Lambda_1^*(t)$ can be obtained by solving the following two estimating equations

$$U_\eta(\eta) = \sum_{i=1}^{n} \int_0^\tau \left\{ \mathbf{X}_i(t) - \bar{X}(t;\eta) \right\} d\widetilde{N}_i(t) = 0 \tag{5}$$

and

$$\sum_{i=1}^{n} \left[d\widetilde{N}_i(t) - e^{\eta'\mathbf{X}_i(t)} d\Lambda_1^*(t) \right] = 0. \tag{6}$$

In the above, τ is the longest follow-up time, $\bar{X}(t;\eta) = S^{(1)}(t;\eta)/S^{(0)}(t;\eta)$ and $S^{(k)}(t;\eta) = n^{-1}\sum_{i=1}^{n} e^{\eta'\mathbf{X}_i(t)}\mathbf{X}_i(t)^{\otimes k}$ with $a^{\otimes 0} = 1$, $a^{\otimes 1} = a$, $\bar{x}(t) = lim_{n\to\infty}\bar{X}(t;\eta_0)$ and $s^{(k)}(t) = lim_{n\to\infty}S^{(k)}(t;\eta_0)$, $k = 0, 1$.

To estimate β, consider

$$\begin{aligned}
&E\{Y_i(t)d\widetilde{N}_i(t)|\mathbf{Z}_i, \mathscr{B}_{it}\} \\
&\quad = E\{I(t \le C_i)Y_i(t)dN_i(t)|\mathbf{Z}_i, \mathscr{B}_{it}\} \\
&\quad = E\{I(t \le C_i)|\mathbf{Z}_i, \mathscr{B}_{it}\}E\{Y_i(t)|\mathbf{Z}_i, \mathscr{B}_{it}\}E\{dN_i(t)|\mathbf{Z}_i, \mathscr{B}_{it}\} \\
&\quad = exp\{-\Lambda_0^*(t) - B_i(t) - \xi'\mathbf{Z}_i^*(t)\} \\
&\Lambda_0(t)\exp\{\beta'\mathbf{Z}_i + b_{1i}(t)\}\exp\{\gamma'\mathbf{Z}_i + b_{2i}(t)\}d\mu_0(t) \\
&\quad = \exp\{(\beta+\gamma)'\mathbf{Z}_i - \xi'\mathbf{Z}_i^*(t)\} \\
&\qquad \exp\{-\Lambda_0^*(t) + b_{1i}(t) + b_{2i}(t) - B_i(t)\}\Lambda_0(t)d\mu_0(t),
\end{aligned}$$

and therefore

$$E\{Y_i(t)d\widetilde{N}_i(t)|\mathbf{Z}_i\} = \exp\{\beta'\mathbf{Z}_i + \eta'\mathbf{X}_i(t)\}d\Lambda_2^*(t), \tag{7}$$

where

$$d\Lambda_2^*(t) = \exp\{-\Lambda_0^*(t)\}\Lambda_0(t)E[exp\{b_{1i}(t) + b_{2i}(t) - B_i(t)\}]d\mu_0(t).$$

Define

$$dM_i(t;\beta,\eta) = Y_i(t)d\widetilde{N}_i(t) - \exp\{\beta'\mathbf{Z}_i + \eta'\mathbf{X}_i(t)\}d\Lambda_2^*(t)$$

and $dM_i(t) = dM_i(t; \beta_0, \eta_0)$, where β_0 denotes the true value of β. Then $M_i(t)$ is a mean-zero stochastic process. This naturally suggests the following estimating equations to estimate β and $d\Lambda_2^*(t)$:

$$U_\beta(\beta; \hat{\eta}) = \sum_{i=1}^{n} \int_0^\tau W(t)\mathbf{Z}_i \left[Y_i(t)d\widetilde{N}_i(t) - e^{\beta'\mathbf{Z}_i + \hat{\eta}'\mathbf{X}_i(t)} d\Lambda_2^*(t) \right] = 0, \tag{8}$$

and

$$\sum_{i=1}^{n} \left[Y_i(t)d\widetilde{N}_i(t) - e^{\beta'\mathbf{Z}_i + \hat{\eta}'\mathbf{X}_i(t)} d\Lambda_2^*(t) \right] = 0, \;\; 0 \le t \le \tau, \tag{9}$$

where $\hat{\eta} = (\hat{\gamma}, \;\; \hat{\xi})'$ and $d\widehat{\Lambda}_1^*(t)$ are the estimators of η and $d\Lambda_1^*(t)$, respectively, solved from (5) and (6), and $W(t)$ is a possibly data-dependent weight function. We denote the estimates of β and $d\Lambda_2^*(t)$ by $\hat{\beta}$ and $d\widehat{\Lambda}_2^*(t)$, respectively, solved from (8) and (9).

To establish the asymptotic properties of $\hat{\beta}$ and $\hat{\eta}$, define

$$\widehat{M}_i^*(t) = \widetilde{N}_i(t) - \int_0^t e^{\hat{\eta}'\mathbf{X}_i(s)} d\widehat{\Lambda}_1^*(s; \hat{\eta}),$$

$$\widehat{M}_i(t) = \int_0^t Y_i(s)d\widetilde{N}_i(s) - \int_0^t e^{\hat{\beta}'\mathbf{Z}_i + \hat{\eta}'\mathbf{X}_i(s)} d\widehat{\Lambda}_2^*(s; \hat{\beta}, \hat{\eta}),$$

$$\widehat{E}_Z(t; \beta, \eta) = \frac{\sum_{i=1}^n \mathbf{Z}_i e^{\beta'\mathbf{Z}_i + \eta'\mathbf{X}_i(t)}}{\sum_{i=1}^n e^{\beta'\mathbf{Z}_i + \eta'\mathbf{X}_i(t)}} \text{ and } e_z(t) = lim_{n\to\infty} \widehat{E}_Z(t; \beta_0, \eta_0).$$

The following theorem gives the consistency and asymptotic normality of $\hat{\beta}$ and $\hat{\eta}$.

Theorem 1. *Assume that the conditions (C1)–(C5) given in the Appendix hold. Then $\hat{\eta}$ and $\hat{\beta}$ are consistent estimators of η_0 and β_0, respectively. The distributions of $n^{1/2}(\hat{\eta} - \eta_0)$ and $n^{1/2}(\hat{\beta} - \beta_0)$ can be asymptotically approximated by the normal distributions with mean zero and covariance matrices $\widehat{\Sigma}_\eta = \widehat{\Omega}_\eta^{-1}\widehat{\Psi}\widehat{\Omega}_\eta^{-1}$ and $\widehat{\Sigma}_\beta = \widehat{A}_\beta^{-1}\widehat{\Sigma}\widehat{A}_\beta^{-1}$, respectively, where $a^{\otimes 2} = aa'$, $\widehat{\Psi} = n^{-1}\sum_{i=1}^n \hat{u}_i^{\otimes 2}$, $\widehat{\Sigma} = n^{-1}\sum_{i=1}^n (\hat{v}_{1i} - \hat{v}_{2i})^{\otimes 2}$,*

$$\hat{u}_i = \int_0^\tau \Big(\mathbf{X}_i(t) - \bar{X}(t; \hat{\eta})\Big) d\widehat{M}_i^*(t),$$

$$\hat{v}_{1i} = \int_0^\tau W(t)\Big(\mathbf{Z}_i - \widehat{E}_Z(t; \hat{\beta}, \hat{\eta})\Big) d\widehat{M}_i(t),$$

$$\hat{v}_{2i} = \int_0^\tau \widehat{A}_\eta \widehat{\Omega}_\eta^{-1}\Big(\mathbf{X}_i(t) - \bar{X}(t; \hat{\eta})\Big) d\widehat{M}_i^*(t),$$

$$\widehat{A}_\beta = n^{-1}\sum_{i=1}^{n}\int_0^\tau W(t)e^{\hat{\beta}'\mathbf{Z}_i+\hat{\eta}'\mathbf{X}_i(t)}\Big(\mathbf{Z}_i - \widehat{E}_Z(t;\hat{\beta},\hat{\eta})\Big)^{\otimes 2} d\widehat{\Lambda}_2^*(t;\hat{\beta},\hat{\eta}),$$

$$\widehat{A}_\eta = n^{-1}\sum_{i=1}^{n}\int_0^\tau W(t)e^{\hat{\beta}'\mathbf{Z}_i+\hat{\eta}'\mathbf{X}_i(t)}\Big(\mathbf{Z}_i - \widehat{E}_Z(t;\hat{\beta},\hat{\eta})\Big)X_i'(t)d\widehat{\Lambda}_2^*(t;\hat{\beta},\hat{\eta})$$

and

$$\widehat{\Omega}_\eta = n^{-1}\sum_{i=1}^{n}\int_0^\tau \{\mathbf{X}_i(t) - \bar{X}(t;\hat{\eta})\}^{\otimes 2} e^{\hat{\eta}'\mathbf{X}_i(t)} d\widehat{\Lambda}_1^*(t;\hat{\eta}).$$

4 A Simulation Study

In this section, we report some results obtained from a simulation study conducted to assess the finite sample behavior of the estimation procedure proposed in the previous sections. For each subject i, the covariate $\mathbf{Z}_i$ was assumed to be a Bernoulli random variable with the probability of success being 0.5. Given $\mathbf{Z}_i$ and some unobserved random effects $\mathbf{b}_i(t) = (b_{1i}(t), b_{2i}(t), b_{3i}(t))'$, the hazard function of the censoring time C_i was assumed to have the form

$$\lambda_i(t|\mathbf{Z}_i, \mathscr{B}_{it}) = \lambda_0 + \xi\mathbf{Z}_i + b_{3i}(t), \tag{10}$$

with the largest follow-up time $\tau = 1$. The number of observations $\widetilde{N}_i(t)$ was assumed to follow a Poisson process on $(0, C_i)$ with the mean function

$$E\{N_i(t)|\mathbf{Z}_i, \mathscr{B}_{it}\} = \int_0^t \exp\{\gamma\mathbf{Z}_i + b_{2i}(s)\}d\mu_0(s)\,. \tag{11}$$

In practice, the exact time of C_i may not be observable and $d\widetilde{N}_i(t)$ is observed instead of $dN_i(t)$, thus we considered $E\{\widetilde{N}_i(t)|\mathscr{B}_{it}\}$ for the observation process. From (10) and (11),

$$E\{d\widetilde{N}_i(t)|\mathbf{Z}_i, \mathscr{B}_{it}\} = \exp\{\gamma\mathbf{Z}_i - \xi\mathbf{Z}_i t\}d\Lambda_1^*(t),$$

where $d\Lambda_1^*(t) = \exp\{-\lambda_0 t + b_{2i}(t) - B_i(t)\}d\mu_0(t)$ and $B_i(t) = \int_0^t b_{3i}(s)ds$. Given $\mathbf{Z}_i$ and $\mathscr{B}_{it}$, $\widetilde{N}_i(t)$ was assumed to follow a nonhomogeneous Poisson process and the total number of observation times m_i was generated with mean $E\{m_i\} = E\{\widetilde{N}_i(\tau)|Z_i, \mathscr{B}_{i\tau}\}$. Then the observation times $\{T_{i,1}, \ldots, T_{i,m_i}\}$ were taken as m_i order statistics from the density function

$$f_{\widetilde{N}}(t) = \frac{\exp\{\gamma\mathbf{Z}_i - \xi\mathbf{Z}_i t\}d\Lambda_1^*(t)}{\int_0^\tau \exp\{\gamma\mathbf{Z}_i - \xi\mathbf{Z}_i t\}d\Lambda_1^*(t)}.$$

The longitudinal response $Y_i(t)$ was generated from a mixed Poisson process with the mean function

$$E\{Y_i(t)|\mathbf{Z}_i, \mathscr{B}_{it}\} = Q_i\Lambda_0(t)\exp\{-\beta\mathbf{Z}_i + b_{1i}(t)\}, \tag{12}$$

where Q_i was generated independently from a gamma distribution with mean 1 and variance 0.5. The results given below are based on the sample size of 100 or 200 with 1000 replications and $W(t) = W_i = 1$.

Table 1 shows the estimation results on β for the situation when b_{1i}, b_{2i} and b_{3i} are time-independent. Note that here $\xi_0 = 0$ or $\gamma_0 = 0$ represents the cases when either censoring or the observation times is independent of covariates, respectively. For the random effects, we took $b_{1i} = b_{2i} = b_{3i} = b_i$, where the $b_i's$ were generated from the uniform distribution over (−0.5, 0.5). It can be seen that the proposed estimates seem unbiased and the estimated standard errors (SEE) are close to the sample standard errors (SSE). Also the empirical 95 % coverage probabilities (CP) are quite accurate.The same conclusions are also obtained for the situation when b_{1i}, b_{2i} and b_{3i} are time-dependent, for which the results are presented in Table 2. Here we took $b_{1i}(t) = b_i t^{1/3}$, $b_{2i}(t) = b_i t^{1/2}$ and $b_{3i} = b_i$ with the same b_i generated as for Table 1. We also considered other set-ups such as using different baselines and with Z_i being a continuous variable and obtained similar results.

Table 1 Estimation results with $\lambda_0 = 2$, $\mu_0(t) = 20t$, $\Lambda_0(t) = 5t$, $b_{1i} = b_{2i} = b_{3i}$

	$n = 100$			$n = 200$		
β_0	0	0.2	0.5	0	0.2	0.5
$(\gamma_0, \xi_0) = (0, 0)$						
Bias	0.007	0.012	0.000	−0.009	−0.005	−0.003
SEE	0.177	0.177	0.179	0.127	0.128	0.129
SSE	0.194	0.188	0.199	0.134	0.129	0.132
CP	0.924	0.934	0.905	0.934	0.946	0.934
$(\gamma_0, \xi_0) = (0, 0.2)$						
Bias	0.036	0.035	0.042	0.036	0.036	0.042
SEE	0.178	0.180	0.182	0.127	0.128	0.130
SSE	0.192	0.186	0.197	0.133	0.134	0.138
CP	0.922	0.937	0.921	0.922	0.932	0.923
$(\gamma_0, \xi_0) = (0.5, 0)$						
Bias	0.006	−0.005	0.004	0.004	−0.003	0.002
SEE	0.173	0.174	0.174	0.123	0.125	0.125
SSE	0.177	0.179	0.183	0.126	0.130	0.130
CP	0.938	0.939	0.937	0.934	0.943	0.927
$(\gamma_0, \xi_0) = (0.5, 0.2)$						
Bias	0.047	0.043	0.035	0.042	0.037	0.041
SEE	0.174	0.173	0.176	0.125	0.125	0.126
SSE	0.181	0.184	0.182	0.128	0.131	0.134
CP	0.918	0.922	0.936	0.929	0.931	0.923

Table 2 Estimation results with $\lambda_0 = 2$, $\mu_0(t) = 20t$, $\Lambda_0(t) = 5t$, $b_{1i}(t) = b_i t^{1/3}$, $b_{2i}(t) = b_i\sqrt{t}$ and $b_{3i}(t) = b_i$

	$n = 100$			$n = 200$		
β_0	0	0.2	0.5	0	0.2	0.5
$(\gamma_0, \xi_0) = (0, 0)$						
Bias	0.003	−0.005	−0.006	−0.003	−0.001	−0.004
SEE	0.172	0.171	0.173	0.123	0.123	0.125
SSE	0.182	0.181	0.181	0.127	0.128	0.130
CP	0.940	0.928	0.933	0.940	0.944	0.942
$(\gamma_0, \xi_0) = (0, 0.2)$						
Bias	0.045	0.038	0.040	0.036	0.044	0.042
SEE	0.173	0.173	0.175	0.123	0.125	0.127
SSE	0.183	0.186	0.185	0.129	0.132	0.133
CP	0.921	0.923	0.927	0.927	0.918	0.926
$(\gamma_0, \xi_0) = (0.5, 0)$						
Bias	0.006	−0.004	−0.002	−0.006	0.006	0.002
SEE	0.168	0.168	0.169	0.120	0.120	0.121
SSE	0.178	0.181	0.173	0.129	0.127	0.122
CP	0.939	0.933	0.944	0.939	0.928	0.944
$(\gamma_0, \xi_0) = (0.5, 0.2)$						
Bias	0.051	0.043	0.035	0.037	0.044	0.036
SEE	0.166	0.169	0.171	0.120	0.120	0.122
SSE	0.182	0.179	0.169	0.126	0.123	0.128
CP	0.911	0.921	0.939	0.922	0.914	0.925

To further investigate the performance of the proposed estimators of β in comparison with those proposed by He et al. (2009) and Sun et al. (2012), we carried out a simulation study and estimated β using all four methods. Note that unlike the proposed estimation procedures, the latter two methods require observing the exact time of a censoring or terminal event C_i. For this, we used the subjects' last observation times as commonly done in practice. With respect to the method given by Sun et al. (2012), we applied it by using C_i as its original terminal event time D_i and τ as its C_i. Note that as mentioned earlier, both He et al. (2009) and Sun et al. (2012) considered the distribution-based random effects for possible correlations. For the comparison, we focus on the performances of their procedures when the random effects follow various distributions besides those assumed. However, since both of them involve covariate effects in forms different from those considered by our proposed models, we fix $\beta_0 = 0$ and $\xi_0 = 0$ in order to avoid unfair comparisons caused by the misspecification of covariate effects. The estimation results are given in Table 3 with three set-ups. In the first set-up, referred to as M_1, we considered the situation as used for Table 1 except $\mu_0(t) = 10t$ and $b_{1i} = -b_{2i} = b_{3i}$. In the second and third set-ups called M_2 and M_3, we generated $b_{1i}(t)$, $b_{2i}(t)$ and $b_{3i}(t)$ from various distributions such that the assumptions required by either Sun et al. (2012)

Table 3 Estimation results on β based on the proposed procedure and the procedures given in Sun et al. (2012) and He et al. (2009) with $\beta_0 = \xi_0 = \gamma_0 = 0$

	Proposed	Sun et al. (2012)	He et al. (2009)
M_1, $n = 100$			
Bias	−0.003	−0.004	0.009
SSE	0.162	0.261	0.206
M_1, $n = 200$			
Bias	−0.003	−0.003	0.007
SSE	0.116	0.184	0.154
M_2, $n = 100$			
Bias	0.004	0.004	0.003
SSE	0.123	0.306	0.184
M_2, $n = 200$			
Bias	−0.001	−0.003	0.011
SSE	0.089	0.227	0.145
M_3, $n = 100$			
Bias	0.001	−0.010	0.000
SSE	0.074	0.221	0.071
M_3, $n = 200$			
Bias	0.002	0.000	−0.003
SSE	0.055	0.150	0.051

Set-up M_1: $\mu_0(t) = 10t$, $\lambda_0 = 2$, $\Lambda_0(t) = 5t$, $b_{1i} = -b_{2i} = b_{3i} = b_i$, where b_i followed a uniform distribution on (−0.5, 0.5)
Set-up M_2: $\mu_0(t) = 10t$, $\lambda_0 = 0$, $\Lambda_0(t) = 5t$, $b_{1i} = -b_{2i} = b_i$, where b_i followed a uniform distribution on (−0.5, 0.5) and b_{3i} followed an extreme value distribution with distribution function $F(t) = 1 - \exp\{-\exp(t)\}$ Set-up M_3: $\mu_0(t) = 4t$, $\lambda_0 = 0$, $\Lambda_0(t) = 5t$, $b_{1i} = 0.2b_{2i} + 0.2b_{2i}$, $b_{2i} = \log(b_{2i}^*)$ and $b_{3i} = \exp(v_i)$, where v_i and b_{2i}^* were generated, respectively, from a normal distribution with mean 0 and standard deviation 0.5 and gamma distribution with mean 4 and variance 8

or He et al. (2009) are satisfied. For example, we took $\lambda_0(t) = 0$ and generated $b_{3i}(t)$ from an extreme-value distribution as assumed by Sun et al. (2012). We also generated $b_{1i}(t)$, $b_{2i}(t)$ and $b_{3i}(t)$ from the assumed distributions required by He et al. (2009).

Note that in all set-ups considered above, our proposed models are correctly specified because there are no assumed distributions on $b_{1i}(t)$, $b_{2i}(t)$ or $b_{3i}(t)$. In contrast, the models from either of He et al. (2009) or Sun et al. (2012) are only correctly specified in one of the set-ups. On the other hand, since there are no covariate effects in all set-ups, we do not expect that the point estimates of β given by He et al. (2009) or Sun et al. (2012) are much biased even if the imposed distributions are misspecified in the estimation. For their variance estimates, we expect that SEE and SSE agree for both, because the former applied bootstrap resampling and the latter did not involve any assumed distribution of random effects in their variance estimation. Therefore, we only compare bias and SSE. It can be seen that all estimation procedures gave comparably small bias as expected. However, it appears that the proposed estimators are more efficient for all cases in general. In comparison, the method given by He et al. (2009) is comparably efficient to the proposed estimators only under M_3 when all its distribution assumptions are satisfied. For the method given by Sun et al. (2012), it is worth noting that when D_i is substituted by the last observation time C_i from subject i, it gives relatively large SSE, especially when C_i's vary much, regardless of whether the assumption about $b_{3i}(t)$ is satisfied (for M_2) or not (for M_3).

5 Concluding Remarks

We proposed a joint model for analyzing longitudinal data with informative censoring and observation times. The mutual correlations are characterized via a shared vector of time-dependent random effects. As mentioned earlier, several procedures have been developed in the literature for longitudinal data when either censoring or observation process is informative. However when both of them are informative, there is limited work that can apply except those given in He et al. (2009) and Sun et al. (2012). In addition, all the existing procedures assumed time-independent or specifically distributed correlation structures. The proposed joint model is flexible in that the shared vector of random effects can be time-dependent and neither of its structure nor distribution are specified. For the parameter estimation, the proposed procedure is simple and easy to implement.

There exist several directions for future research. One is that as mentioned above, one may want to consider other models rather than models (1)–(3) and develop similar estimation procedures. Of course, a related problem is model selection and one may want to develop some model selection techniques to choose the optimal model among several candidate models (Tong et al. 2009; Wang et al. 2014). Note that in the proposed method, we have employed a weight function $W(t)$ and it would be desirable to develop some procedures for the selection of an optimal $W(t)$. As in most similar situations, this is clearly a difficult problem as it requires the specification of the covariance function of $Y_i(t)$ and $\widetilde{N}_i(t)$ (Sun et al. 2012). Finally in the above, we have focused on regression analysis of $Y_i(t)$ with time-independent covariates. Sometimes one may face time-dependent covariates and thus it would be helpful to generalize the proposed method to this latter situation. Also sometimes nonparametric estimation of $Y_i(t)$ or the baseline functions may be of interest. For those purposes, some constraints should be imposed on $\mathbf{b}_i(t)$ for identifiability, for example, $E\{\mathbf{b}_i(t)\} = \mathbf{0}$. When panel count data arise (Sun and Zhao, 2013), the generalization of existing nonparametric estimation procedures to cases with informative observation or censoring times is a challenging direction for future work too.

Appendix

Proof of Theorem 1

To derive the asymptotic properties of the proposed estimators $\hat{\beta}$ and $\hat{\eta}$, we need the following regularity conditions:

(C1) $\{\widetilde{N}_i(\cdot), Y_i(\cdot), C_i, \mathbf{Z}_i\}_{i=1}^n$ are independent and identically distributed.
(C2) There exists a $\tau > 0$ such that $P(C_i \geq \tau) > 0$.
(C3) Both $\widetilde{N}_i(t)$ and $Y_i(t)$ $(0 \leq t \leq \tau, i = 1, \ldots, n)$ are bounded.
(C4) $W(t)$ and $\mathbf{Z}_i$, $i = 1, \ldots, n$, have bounded variations and $W(t)$ converges almost surely to a deterministic function $w(t)$ uniformly in $t \in [0, \tau]$.
(C5) $A_\beta = E\{\int_0^\tau w(t)e^{\beta_0'\mathbf{Z}_i+\eta_0'\mathbf{X}_i(t)}[\mathbf{Z}_i - e_z(t)]^{\otimes 2}d\Lambda_2^*(t)\}$ and $\Omega_\eta = E\Big[\int_0^\tau \{\mathbf{X}_i(t) - \bar{x}(t)\}^{\otimes 2} e^{\eta_0'\mathbf{X}_i(t)}d\Lambda_1^*(t)\Big]$ are both positive definite.

Under condition (C2), we define

$$U_1(\beta; \hat{\eta}) = \sum_{i=1}^n \int_0^\tau W(t)\mathbf{Z}_i\Big[Y_i(t)d\widetilde{N}_i(t) - e^{\beta'\mathbf{Z}_i+\hat{\eta}'\mathbf{X}_i(t)}d\widehat{\Lambda}_2^*(t)\Big],$$

which is integrable under conditions (C3) and (C4). Also note that $d\widehat{\Lambda}_2^*(t)$ satisfies

$$\sum_{i=1}^n \Big[Y_i(t)d\widetilde{N}_i(t) - e^{\beta'\mathbf{Z}_i+\hat{\eta}'\mathbf{X}_i(t)}d\widehat{\Lambda}_2^*(t)\Big] = 0, \;\; 0 \leq t \leq \tau. \tag{13}$$

Let

$$\widehat{A}_\beta(\beta) = -n^{-1}\partial U_1(\beta, \hat{\eta})/\partial\beta', \widehat{A}_\eta(\eta) = -n^{-1}\partial U_1(\beta_0, \eta)/\partial\eta',$$

and under (C1), let

$$A_\beta = \lim_{n\to\infty} \widehat{A}_\beta(\beta_0), \; A_\eta = \lim_{n\to\infty} \widehat{A}_\eta(\eta_0).$$

The consistency of $\hat{\beta}$ and $\hat{\eta}$ follows from the facts that $U_1(\beta_0; \hat{\eta})$ and $U_\eta(\eta_0)$ both tend to 0 in probability as $n \to \infty$, and that under condition (C5), $\widehat{A}_\beta(\beta)$ and $-n^{-1}\partial U_\eta(\eta)/\partial\eta'$ both converge uniformly to the positive definite matrices A_β and Ω_η over β and η, respectively, in neighborhoods around the true values β_0 and η_0. Then the Taylor series expansions of $U_1(\hat{\beta}; \hat{\eta})$ at $(\beta_0; \hat{\eta})$ and (β_0, η_0) yield $n^{1/2}(\hat{\beta} - \beta_0) = A_\beta^{-1}n^{-1/2}U_1(\beta_0; \hat{\eta}) + o_p(1) = A_\beta^{-1}\Big\{n^{-1/2}U_1(\beta_0; \eta_0) - A_\eta n^{1/2}(\hat{\eta} - \eta_0)\Big\} + o_p(1)$.

The proof of Theorem 1 is sketched as follows:

(1) First, using some derivation operation to $U_1(\beta;\hat{\eta})$ and (13), we can get

$$\widehat{A}_\beta(\beta) = n^{-1}\sum_{i=1}^{n}\int_0^\tau W(t)\{\mathbf{Z}_i - \widehat{E}_Z(t;\beta,\hat{\eta})\}^{\otimes 2} e^{\beta'\mathbf{Z}_i+\hat{\eta}'\mathbf{X}_i(t)} d\widehat{\Lambda}_2^*(t;\beta,\hat{\eta}).$$

(2) Solving $d\widehat{\Lambda}_2^*(t;\beta_0,\eta_0)$ from (13) and applying to $U_1(\beta_0;\eta_0)$ yields

$$U_1(\beta_0;\eta_0) = \sum_{i=1}^{n}\int_0^\tau w(t)\Big(\mathbf{Z}_i - e_z(t)\Big)dM_i(t) + o_p(n^{1/2}),$$

where $e_z(t) = lim_{n\to\infty}\widehat{E}_Z(t;\beta_0,\eta_0)$ as defined earlier in Sect. 3 and $w(t)$ is a deterministic function defined under (C5).

(3) Differentiation of $U_1(\beta_0,\eta)$ and (13) with respect to η yields

$$\widehat{A}_\eta(\eta) = n^{-1}\sum_{i=1}^{n}\int_0^\tau W(t)\big[\mathbf{Z}_i - \widehat{E}_Z(t;\beta_0,\eta)\big] e^{\beta_0'\mathbf{Z}_i+\eta'\mathbf{X}_i(t)} X_i'(t) d\widehat{\Lambda}_2^*(t;\beta_0,\eta)\,.$$

(4) According to Eq. (5) and by using the asymptotic results in Lin et al. (2000) (A.5), one can show that

$$n^{1/2}\{\hat{\eta}-\eta_0\} = \Omega_\eta^{-1} n^{-1/2}\sum_{i=1}^{n}\left[\int_0^\tau\Big(\mathbf{X}_i(t) - \frac{s^{(1)}(t)}{s^{(0)}(t)}\Big)dM_i^*(t)\right] + o_p(1),$$

where $\Omega_\eta = E\Big[\int_0^\tau\{\mathbf{X}_i(t) - \bar{x}(t)\}^{\otimes 2} e^{\eta_0'\mathbf{X}_i(t)} d\Lambda_1^*(t)\Big]$, which is invertible under (C5).

Combining the results in steps (1)–(4), we have

$$\begin{aligned} U_1(\beta_0;\hat{\eta}) = &\sum_{i=1}^{n}\left[\int_0^\tau w(t)\{\mathbf{Z}_i - e_z(t)\}dM_i(t)\right] \\ &- A_\eta\Omega_\eta^{-1}\sum_{i=1}^{n}\left[\int_0^\tau\{\mathbf{X}_i(t) - \bar{x}(t)\}dM_i^*(t)\right] + o_p(n^{1/2}). \end{aligned}$$

Since A_β is also invertible under (C5), it then follows from the multivariate central limit theorem that the conclusions hold.

References

Cheng, S. C., & Wei, L. J. (2000). Inferences for a semiparametric model with panel data. *Biometrika, 87*, 89–97.

Gandy, A., & Jensen, U. (2005). Checking a semiparametric additive hazards model. *Lifetime Data Analysis, 11*, 451–472.

Ghosh, D. (2003). Goodness-of-fit methods for additive-risk models in tumorignenicity experiments. *Biometrics, 59*, 721–726.

He, X., Tong, X., & Sun, J. (2009). Semiparametric analysis of panel count data with correlated observation and follow-up times. *Lifetime Data Analysis, 15*, 177–196.

Hu, X. J., Sun J., & Wei, L. J. (2003). Regression parameter estimation from panel counts. *Scandinavian Journal of Statistics, 30*, 25–43.

Huang, C. Y., Wang, M. C., & Zhang, Y. (2006). Analysing panel count data with informative observation times. *Biometrika, 93*, 763–775.

Kalbfleisch, J. D., & Prentice, R. L. (2002). *The statistical analysis of failure time data*. New York: Wiley.

Kim, J., & Lee, S.Y. (1998). Two-sample goodness-of-fit tests for additive risk models with censored observations. *Biometrika, 85*, 593–603.

Kim, S., Zeng, D., Chambless, L., & Li, Y. (2012). Joint models of longitudinal data and recurrent events with informative terminal event. *Statistics in Biosciences, 4*, 262–281.

Li, N., Zhao, H., & Sun, J. (2013). Semiparametric transformation models for panel count data with correlated observation and follow-up times. *Statistics in Medicine, 32*(17), 3039–3054.

Lin, D. Y., Oaks, D., & Ying, Z. (1998). Additive hazards regression with current status data. *Biometrika, 85*(2), 289–298.

Lin, D. Y., & Ying, Z. (2001). Semiparametric and Nonparametric Regression Analysis of Longitudinal Data (with discussion). *Journal of the American Statistical Association, 96*(453), 103–113.

Sun, J., & Kalbfleisch, J. D. (1995). Estimation of the mean function of point processes based on panel count data. *Statistica Sinica, 5*, 279–289.

Sun, J., Tong, X., & He, X. (2007). Regression analysis of panel count data with dependent observation times. *Biometrics, 63*, 1053–1059.

Sun, J., & Wei, L. J. (2000). Regression analysis of panel count data with covariate-dependent observation and censoring times. *Journal of the Royal Statistical Society, Series B, 62*, 293–302.

Sun, J., & Zhao, X., (2013). *The statistical analysis of panel count data*. New York: Springer.

Sun, L., Song, X., Zhou, J., & Liu, L. (2012). Joint analysis of longitudinal data with informative observation times and a dependent terminal event. *Journal of the American Statistical Association, 107*(498), 688–700.

Tong, X., Sun, L., He, X., & Sun, J. (2009). Variable selection for panel count data via non-concave penalized estimating function. *Scandinavian Journal of Statistics, 36*, 620–635.

Wang, H., Li, Y., & Sun, J. (2014). Focused and model average estimation for regression analysis of panel count data. *Scandinavian Journal of Statistics*. doi:10.1002/sjos.12133.

Wellner, J. A., & Zhang, Y. (2000). Two estimators of the mean of a counting process with panel count data. *Annals of Statistics, 28*, 779–814.

Wellner, J. A., & Zhang, Y. (2007). Two likelihood-based semiparametric estimation methods for panel count data with covariates. *Annals of Statistics, 35*, 2106–2142.

Yuen, K.C., & Burke, M.D. (1997). A test of fit for a semiparametric additive risk model. *Biometrika, 84*, 631–639.

Zhang, Y. (2002). A semiparametric pseudolikelihood estimation method for panel count data. *Biometrika, 89*, 39–48.

Zhang, Z., Sun, J., & Sun, L. (2005). Statistical analysis of current status data with informative observation times. *Statistics in Medicine, 24*, 1399–1407.

Zhao, X., & Tong, X. (2011). Semiparametric regression analysis of panel count data with informative observation times. *Computational Statistics and Data Analysis, 55*(1), 291–300.

Zhao, X., Tong, X., & Sun, J. (2013). Robust estimation for panel count data with informative observation times. *Computational Statistics and Data Analysis, 57*, 33–40.

Zhou, J., Zhao, X., & Sun, L. (2013). A new inference approach for joint models of longitudinal data with informative observation and censoring times. *Statistica Sinica, 23*, 571–593.

A Markov Switching Model with Stochastic Regimes with Application to Business Cycle Analysis

Haipeng Xing, Ning Sun, and Ying Chen

Abstract Since the publication of Hamilton's seminal work on Markov switching model, a large amount of its applications have been found in economics and finance. As existing Markov switching models describe the regimes or parameter values in a categorical way, it is restrictive in practical analysis. In this paper, we consider a Markov switching model with stochastic regimes, in which the regimes and model parameters are represented both categorically and continuously. Assuming conjugate priors, we develop closed-form recursive Bayes estimates of the regression parameters, an approximation scheme that has much lower computational complexity and yet are comparable to the Bayes estimates in statistical efficiency, and an expectation-maximization procedure to estimate the unknown hyperparameters. We conduct intensive simulation studies to evaluate the performance of our estimators. We also use our model to analyze the series of the U.S. monthly total nonfarm employee.

1 Introduction

Many economic time series occasionally exhibit Markov switching and dynamical instability in their behavior. After Hamilton (1989, 1990) used Markov switching regressions to characterize time-varying parameters in an autoregressive process as a finite-state hidden Markov chain for business cycles, the idea of Markov switching among finite regimes has been used to study various problems in economics and finance. For instance, to make state transition probabilities dependent on economic

H. Xing (✉)
Department of Applied Mathematics and Statistics, State University of New York, Stony Brook, NY 11794, USA
e-mail: xing@ams.sunysb.edu

N. Sun
IBM Research Center, Beijing, China
e-mail: sunning1023@gmail.com

Y. Chen
QFR Capital Management, L.P., New York, NY 10036, USA
e-mail: yingemma.chen@gmail.com

Z. Jin et al. (eds.), *New Developments in Statistical Modeling, Inference and Application*, ICSA Book Series in Statistics, DOI 10.1007/978-3-319-42571-9_3

variables, finite-state Markov switching regression models have been extended to allow economic variables (Diebold and Rudebusch 1996; Durland and McCurdy 1994; Filardo and Gordon 1998; Kim et al. 2008). In more complicated applications, the idea of Markov switching with finite regimes is combined with other state-of-the-art models in finance, economics, and statistics. This, for example, includes volatility models of stock returns and interest rates (Ang and Bekaert 2002a,b; Cai 1994; Gray 1996; Hamilton and Susmel 1994; So et al. 1998), term structure models of interest rates (Smith 2002), state space models (Kim 1994), and others.

In classical Markov switching models with finite regimes, an essential assumption is that the unobserved model parameters follow a hidden Markov chain with finite categorical states, and hence the behavior of interested economic variables can be described by the dynamical system with regime-dependent parameters. Then using the developed statistical inference procedures such as likelihood-based or Bayesian estimates of finite state regimes and switching times, one is able to make inference on the switching times among finite categorical regimes, the probability of each categorical regime, and the parameter values of the dynamic system in each period, and hence provides an interpretation for the mechanism of the dynamical system within and across economic cycles. Such treatment brings much convenience into business cycle analysis, however, as pointed out by Hamilton (1996) and many others, the approach is challenged by the difficulty of making proper inference on the number of regimes and their corresponding numerical values in real data analysis.

Intuitively, this difficulty is due to the categorical specification of regimes in the model, for example, model parameters in different economic recessions are usually different. To account for this difficulty, we consider another type of Markov switching regression model with stochastic regimes that have both categorical and continuous representations of regimes for interested business-cycle-related variables. In particular, we assume a finite-state hidden Markov chain to represent categorically economic regimes at each period and a regime-dependent continuous prior distribution for model parameters in each categorical regime. In this way, the model parameters may take different numerical values at two different periods with same categorical regimes. Such specification not only shares the original motivation of analyzing economic cycles with finite categorical regimes, but also describe numerically variations of the parameter values over time. Therefore, the proposed model gets around the issue of testing the number of categorical regimes and provide more intuitive inference on dynamics of both economic cycles and their corresponding parameter values over time.

Since the proposed model has both categorical and continuous components in regime-dependent parameters, we consider an inference framework that has attractive statistical and computational properties. In particular, we derive the explicit filters and smoothers and provide nonlinear inference for both the categorical and continuous representations of regime-dependent parameters in the model. The derived explicit filter and smoother for continuous representation of regimes at a given time are mixtures of posterior distributions, and the weight of mixture components can be computed recursively. Furthermore, the filters and smoothers for the probabilities of categorical regimes are expressed as sums of mixture weights. Computationally, the derived filter and smoother yield a Bayes algorithm with quadratic and cubic computational complexity, respectively. To further reduce the computational complexity, we develop an efficient approximation scheme whose computational complexity is only linear, for the Bayes filter and smoother. To estimate the hyperparameters in the proposed model, which consist of the transition matrix and the parameters of prior distribution of regimes, we develop an expectation-maximization (EM) procedure, and discuss how the estimation procedures for hyperparameters relates to the identification issues of categorical regimes via some simulation examples.

We then use the model to analyze the U.S. monthly total nonfarm employee from February 1968 to June 2011. We show that, while a Markov switching model with categorical regimes don't provide a satisfactory analysis, the proposed model does catch the categorical and continuous features of regime-dependent parameters during economic cycles. The estimated categorical representations of regimes are economically meaningful and the recession periods inferred from our model match well with the ones announced by NBER. The estimated model parameters show indeed different values over different periods even when the parameters belong to the same categorical regime.

The rest of the paper is organized as follows. Section 2 specifies the model and derives the filtering and smoothing estimates of model parameters. Bounded complexity of mixtures approximation and hyperparameter estimation are also introduced there. In Sect. 3, we study the performance of our estimators and issues on hyperparameter estimation via extensive simulation studies. Section 4 analyze the U.S. monthly total nonfarm employee data using the proposed model, and compare the result with the one obtained from a Markov switching model with categorical regimes. Some concluding remarks are given in Sect. 5.

2 A Markov Switching Regression Model with Both Categorical and Continuous Regimes

2.1 Model Specification

We assume that observations $\{y_t\}$ follow the stochastic regression model

$$y_t = \beta_t' x_t + \epsilon_t, \qquad t = 1, \ldots, T, \tag{1}$$

where ϵ_t are independent and identically distributed normal random variables with mean 0 and variance σ^2, $x_t \in \mathbb{R}^d$ are stochastic regressor consisting of the historical observations $y_{t-1}, y_{t-2}, \ldots$ and exogenous variables, β_t is a continuous state Markov chain that is determined by an unobserved finite state Markov chain $\{s_t\}$ with the following constraints

(A1) The Markov chain $\{s_t \in \{1, \ldots, K\} | t \geq 0\}$ is irreducible, and follows the transition probability matrix $Q = (q_{ij})_{1 \leq i,j \leq K}$, i.e., $q_{ij} = P(s_t = j | s_{t-1} = i)$.

(A2) The Markov chain $\{s_t, t \geq 0\}$ has a stationary distribution $\pi = (\pi_1, \ldots, \pi_K)^T$.

Assumption (A2) is appropriate in practical analysis, as it provides distribution of s_t when the economy with business cycles reaches equilibrium. Furthermore, if $\{s_t\}$ is initialized at the stationary distribution π, a time-reversed Markov chain can be defined, which has transition matrix $\widetilde{Q} = (\tilde{q}_{ij})_{1 \leq i,j \leq K}$ with

$$\tilde{q}_{ij} = P(s_t = j | s_{t+1} = i) = q_{ji}\pi_j / \pi_i. \tag{2}$$

To specify the dynamics of β_t. We assume that, at time t, if there is no regime switching, i.e., $s_t = s_{t-1}$, then $\beta_t = \beta_{t-1}$; if regime switching occurs, i.e., $s_t \neq s_{t-1}$, then β_t will jump to a new value which follows a regime-dependent normal prior distribution. This specification allows β_t take new values that are different from those in the same categorical regime before time $t-1$, and introduces more flexibility to the dynamics of β_t. We summarize this as the following assumption

(A3) The dynamics of β_t is given by $\beta_t = 1_{\{s_t = s_{t-1}\}}\beta_{t-1} + 1_{\{s_t \neq s_{t-1}\}} z_t$, in which z_t are independent and identically distributed normal random variables with mean $z^{(s_t)}$ and covariance matrix $V^{(s_t)}$. For convenience, we assume $s_1 \neq s_0$.

2.2 *Filtering Estimate*

Denote that $\mathscr{Y}_t = (y_1, \ldots, y_t)$, $1 \leq t \leq T$, and $\mathscr{Y}_{ij} = (y_i, \ldots, y_j)$, $1 \leq i < j \leq T$. Let $J_t^{(k)} = \max\{i \leq t : s_{i-1} \neq s_i = \cdots = s_t = k\}$ be the most recent switching time up to time t. Then at $J_t^{(k)}$, s_t switches to regime k from another regime. Let

$$\xi_t^{(k)} = P(s_t = k | \mathscr{Y}_t), \qquad \xi_{i,t}^{(k)} = P(J_t^{(k)} = i | \mathscr{Y}_t), \tag{3}$$

for $1 \leq i \leq t$ and $1 \leq k \leq K$. By definition, $\xi_t^{(k)} = \sum_{i=1}^{t} \xi_{i,t}^{(k)}$. Since the conditional distribution of β_t given $\mathscr{Y}_t$ and $J_t^{(k)} = i$ is Normal$(z_{i,t}^{(k)}, V_{i,t}^{(k)})$, where

$$V_{i,j}^{(k)} = \left(\left[V^{(k)} \right]^{-1} + \frac{1}{\sigma^2} \sum_{u=i}^{j} x_u x_u' \right)^{-1}, \quad z_{i,j}^{(k)} = V_{i,j}^{(k)} \left(\left[V^{(k)} \right]^{-1} z^{(k)} + \frac{1}{\sigma^2} \sum_{u=i}^{j} x_u y_u \right),$$

for $j \geq i$, it follows that the posterior distribution of β_t given $\mathscr{Y}_t$ is a mixture of normal distributions:

$$\beta_t | \mathscr{Y}_t \sim \sum_{k=1}^{K} \sum_{i=1}^{t} \xi_{i,t}^{(k)} \text{Normal}(z_{i,t}^{(k)}, V_{i,t}^{(k)}). \tag{4}$$

Denote $g_{i,j}^{(k)}(u)$ the density function of Normal$(z_{i,t}^{(k)}, V_{i,t}^{(k)})$ distribution at point u, i.e., $g_{i,j}^{(k)}(u) = (2\pi)^{-d/2}|V_{i,j}^{(k)}|^{-1/2}\exp\{-\frac{1}{2}(u - z_{i,t}^{(k)})'[V^{(k)}]^{-1}(u - z_{i,t}^{(k)})\}$. Making use of $\sum_{k=1}^{K}\sum_{i=1}^{t}\xi_{i,t}^{(k)} = 1$, we can show that conditional probabilities $\xi_{i,t}^{(k)}$ are determined by $\xi_{i,t}^{(k)} = \xi_{i,t}^{(k)*}\Big/\Big[\sum_{h=1}^{K}\sum_{j=1}^{t}\xi_{j,t}^{(h)*}\Big]$, in which

$$\xi_{i,t}^{(k)*} := \begin{cases} \left(\sum_{l\neq k}\xi_{t-1}^{(l)}q_{lk}\right)\psi_{0,0}^{(k)}/\psi_{t,t}^{(k)} & i = t, \\ q_{kk}\xi_{i,t-1}^{(k)}\psi_{i,t-1}^{(k)}/\psi_{i,t}^{(k)} & i < t, \end{cases} \tag{5}$$

$\psi_{0,0}^{(k)} = g_{0,0}^{(k)}(0)$, and $\psi_{i,j}^{(k)} = g_{i,j}^{(k)}(0)$. Then expressions (3) and (4) implies

$$P(s_t = k|\mathcal{Y}_t) = \sum_{i=1}^{t}\xi_{i,t}^{(k)}, \qquad E(\beta_t|\mathcal{Y}_t) = \sum_{k=1}^{K}\sum_{i=1}^{t}\xi_{i,t}^{(k)}z_{i,t}^{(k)}. \tag{6}$$

2.3 Smoothing Estimate

Assumptions (A1)–(A3) imply that, a stationary distribution of β_t exists and is expressed as $\sum_{k=1}^{K}\pi_k$ Normal$(z^{(k)}, V^{(k)})$. Then if β_t is initialized at the stationary distribution, its time-reversed Markov chain $\widetilde{Q} = (\tilde{q}_{lk})$ is defined by (2). Note that this also imposes stationarity conditions for y_t, for instance, if the regression model has an autoregressive component, the stationarity condition for components of β_t should be imposed. In such case, we shall replace the Normal distribution in the stationary distribution $\sum_{k=1}^{K}\pi_k$ Normal$(z^{(k)}, V^{(k)})$ by a truncated Normal distribution that has support in stability region. Such treatment also applies for the smoothing estimates of β_t. For notational convenience, we still use Normal (instead of truncated Normal) in the sequel.

We then use the time-reversed chain of β_t to obtain a backward analog of (4),

$$\beta_{t+1}|\mathcal{Y}_{t+1,T} \sim \sum_{k=1}^{K}\sum_{j=t+1}^{T}\eta_{t+1,j}^{(k)}\text{Normal}(z_{t+1,j}^{(k)}, V_{t+1,j}^{(k)}), \tag{7}$$

in which the weights $\eta_{t+1,j}^{(k)}$ can be obtained by backward induction using the time-reversed analog of (5):

$$\eta_{t+1,j}^{(k)} \propto \eta_{t+1,j}^{(k)*} := \begin{cases} \left(\sum_{l\neq k}\eta_{t+2}^{(l)}\tilde{q}_{lk}\right)\psi_{0,0}^{(k)}/\psi_{t+1,t+1}^{(k)} & j = t+1, \\ \tilde{q}_{kk}\eta_{t+2,j}^{(k)}\psi_{t+2,j}^{(k)}/\psi_{t+1,j}^{(k)} & j > t+1. \end{cases} \tag{8}$$

Since for $B \subset \mathbb{R}^d$, $P(\beta_t \in B|\mathcal{Y}_{t,T}) = \int P(\beta_t \in B|\beta_{t+1})dP(\beta_{t+1}|\mathcal{Y}_{t,T})$, it follows from (7) that

$$\beta_t|\mathscr{Y}_{t+1,T} \sim \sum_{k=1}^{K}\Big\{\tilde{q}_{kk}\sum_{j=t+1}^{T}\eta_{t+1,j}^{(k)}\text{Normal}(z_{t+1,j}^{(k)}, V_{t+1,j}^{(k)})$$
$$+\Big(\sum_{l\neq k}\tilde{q}_{lk}\eta_{t+1}^{(l)}\Big)\text{Normal}(z^{(k)}, V^{(k)})\Big\}. \tag{9}$$

Next, we shall use Bayes' theorem to combine the forward filter (4) with its backward variant (9) to derive the posterior distribution of β_t given $\mathscr{Y}_T$ $(1 \le t < T)$, which is expressed as the following mixture of normal distributions

$$\beta_t|\mathscr{Y}_T \sim \sum_{k=1}^{K}\sum_{1\le i\le t\le j\le T}\alpha_{ij,t}^{(k)}\text{Normal}(z_{i,j}^{(k)}, V_{i,j}^{(k)}), \tag{10}$$

in which the mixture weights $\alpha_{ij,t}^{(k)}$ are posterior probabilities explained below. Consider the event $C_{ij}^{(k)} = \{s_i = \cdots = s_j = k, s_i \neq s_{i-1}, s_j \neq s_{j+1}\}$, We can show that, for $i \le t \le j$, $\alpha_{ijt}^{(k)} = P(C_{ij}^{(k)}|\mathscr{Y}_n)$ and $\alpha_{ij,t}^{(k)}$ can be calculated by

$$\alpha_{ijt}^{(k)} = \alpha_{ijt}^{(k)*}\Big/D_t, \qquad D_t = \sum_{k=1}^{K}\sum_{1\le i\le t\le j\le T}\alpha_{ijt}^{(k)*},$$
$$\alpha_{ijt}^{(k)*} = \begin{cases}\xi_{i,t}^{(k)}\big(\sum_{l\neq k}\eta_{t+1}^{(l)}q_{kl}/\pi_l\big) & i \le t = j,\\ q_{kk}\xi_{i,t}^{(k)}\eta_{t+1,j}^{(k)}\psi_{i,t}^{(k)}\psi_{t+1,j}^{(k)}\big/(\pi_k\psi_{i,j}^{(k)}\psi_{0,0}^{(k)}) & i \le t < j.\end{cases} \tag{11}$$

Therefore, the smoothing estimates of β_t and s_t given $\mathscr{Y}_T$ are given by

$$E(\beta_t|\mathscr{Y}_T) = \sum_{k=1}^{K}\sum_{1\le i\le t\le j\le T}\alpha_{ijt}^{(k)}z_{i,j}^{(k)}. \tag{12}$$

$$P(s_t = k|\mathscr{Y}_T) = \sum_{1\le i\le t\le j\le T}\alpha_{ijt}^{(k)}. \tag{13}$$

One concern here is that, since (12) are represented as K mixtures of mixtures of normals, it is questionable whether the smoothing formula could differentiate the values of β_t when K regimes are close to each other. Such identification issue is closed related to the choice of appropriate hyperparameters, and will be discussed in Sect. 3.

2.4 Bounded Complexity Mixture Approximation

Although the Bayes filter (4) uses a recursive updating formula (5) for weights $\xi_{i,t}^{(k)}$ $(1 \leq i \leq t, 1 \leq k \leq K)$, the number of weights increases dramatically with t, resulting in rapidly increasing computational complexity and memory requirements in estimating β_t as t keeps increasing. To address the issue of computational efficiency, we follow Lai and Xing (2011) and consider a *bounded complexity mixture* (BCMIX) approximation procedure with much lower computational complexity yet comparable to the Bayes estimates in statistical efficiency. The idea of BCMIX approximation is to keep only a fixed number M of weights at every stage t, in particular, the most recent m $(1 \leq m < M)$ weights $\xi_{i,t}^{(k)}$ (with $t-m < i \leq t$) and the largest $M - m$ of the remaining weights.

Denote $\mathscr{K}_{t-1}^{(k)}$ the set of indices i for which $\xi_{i,t-1}^{(k)}$ in (5) is kept at stage $t-1$ for regime k. Note that there are at most M indices in $\mathscr{K}_{t-1}^{(k)}$ and $\mathscr{K}_{t-1}^{(k)} \supset \{t-1, \cdots, t-m\}$. When a new observation arrives at time t, we still define $\xi_{i,t}^{(k)*}$ by (5) for $i \in \{t\} \cup \mathscr{K}_{t-1}^{(k)}$ and denote i_t the index not belonging to the most recent m stages, $\{t, t-1, \ldots, t-m+1\}$, such that

$$\xi_{i_t,t}^{(k)*} = \min\{\xi_{i,t}^{(k)*} : i \in \mathscr{K}_{t-1}^{(k)} \quad \text{and} \quad i \leq t-m\}, \tag{14}$$

choosing $i_t^{(k)}$ to be the one farthest from t if the minimizing set in (14) has more than one element. Define $\mathscr{K}_t^{(k)} = \{t\} \cup (\mathscr{K}_{t-1}^{(k)} - \{i_t^{(k)}\})$, and then

$$\xi_{i,t}^{(k)} = \Bigg(\xi_{i,t}^{(k)*} \Bigg/ \sum_{j \in \mathscr{K}_t^{(k)}} \xi_{j,t}^{(k)*}\Bigg), \qquad i \in \mathscr{K}_t^{(k)}, \tag{15}$$

yields a BCMIX approximation to the forward filter.

Similarly, to obtain a BCMIX approximation to the backward filter (8), let $\widetilde{\mathscr{K}}_{t+1}^{(k)}$ denote the set of indices j for which $\eta_{j,t+1}^{(k)}$ in (8) is kept at stage $t+1$ for regime k; thus, $\widetilde{\mathscr{K}}_{t+1}^{(k)} \supset \{t+1, \cdots, t+m\}$. At time t, define $\eta_{j,t}^{(k)}$ by (8) for $j \in \{t\} \cup \mathscr{K}_{t+1}^{(k)}$ and let j_t be the index not belonging to the most recent m stages, $\{t, t+1, \cdots, t+m-1\}$ such that

$$\eta_{j_t,t}^{(k)*} = \min\{\eta_{j,t}^{(k)*} : j \in \widetilde{\mathscr{K}}_{t+1}^{(k)} \quad \text{and} \quad j \geq t+m\}, \tag{16}$$

choosing $j_t^{(k)}$ to be the one farthest from t if the minimizing set in (16) has more than one element. Define $\widetilde{\mathscr{K}}_t^{(k)} = \{t\} \cup (\mathscr{K}_{t+1}^{(k)} - \{i_t^{(k)}\})$, and then

$$\eta_{j,t}^{(k)} = \Bigg(\eta_{j,t}^{(k)*} \Bigg/ \sum_{j \in \widetilde{\mathscr{K}}_t^{(k)}} \eta_{j,t}^{(k)*}\Bigg), \qquad j \in \widetilde{\mathscr{K}}_t^{(k)}, \tag{17}$$

yields a BCMIX approximation to the backward filter.

For the smoothing estimate $E(\beta_t|\mathscr{Y}_T)$ and its associated posterior distribution, we construct BCMIX approximations by combining the preceding forward and backward BCMIX filters with index sets $\mathscr{K}_t^{(k)}$ and $\widetilde{\mathscr{K}}_{t+1}^{(k)}$, respectively, at time t. Then the BCMIX approximations to (11) are given as

$$\tilde{\alpha}_{ijt} = \alpha^*_{ijt}/\widetilde{D}_t, \qquad \widetilde{D}_t = \sum_{i\in\mathscr{K}_t^{(k)},\, j\in\{t\}\cup\widetilde{\mathscr{K}}_{t+1}^{(k)}} \alpha^*_{ijt},$$

$$\alpha_{ijt}^{(k)*} = \begin{cases} \xi_{i,t}^{(k)}\left(\sum_{l\neq k}\eta_{t+1}^{(l)}q_{kl}/\pi_l\right) & i\in\mathscr{K}_t^{(k)}, \\ q_{kk}\xi_{i,t}^{(k)}\eta_{t+1,j}^{(k)}\psi_{i,t}^{(k)}\psi_{t+1,j}^{(k)}/(\pi_k\psi_{i,j}^{(k)}\psi_{0,0}^{(k)}) & i\in\mathscr{K}_t^{(k)}, j\in\{t\}\cup\widetilde{\mathscr{K}}_{t+1}^{(k)}. \end{cases}$$

Therefore, the BCMIX smoother for β_t and s_t given $\mathscr{Y}_T$ are expressed as

$$E(\beta_t|\mathscr{Y}_T) \approx \sum_{k=1}^{K}\sum_{i\in\mathscr{K}_t^{(k)},\, j\in\{t\}\cup\widetilde{\mathscr{K}}_{t+1}^{(k)}} \tilde{\alpha}_{ijt}^{(k)} z_{i,j}^{(k)}, \tag{18}$$

$$P(s_t = k|\mathscr{F}_T) \approx \sum_{k=1}^{K}\sum_{i\in\mathscr{K}_t^{(k)},\, j\in\{t\}\cup\widetilde{\mathscr{K}}_{t+1}^{(k)}} \tilde{\alpha}_{ijt}^{(k)}. \tag{19}$$

The BCMIX approximation fixes the number of filters as M at each time, and keeps the m closest weights and the other $M - m$ largest weights. This greatly reduces the computational complexity $O(T^2)$ of the filter in Sect. 2.2 and $O(T^3)$ of the smoother in Sect. 2.3 to $O(T)$. The specification of M and m are discussed in Sect. 3.

2.5 Hyperparameter Estimation

The above inference procedure involve hyperparameters $\Phi = \{Q, z^{(1)}, V^{(1)}, \ldots, z^{(K)}, V^{(K)}, \sigma^2\}$, which can be replaced by their estimates in practice. Since Φ contains $[(K-1)K + d(d+1)K + 1]$ unknown parameters, we use an EM algorithm to estimate Φ. Specifically, we note that the log likelihood $l_c(\Phi)$ of the complete data $\{(y_t, s_t, \beta_t), 1 \le t \le T\}$ is given as

$$l_c(\Phi|s_0) = \sum_{t=1}^{T} f(y_t, \beta_t, s_t|\{y_i, \beta_i, s_i; i = 0, \ldots, t-1\})$$

$$= \sum_{t=1}^{T}\left\{\log f(y_t|\beta_t) + \sum_{k=1}^{K} f(\beta_t|s_t = k)1_{\{s_t=k\}} + \sum_{k,l=1}^{K}\log(q_{kl})1_{\{s_{t-1}=k, s_t=l\}}\right\}$$

$$= -\frac{1}{2}\sum_{t=1}^{T}\left\{\frac{(y_t-\beta_t'x_t)^2}{\sigma^2}+\log(2\pi\sigma^2)\right\}+\sum_{t=1}^{T}\sum_{k,l=1}^{K}\log(q_{kl})1_{\{s_{t-1}=k,s_t=l\}}$$

$$-\frac{1}{2}\sum_{t=1}^{T}\sum_{k=1}^{K}\left\{(\beta_t-z^{(k)})'\left[V^{(k)}\right]^{-1}(\beta_t-z^{(k)})+\log((2\pi)^d|V^{(k)}|)\right\}1_{\{s_t=k,s_t\neq s_{t-1}\}} \tag{20}$$

The E-step of the EM algorithm involves the computation of the conditional probabilities, $P(s_t = k|\mathscr{Y}_T)$ and $P(s_{t-1} = k, s_t = l|\mathscr{Y}_T)$, and the conditional expectations, $E[(y_t-\beta_t'x_t)^2|\mathscr{Y}_T]$ and $E[(\beta_t-z^{(k)})'\left[V^{(k)}\right]^{-1}(\beta_t-z^{(k)})1_{\{s_t=k\}}|\mathscr{Y}_T]$. The M-step of the EM algorithm involves calculating the partial derivatives of (20) with respect to Φ. Simple algebra yields the following updating formulas for Φ.

$$\hat{q}_{kl,\text{new}} = \frac{\sum_{t=2}^{T}P(s_{t-1}=k,s_t=l|\mathscr{Y}_T,\widehat{\Phi}_{\text{old}})}{\sum_{t=2}^{T}P(s_{t-1}=k|\mathscr{Y}_T,\widehat{\Phi}_{\text{old}})}, \tag{21}$$

$$\hat{z}^{(k)}_{\text{new}} = \frac{\sum_{t=1}^{T}E(\beta_t 1_{\{s_t=k\}}|\mathscr{Y}_T,\widehat{\Phi}_{\text{old}})}{\sum_{t=1}^{T}P(s_t=k|\mathscr{Y}_T,\widehat{\Phi}_{\text{old}})}, \tag{22}$$

$$\widehat{V}^{(k)}_{\text{new}} = \frac{\sum_{t=1}^{T}E[(\beta_t-\hat{z}^{(k)}_{\text{old}})(\beta_t-\hat{z}^{(k)}_{\text{old}})'1_{\{s_t=k\}}|\mathscr{Y}_T,\widehat{\Phi}_{\text{old}}]}{\sum_{t=1}^{T}P(s_t=k|\mathscr{Y}_T,\widehat{\Phi}_{\text{old}})}, \tag{23}$$

$$\hat{\sigma}^2_{\text{new}} = \frac{1}{T}\sum_{t=1}^{T}E[(y_t-\beta_t'x_t)^2|\mathscr{Y}_T,\widehat{\Phi}_{\text{old}}]. \tag{24}$$

In above, $P(s_t = k|\mathscr{Y}_T)$ can be computed by (13), and other items are given as follows,

$$P(s_{t-1}=k,s_t=l|\mathscr{Y}_T) = \frac{f^{(l)}_{t,t}/f^{(l)}_{0,0}q_{kl}\widetilde{Q}_l'\eta_{t+1}/\pi_l}{\sum_{i=1}^{K}\left[f^{(i)}_{t,t}/f^{(i)}_{0,0}q_{ki}\widetilde{Q}_i'\eta_{t+1}/\pi_i\right]}\sum_{1\le i\le t-1\le j\le T}\alpha^{(k)}_{i,j,t-1}. \tag{25}$$

$$E(\beta_t 1_{\{s_t=k\}}|\mathscr{Y}_T) = \sum_{1\le i\le t\le j\le T}\alpha^{(k)}_{ijt}z^{(k)}_{i,j}, \tag{26}$$

$$E\left[(\beta_t-z^{(k)})'(\beta_t-z^{(k)})1_{\{s_t=k\}}|\mathscr{Y}_T\right]$$
$$= \sum_{1\le i\le t\le j\le T}\alpha^{(k)}_{ijt}\left[\left[z^{(k)}_{i,j}\right]'z^{(k)}_{i,j}+V^{(k)}_{i,j}-2z^{(k)}_{i,j}z^{(k)}+\left[z^{(k)}\right]'z^{(k)}\right] \tag{27}$$

$$E[(y_t-\beta_t'x_t)^2|\mathscr{Y}_T] = \sum_{t=1}^{T}\sum_{k=1}^{K}\alpha^{(k)}_{ijt}\left[(y_t-x_t'z^{(k)}_{i,j})^2+x_t'V^{(k)}_{i,j}x_t\right]. \tag{28}$$

The iteration schemes (21)–(24) are carried out until convergence or until some prescribed upper bound on the number of iterations is reached.

To speed up the computations involved in the EM algorithm, one can use the BCMIX approximations in Sect. 2 instead of the full recursions to compute (25)–(28). Our simulation studies show that the EM procedure converges vary fast.

3 Numerical Studies

We now present some simulation studies on the performance of Bayes and BCMIX estimates from both frequentist and Bayesian viewpoints. We consider the four measures for different purpose. The mean *Kullback-Leibler* (KL) divergence measures the mean error between the estimates $\hat{\beta}_t$ and the true β_t, i.e., $\kappa := \frac{1}{T}\sum_{t=1}^{T} \text{KL}(\beta_t, \hat{\beta}_t) = \frac{1}{2\sigma^2 T}\sum_{t=1}^{T}\left[(\hat{\beta}_t - \beta_t)'x_t\right]^2$. The mean *residual sum of squares* (RSS) measures the goodness of fit using an estimation procedure, i.e., $\chi := \frac{1}{T}\sum_{t=1}^{T}(y_t - \hat{\beta}'x_t)^2$. The l_2 distance of β_t and $\hat{\beta}_t$ measures the Euclidean distance between the true β_t and their estimates, $l_2 := \frac{1}{T}\sum_{t=1}^{T}||\hat{\beta}_t - \beta_t||^2$. The fourth measure is to measure the accuracy of our inference on the underlying regimes s_t. Since our model only computes the posterior probability of s_t given $\mathscr{Y}_T$, we estimate the regime of time t as the one whose posterior probability of s_t given $\mathscr{Y}_T$ exceeds 0.5, i.e,

$$\hat{s}_t := \max\{k|k \in \{1,\ldots,K\}, P(s_t = k|\mathscr{Y}_T) > 0.5\}. \tag{29}$$

Based on $\hat{s}_t$, we define the mean misclassification ratio as $\nu = \frac{1}{T}\sum_{t=1}^{T} 1_{\{s_t \neq \hat{s}_t\}}$.

3.1 Performance of Bayes and BCMIX Estimates in Frequentist Scenarios

We first evaluate the performance of Bayes estimates (12) and (13) and BCMIX estimates (18) and (19) via simulations. For illustration purpose, we consider an AR(1) model with time-varying autoregressive coefficients,

$$y_t = \alpha_t y_{t-1} + \epsilon_t, \tag{30}$$

in which ϵ_t are independent and identically distributed normal random variables with mean 0 and variance σ^2, and α_t are time-varying parameters with two regimes, i.e., $K = 2$ and $s_t \in \{1, 2\}$. We consider four scenarios which have one, two or three regime switchings, respectively.

S1. $s_t = 1$ for $t/T \in (0, 0.3]$ and $s_t = 2$ for $t/T \in (0.3, 1]$.
S2. $s_t = 1$ for $t/T \in (0, 0.5]$ and $s_t = 2$ for $t/T \in (0.5, 1]$.
S3. $s_t = 1$ for $t/T \in (0, 0.35] \cup (0.7, 1]$ and $s_t = 2$ for $t/T \in (0.35, 0.7]$.
S4. $s_t = 1$ for $t/T \in (0, 0.2] \cup (0.5, 0.6]$ and $s_t = 2$ for $t/T \in (0.2, 0.5] \cup (0.6, 1]$.

Then given the period segmented by the piecewise constant $s_t = k \in \{1, 2\}$, the AR coefficient α_t are also piecewise constant and sampled from the prior distribution Normal$(z^{(k)}, V^{(k)})$ with $z^{(1)} = 0.5$, $z^{(2)} = -0.5$, $V^{(1)} = V^{(2)} = 0.16$, and $\sigma^2 = 1$. Note that the parameter α_t with the same s_t over different periods are not same. For example, regime 1 in Scenario 4 suggest that β_t are constant in the period $(0, 0.2T]$ and $(0.5T, 0.6T]$, respectively, but $\alpha_1 = \cdots = \alpha_{200} \neq \alpha_{501} = \cdots = \alpha_{600}$ although there are in the same categorical regime. To avoid the nonstationarity issue, we impose the restriction $|\alpha_t| < 1$.

We then fit our model to the data by letting $x_t = y_{t-1}$ and $\beta_t = \alpha_t$ in (1), and apply the EM algorithm for hyperparameter and the Bayes and BCMIX smoothers for α_t and s_t in Sect. 2. For each scenario, 500 samples of size $T = 1000$ were generated to evaluate the performance of Bayes and BCMIX estimates. To demonstrate the performance, we also consider a much simpler benchmark in which the regime switching times are known so that the Bayes estimates of β_t between two switching times are given by the standard Bayesian formulas for normal populations. We call this benchmark "oracle" estimate. For BCMIX smoother, since its performance seems to relate to the choice of M and m, we compare BCMIX smoothers with $(M, m) = (10, 5), (20, 10), (30, 15), (40, 20)$. We first estimate the hyperparameters by the EM algorithm and then apply Bayes and BCMIX estimation formulas derived in Sect. 2. Table 1 compares the oracle smoother (Oracle), Bayes smoother (Bayes), and BCMIX smoothers (BCMIX) in terms of RSS, KL and l_2 measures. The average of RSS computed by different methods are very close to each other in each scenario, indicating that the Bayes and BCMIX smoothers all gives good fit to the data. The average of KL and l_2 distance between the true and estimated autoregression coefficients and the misclassification rate of regimes show that the Bayes and BCMIX smoothers are very close, and both provide good estimates of autoregression coefficients and regimes. Actually, with slight modification of the proofs in Lai and Xing (2011), we can show that the BCMIX smoother converges to the true value under certain regularity conditions. Therefore, in the rest of the paper, we only present the result based on BCMIX smoother (in particular, we use $(M, m) = (20, 10)$).

3.2 Performance of the BCMIX Smoother Under Bayesian Scenarios

We then study the performance of the BCMIX smoother for series that are simulated from the following AR(1) model with intercept

$$y_t = \mu_t + \alpha_t y_{t-1} + \epsilon_t, \tag{31}$$

in which ϵ_t are independent and identically distributed normal random variables with mean 0 and variance σ^2, and the dynamics of the regression coefficient $\beta_t = (\mu_t, \alpha_t)'$ follow (A1)–(A3) with $K = 2$, $\sigma^2 = 1$ and

Table 1 Performance of Oracle, Bayes and BCMIX estimates under four scenarios (standard errors are shown in parenthesis)

				BCMIX							BCMIX			
		Oracle	Bayes	(10,5)	(20,10)	(30,15)	(40,20)		Oracle	Bayes	(10,5)	(20,10)	(30,15)	(40,20)
$10^3\kappa$	S1	2.019	3.963	3.945	3.934	3.934	3.932	$10^3 l_2$	1.023	1.778	1.777	1.770	1.770	1.770
		(0.091)	(0.140)	(0.139)	(0.141)	(0.141)	(0.140)		(0.026)	(0.032)	(0.032)	(0.032)	(0.032)	(0.032)
	S2	2.031	4.053	4.045	4.025	4.021	4.023		1.018	1.766	1.770	1.758	1.757	1.758
		(0.093)	(0.160)	(0.160)	(0.161)	(0.161)	(0.160)		(0.026)	(0.034)	(0.033)	(0.034)	(0.034)	(0.034)
	S3	3.025	6.580	6.860	6.610	6.571	6.568		1.307	2.389	2.438	2.395	2.388	2.387
		(0.107)	(0.189)	(0.200)	(0.190)	(0.189)	(0.190)		(0.027)	(0.033)	(0.034)	(0.033)	(0.033)	(0.033)
	S4	3.925	9.985	10.780	10.292	10.151	10.096		1.538	3.022	3.121	3.054	3.037	3.031
		(0.125)	(0.280)	(0.330)	(0.310)	(0.302)	(0.298)		(0.027)	(0.040)	(0.043)	(0.042)	(0.041)	(0.041)
χ	S1	0.998	0.995	0.995	0.996	0.996	0.996	$10^2\nu$		2.7	3.0	2.7	2.7	2.7
		(0.002)	(0.002)	(0.002)	(0.002)	(0.002)	(0.002)			(0.6)	(0.7)	(0.6)	(0.6)	(0.6)
	S2	0.998	0.995	0.996	0.996	0.996	0.996			2.9	2.7	2.8	2.8	2.7
		(0.002)	(0.002)	(0.002)	(0.002)	(0.002)	(0.002)			(0.7)	(0.7)	(0.7)	(0.6)	(0.6)
	S3	0.997	0.993	0.993	0.993	0.993	0.993			2.6	2.5	2.3	2.4	2.5
		(0.002)	(0.002)	(0.002)	(0.002)	(0.002)	(0.002)			(0.5)	(0.5)	(0.5)	(0.5)	(0.5)
	S4	0.996	0.990	0.990	0.990	0.990	0.990			2.8	3.4	3.0	2.9	2.6
		(0.002)	(0.002)	(0.002)	(0.002)	(0.002)	(0.002)			(0.4)	(0.5)	(0.4)	(0.4)	(0.4)

$$z^{(1)} = \begin{pmatrix} 0.2 \\ -0.3 \end{pmatrix}, \quad z^{(2)} = \begin{pmatrix} 0.5 \\ -0.5 \end{pmatrix}, \quad V^{(1)} = V^{(2)} = \begin{pmatrix} 0.16 & 0 \\ 0 & 0.16 \end{pmatrix}.$$

To make $\{y_t\}$ stationary in each regime, α_t is restricted by $|\alpha_t| < 1$. The transition matrix has the structure

$$P = \begin{pmatrix} 1-p & p \\ q & 1-q \end{pmatrix},$$

in which p and q takes the following four sets of values: $(p, q) = (0.002, 0.001)$, $(0.004, 0.001)$, $(0.016, 0.008)$, and $(0.016, 0.016)$, we will number them as Case 1 to 4, respectively. For each case, 500 samples of size $T = 3000$, 4000, 5000, 6000, 7000 and 8000 were generated to evaluate the performance of the BCMIX(20,10) smoother. In all simulations, the hyperparameters are assumed unknown and estimated by the EM algorithm in Sect. 2.5. Figure 1 shows one of 500 simulated series of $T = 3000$ and its estimates in the 9th case. We notice that the regression coefficients β_t has only two regimes but could take different values over time even β_t are in the same regime. Table 2 shows the averaged KL and l_2 distance of the true and estimated regression coefficients, the averaged RSS and total misclassification ratio. In each case, as T increases, κ and l_2 seem to converge to certain values, and the limiting value are different in each case. On the other hand, κ and l_2 get larger when the values of p and/or q increase (i.e., regime switching happens more frequently). The averaged RSS are similar in all cases, and the misclassification rate decreases when the sample size T increases.

3.3 *Identification Issues and Sensitivity Analysis*

As shown in Sect. 2.3, the smoothing estimate (12) is K mixtures of mixture distributions, which indicates that the smoothing estimates largely depend on the specification of the prior distribution Normal($z^{(k)}$, $V^{(k)}$) of each regime. When regimes are not very close or their prior distributions don't have much overlap, the EM procedure of estimating hyperparameters can gradually learn the true regimes through iterations, whether one has knowledge or information on the true regimes or not. Sections 3.1 and 3.2 have shown the good performance of the Bayes and BCMIX smoother of our model under this circumstance. When two regimes (or their prior distributions) overlaps a lot, a natural question is whether the EM algorithm can learn (or calibrate) the right prior parameters so that the model still gives good estimates. We now discuss this issue via two numerical examples.

Example 1. Assume that the observations y_t are generated by the AR(1) model (30) of Scenario 4 with fixed regime switching times in Sect. 3.1 with different ($z^{(k)}$, $V^{(k)}$), $1 \leq k \leq K = 2$ and $T = 1000$. The autoregression coefficients α_t are generated by the priors with $z^{(1)} = 0.5$, $z^{(2)} = 0.4$, and $V^{(1)} = V^{(2)} = 0.16$.

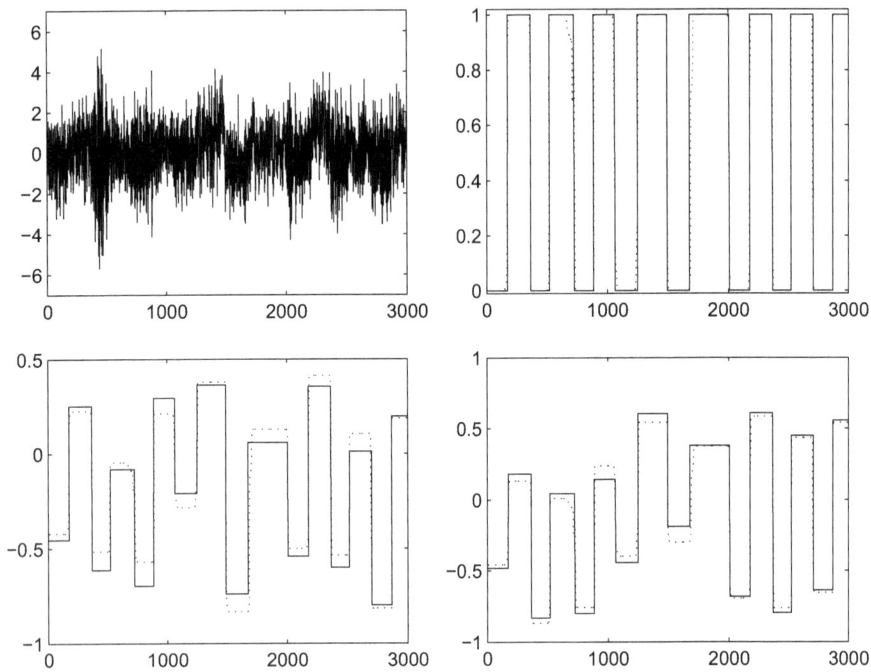

Fig. 1 A simulation example in Case 9 (x-axis: time; y-axis: numerical values): simulated series (*top left*), true and estimated s_t (*top right*), μ_t (*bottom left*), and α_t (*bottom right*)

Note that these two regimes cannot be easily distinguished as the standard deviation of each regime is large ($\sqrt{V^{(1)}} = \sqrt{V^{(2)}} = 0.4$), compare to the distance between $z^{(1)}$ and $z^{(2)}$. We use our model as a working model and $z_0^{(1)} = 0.2$, $z_0^{(2)} = 0.6$, and $V_0^{(1)} = V_0^{(2)} = 0.2$ to initialize the EM algorithm for hyperparameter estimation. We then use the estimated hyperparameter and apply the smoother in Sect. 3.3. The left panel in Fig. 2 shows the simulated y_t and our estimates. We notice that the probabilities of regimes over time are poorly estimated, and the regime shift in $t/T \in (0.5, 0.6)$ are completely missed. The reason of such poor estimation is that the EM algorithm doesn't give (or learn) the right prior on regimes since the regimes themselves are undistinguishable.

Example 2. The y_t and α_t are generated in the same way as in Example 1. We still use our model as the working model, but different from the initial value specification of the EM estimation in Example 1, we use $z_0^{(1)} = 0.6$, $z_0^{(2)} = 0.2$, and $V_0^{(1)} = V_0^{(2)} = 0.2$ as initial values of the EM algorithm. The right panel of Fig. 2 shows the simulated y_t and our estimates. We notice that the regime switching of α_t are nicely caught by our estimation procedure. The estimated probabilities of $s_t = 1$, though not perfectly 0 and 1, shows the regime shifts as well. This indicates that some misspecified hyperparameter can provide nice results even when the regimes are undistinguishable.

Table 2 Averaged KL, l_2, RSS, misclassification ratio and their standard errors (in parenthesis) of BCMIX(20,10) estimates

	Case	3000	4000	5000	6000	7000	8000
$10^3\kappa$	2	4.837	4.563	4.473	4.474	4.414	4.408
		(0.148)	(0.109)	(0.096)	(0.096)	(0.083)	(0.083)
	4	5.605	5.228	5.307	5.086	5.105	5.074
		(0.151)	(0.130)	(0.114)	(0.100)	(0.092)	(0.087)
	8	15.371	15.244	15.083	15.239	14.991	15.088
		(0.204)	(0.176)	(0.149)	(0.147)	(0.126)	(0.118)
	9	17.750	17.361	17.414	17.331	17.313	17.267
		(0.212)	(0.173)	(0.160)	(0.144)	(0.138)	(0.120)
χ	2	0.994	0.994	0.994	0.994	0.994	0.994
		(1.2e−3)	(1.0e−3)	(9.6e−4)	(8.7e−4)	(7.7e−4)	(7.3e−4)
	4	0.994	0.994	0.993	0.993	0.994	0.994
		(1.2e−3)	(1.0e−3)	(9.5e−4)	(8.7e−4)	(7.8e−4)	(7.3e−4)
	8	0.984	0.984	0.984	0.983	0.984	0.984
		(1.2e−3)	(1.0e−3)	(9.6e−4)	(8.7e−4)	(7.7e−4)	(7.3e−4)
	9	0.982	0.982	0.981	0.981	0.982	0.982
		(1.2e−3)	(1.0e−3)	(9.4e−4)	(8.7e−4)	(7.6e−4)	(7.3e−4)
$10^3 l_2$	2	1.284	1.111	0.991	0.918	0.841	0.786
		(0.022)	(0.015)	(0.012)	(0.011)	(0.009)	(0.008)
	4	1.401	1.196	1.073	0.980	0.905	0.842
		(0.021)	(0.017)	(0.013)	(0.010)	(0.009)	(0.008)
	8	2.475	2.118	1.877	1.730	1.585	1.484
		(0.018)	(0.013)	(0.010)	(0.009)	(0.007)	(0.006)
	9	2.635	2.259	2.023	1.846	1.699	1.593
		(0.016)	(0.012)	(0.010)	(0.008)	(0.007)	(0.006)
$10^2\nu$	2	3.1	1.8	1.2	1.5	1.1	1.0
		(0.690)	(0.471)	(0.325)	(0.388)	(0.305)	(0.226)
	4	3.0	1.6	1.2	1.8	1.2	0.8
		(0.677)	(0.464)	(0.339)	(0.452)	(0.306)	(0.182)
	8	1.3	1.1	1.1	1.1	1.1	0.9
		(0.140)	(0.090)	(0.089)	(0.075)	(0.068)	(0.025)
	9	1.3	1.2	1.2	1.2	1.2	1.1
		(0.085)	(0.068)	(0.059)	(0.045)	(0.047)	(0.026)

The above examples shows that, when regimes are close to each other, the EM or purely data-driven statistical procedure might not work well, or the performance of the smoothing estimates (13) on regimes may depends on the specification of the prior distributions Normal($z^{(k)}$, $V^{(k)}$). For example, the numerical estimates can be improved if the variances (or covariance matrices) $V^{(k)}$ are specified small enough

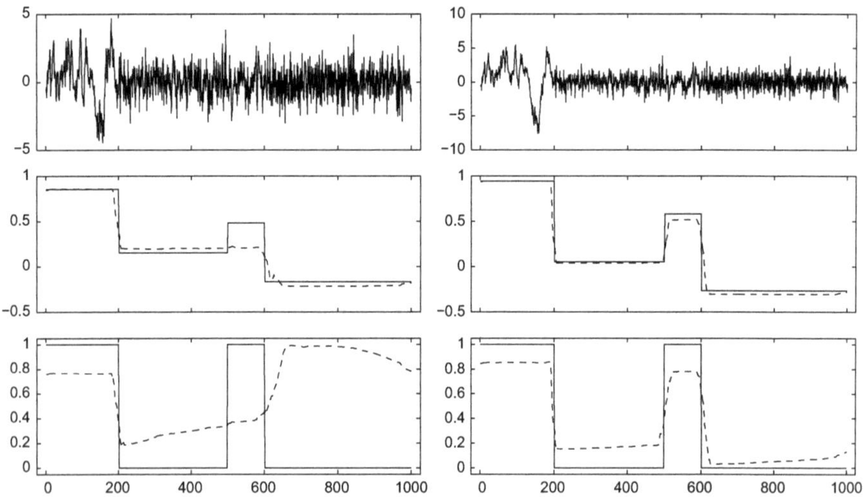

Fig. 2 The simulated series and estimates by our model in Examples 1 and 2 (x-axis: time; y-axis: numerical values). *Top*: simulated y_t; *Middle*: α_t (*solid line*) their BCMIX estimates (*dashed line*); *Bottom*: the probability of regime 1 (*solid line*) and their estimates (*dashed line*)

so that the prior distributions $N(z^{(k)}, V^{(k)})$ has small overlap. This also corresponds to specifying informative prior in statistics or having knowledge on regimes in economics before the data analysis.

4 Real Data Analysis

We now use our model to study the series of U.S. monthly total nonfarm employee (in millions) from February 1968 and June 2011. Released by the U.S. Department of Labor every month, the total nonfarm employee is an important labor statistic used to determine the health of the job market due to its large sample size and historical significance in relation to interpreting business cycles accurately. The data we used here has been deseasonalized and can be downloaded from the Federal Reserve Bank of St. Louis. The top panel of Fig. 3 show the series of monthly total nonfarm employee, denoted by w_t, in solid curve, and the recession periods announced by NBER in shaded areas. We can see that the total nonfarm employee increases almost exponentially during the non-recession periods, and decreases during all recessions, indicating a rising unemployment rate during recessions.

Since the series w_t is clearly nonstationary, we consider the differenced series $y_t = w_t - w_{t-1}$, $t =$ January 1970, ..., June 2011, as shown in the bottom panel of Fig. 3. An augmented Dickey-Fuller test yields a p-value less than 0.001, indicating the differenced series is stationary. In the sequel, we analyze the differenced series

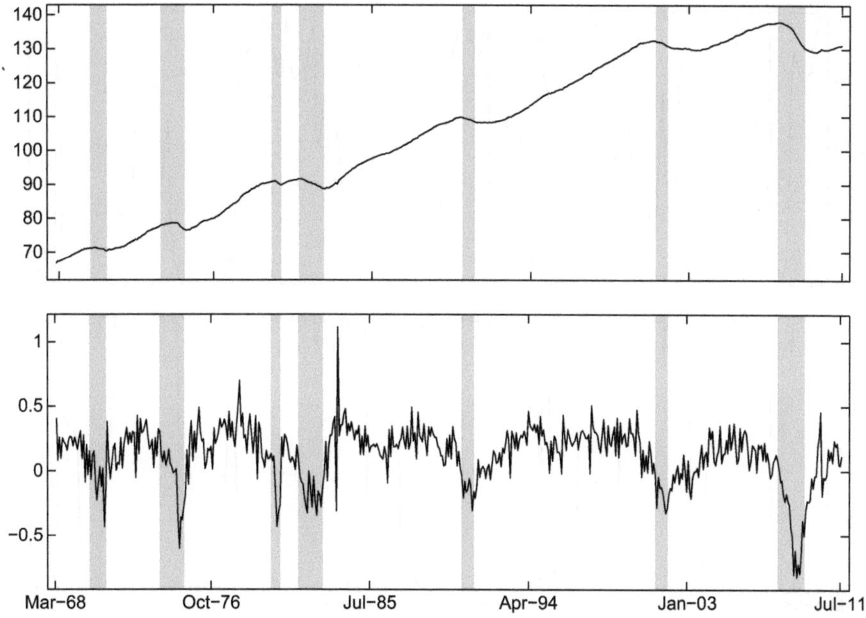

Fig. 3 The U.S. monthly total nonfarm employee (*top*) and its differenced series (*bottom*) from February 1968 to June 2011 (unit: millions)

y_t using the classic Markov switching models in Sect. 2 and the proposed model in Sect. 3, respectively. Both models assume a first-order autoregressive model with time-varying coefficient.

$$y_t = \mu_t + \alpha_t y_{t-1} + \epsilon_t, \tag{32}$$

where ϵ_t are independent and identically distributed normal random variables with mean 0 and variance σ^2, and the regression coefficient $\beta_t = (\mu_t, \alpha_t)'$ are time-varying and their dynamics are specified later. The model can be viewed as a stochastic regression model (1) with $x_t = (1, y_{t-1})'$. Since the series is closely related to economic expansion and contraction, we assume only two regimes, i.e., $K = 2$, and denote 1 and 2 for booming and recession regimes, respectively.

We first analyze y_t using the classic regime switching model [denoted as model (A)]. In this model, the coefficient $\{\beta_t\}$ is a two-state hidden Markov chain with state space $\{\beta^{(1)}, \beta^{(2)}\}$ and a probability transition matrix $Q_A = \{a_{ij}\}_{\{1\le i,j\le 2\}}$, where $a_{12} = 1 - a_{11}$ and $a_{21} = 1 - a_{22}$. We then use the method in Hamilton (1989) to compute the ML estimates, which are given as follows (standard errors are given in brackets):

$$\hat{a}_{11} = 0.9051(0.0320), \quad \hat{a}_{22} = 0.9370(0.0430), \quad \hat{\sigma}^2 = 0.0162(0.0011),$$

$$\hat{\beta}^{(1)} = \begin{pmatrix} 0.2891(0.0211) \\ -0.2258(0.0662) \end{pmatrix}, \quad \hat{\beta}^{(2)} = \begin{pmatrix} 0.0014(0.0076) \\ 0.8331(0.0344) \end{pmatrix}.$$

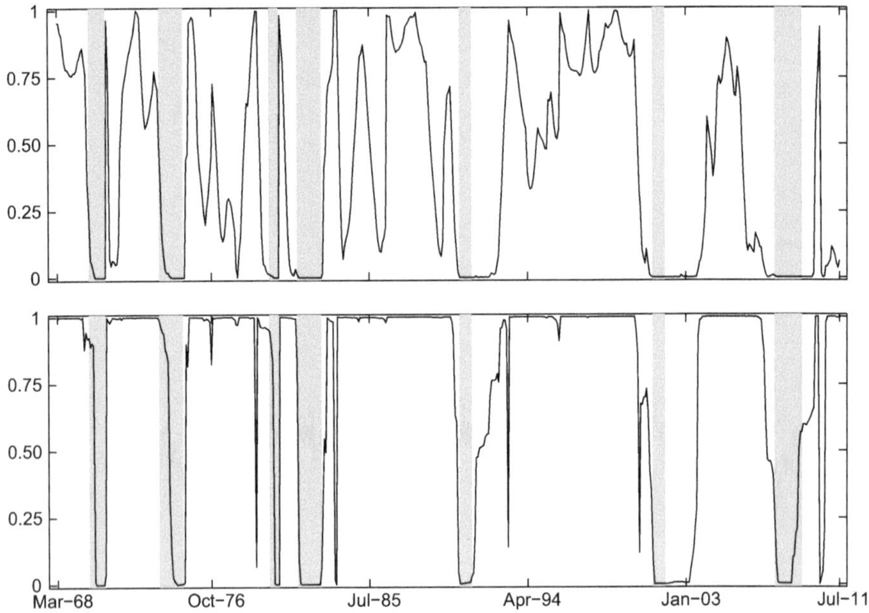

Fig. 4 Estimated probabilities of booming states in the classic Markov switching regression model (*top*) and in our model (*bottom*)

The top panel of Fig. 4 shows the estimated probability $\widehat{P}_A(s_t = 1|\mathscr{Y}_T)$ of booming states using the estimated parameter above. Note that, although the recession regimes inferred from $\widehat{P}_A(s_t = 1|\mathscr{Y}_T)$ overlap with the ones announced by NBER, the booming states are a little blurred among the recessions and such indistinction cannot be simply explained as a long transition period. For example, $\widehat{P}_A(s_t = 1|\mathscr{Y}_T)$ have several ups and downs between the July 1981–November 1982 and July 1990–March 1991 recessions, and similar patterns are found in the periods between two recessions.

We then fit our model [denoted as model (B)] to the differenced series. Note that the proposed model also admits a two-state hidden Markov chain with the probability transition matrix $Q_B = \{b_{ij}\}_{\{1\le i,j\le 2\}}$, where $b_{12} = 1 - b_{11}$ and $b_{21} = 1 - b_{22}$, and each regime $k \in \{1, 2\}$ is associated with a regime-dependent Normal prior distribution with mean $z^{(k)}$ and covariance $V^{(k)}$. We use the EM algorithm to estimate hyperparameters in the model and obtain

$$\hat{b}_{11} = 0.8747, \quad \hat{b}_{22} = 0.6334, \quad \hat{\sigma}^2 = 0.006518,$$

$$\hat{z}^{(1)} = \begin{pmatrix} 0.1866 \\ 0.1514 \end{pmatrix}, \qquad 100\widehat{V}^{(1)} = \begin{pmatrix} 0.2704 & 0.0535 \\ 0.0535 & 5.3052 \end{pmatrix},$$

$$\hat{z}^{(2)} = \begin{pmatrix} -0.0639 \\ 0.2285 \end{pmatrix}, \qquad 100\widehat{V}^{(2)} = \begin{pmatrix} 0.1230 & -0.0887 \\ -0.0887 & 21.614 \end{pmatrix}.$$

Then we use the above hyperparameters and apply the smoothing formulas in Sect. 2.3 to compute the estimates of coefficients μ_t, α_t, and probabilities of booming states $P_B(s_t = 1|\mathscr{Y}_T)$ (Our result shows almost no difference between the Bayes and BCMIX estimates, so we only present the BCMIX results with $(M, m) = (20, 10)$).

The bottom panel of Fig. 4 shows the estimated probabilities of the booming states, $\widehat{P}_B(s_t = 1|\mathscr{Y}_T)$. Comparing to those computed from the Markov switching model with two categorical regimes in the top panel of Fig. 4, the proposed model provides a much more distinctive representation of booming and recessions states. Not only the recession periods announced by NBER are clearly shown, but the booming periods as well. Figure 5 shows the estimated regression coefficients μ_t and α_t in the top and bottom panels, respectively. Note that the estimated μ_t and α_t in Fig. 5 show clear time variations that cannot be solely explained by two categorical regimes, suggesting that the categorical description of Markov switching is too restrictive, while the proposed model removes such restriction.

To study the dates of booming and recession regimes inferred from models (A) and (B), we use the rule (29) to define the inferred regimes. We notice that both models (A) and (B) estimate the dates of recessions very well, while model (B)

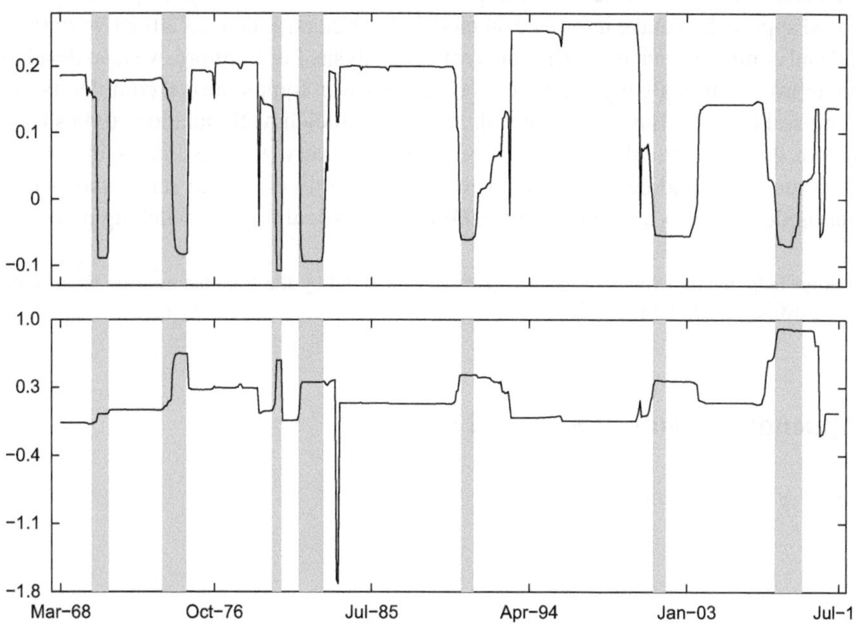

Fig. 5 The smoothing estimates of regression coefficient in the proposed model: $\hat{\mu}_t$ (*top*) and $\hat{\alpha}_t$ (*bottom*)

gives a clearer cut on the boundaries between booming and recession. In fact, if we use the booming and recession periods announced by NBER as a benchmark and denote $\tau_{A,k}$ and $\tau_{B,k}$ the misclassification rate for the kth regime in models (A) and (B), respectively, we obtain that $\tau_{A,1} = 0.469$, $\tau_{A,2} = 0.011$, and $\tau_{B,1} = 0.104$, $\tau_{B,2} = 0.2$. This result is consistent with the blurred boundaries between booming and recessions in the top panel of Fig. 4. We further summarize the dates of recessions given by NBER and estimated models (A) and (B) and the estimated regression coefficients by model (B) in Table 3. We first notice that the regression coefficients in model (B) varies significantly, even all of them are in the recession regime. Furthermore, the estimated coefficients in Fig. 5 shows that the autoregressive coefficients α_t in recessions are generally larger than those in booming periods, indicating a high persistence of the series during the recessions (or the bad employment situation is lingering around).

5 Conclusion

We consider herein a class of regime switching models with both categorical and continuous states to analyze economic variables related to business cycles. Our model is different from the classic Markov switching models with categorical regimes as it allows both categorical and continuous descriptions of model parameters, and provides more flexibility in practical analysis. We also developed a filtering based approach to make inference on model parameters, which has attractive statistical and computational properties in practical analysis. Furthermore, we also develop an approximation algorithm, which has much lower computational complexity yet comparable to the Bayes estimates in statistical efficiency. Simulation studies have shown that the smoothers in our model can give very good estimates in various situations. Our real data analysis of the U.S. monthly employee series shows that our model provides a better interpretation than classical regime switching models.

Acknowledgements Xing's research is partially supported by the National Science Foundation DMS-0906593 and DMS-1206321.

Appendix: Proofs in Sects. 2.2 and 2.3

Proof of (5). First note that

Table 3 Recessions given by NBER, the classic Markov switching (Model A) and the proposed (Model B) models

NBER		Model A		Model B			
Peak	Trough	Peak	Trough	Peak	Trough	μ_t	α_t
December-1969	November-1970	November-1969	November-1970	March-1970	November-1970	−0.0878	0.0257
November-1973	March-1975	December-1973	June-1975	May-1974	March-1975	−0.0709	0.6262
January-1980	July-1980	June-1979	June-1980	March-1980	June-1980	−0.1078	0.5776
July-1981	November-1982	November-1980	January-1983	July-1981	January-1983	−0.0878	0.3522
July-1990	March-1991	February-1990	December-1992	May-1990	June-1991	−0.0477	0.4225
March-2001	Nov-2001	May-2000	January-2004	December-2000	July-2003	−0.0462	0.3521
December-2007	June-2009	March-2006	January-2010	June-2007	February-2009	−0.0383	0.8188

$$f(\beta_t, y_t, s_{t-1} = k|\mathscr{Y}_{t-1}) = \sum_{l=1}^{K} f(\beta_t, y_t, s_{t-1} = k, s_t = l|\mathscr{Y}_{t-1})$$

$$= \sum_{l \neq k} f(\beta_t, y_t|\mathscr{Y}_{t-1}, s_{t-1} = k, s_t = l) P(s_{t-1} = k, s_t = l|\mathscr{Y}_{1,t-1})$$

$$+ \sum_{i=1}^{t-1} f(J_{t-1} = i, s_{t-1} = s_t = k, \beta_t, y_t|\mathscr{Y}_{t-1})$$

$$= p_{t-1}^{(k)} \sum_{l \neq k} a_{kl} f(y_t|s_t = l, J_t = t) f_{t,t}^{(l)}(\beta_t) + \sum_{i=1}^{t-1} p_{i,t-1}^{(k)} a_{kk} f(\beta_t, y_t|\mathscr{Y}_{t-1}, s_t = k, J_t = i)$$

$$= p_{t-1}^{(k)} \sum_{l \neq k} a_{kl} f(y_t|s_t = l, J_t = t) f_{t,t}^{(l)}(\beta_t) + a_{kk} \sum_{i=1}^{t-1} p_{i,t-1}^{(k)} f(y_t|\mathscr{Y}_{t-1}, s_t = k, J_t = i) f_{i,t}^{(k)}(\beta_t)$$

$$= \sum_{l \neq k} p_{t-1}^{(k)} a_{kl} f(y_t|s_t = l, J_t = t) f_{t,t}^{(l)}(\beta_t) + \sum_{i=1}^{t-1} p_{i,t}^{(k)*} f_{i,t}^{(k)}(\beta_t).$$

Then

$$f(\beta_t|\mathscr{Y}_t) \propto \sum_{k=1}^{K} f(\beta_t, y_t, s_{t-1} = k|\mathscr{Y}_{t-1})$$

$$= \sum_{k=1}^{K} \sum_{l \neq k} p_{t-1}^{(k)} a_{kl} f(y_t|s_t = l, J_t = t) f_{t,t}^{(l)}(\beta_t) + \sum_{k=1}^{K} \sum_{i=1}^{t-1} p_{i,t}^{(k)*} f_{i,t}^{(k)}(\beta_t)$$

$$= \sum_{l=1}^{K} \sum_{k \neq l} p_{t-1}^{(l)} a_{lk} f(y_t|s_t = k, J_t = t) f_{t,t}^{(k)}(\beta_t) + \sum_{k=1}^{K} \sum_{i=1}^{t-1} p_{i,t}^{(k)*} f_{i,t}^{(k)}(\beta_t)$$

$$= \sum_{k=1}^{K} p_{t,t}^{(k)*} f_{t,t}^{(k)}(\beta_t) + \sum_{k=1}^{K} \sum_{i=1}^{t-1} p_{i,t}^{(k)*} f_{i,t}^{(k)}(\beta_t).$$

Proof of (9). We first note that

$$f(\beta_t|\mathscr{Y}_{t+1,T}) = \sum_{k=1}^{K} f(\beta_t, s_{t+1} = k|\mathscr{Y}_{t+1,T})$$

$$= \sum_{k=1}^{K} P(s_{t+1} = k|\mathscr{Y}_{t+1,T}) f(\beta_t|s_{t+1} = k, \mathscr{Y}_{t+1,T})$$

$$= \sum_{k=1}^{K} \sum_{l=1}^{K} P(s_{t+1} = k|\mathscr{Y}_{t+1,T}) \tilde{q}_{kl} f(\beta_t|s_{t+1} = k, s_t = l, \mathscr{Y}_{t+1,T}).$$

Then using the fact

$$\tilde{q}_{kk}P(s_{t+1} = k|\mathcal{Y}_{t+1,T})f(\beta_t|s_{t+1} = k, s_t = k, \mathcal{Y}_{t+1,T})$$

$$= \tilde{q}_{kk}f(\beta, s_{t+1} = i|\mathcal{Y}_{t+1,T})\Big|_{\beta=\beta_t} = \tilde{q}_{kk}\sum_{j=t+1}^{T} q^{(k)}_{t+1,j}f^{(k)}_{t+1,j}(\beta)\Big|_{\beta=\beta_t}.$$

for the case $k = l$, and For the case $k \neq l$,

$$\tilde{q}_{kl}P(s_{t+1} = k|\mathcal{Y}_{t+1,T})f(\beta_t|s_{t+1} = k, s_t = l, \mathcal{Y}_{t+1,T}) = \tilde{q}_{kl}q^{(k)}_{t+1}f(\beta|s_t = l)\Big|_{\beta=\beta_t},$$

for the case $k \neq l$, we can show (9).

Proofs of (10) *and* (11). Let $f_t(\cdot|\mathcal{Y}_T)$, $f_t(\cdot|\mathcal{Y}_t)$, and $f_t(\cdot|\mathcal{Y}_{t+1,T})$ denote the density functions of the absolutely continuous components of β_t given $\mathcal{Y}_T$, $\mathcal{Y}_t$, and $\mathcal{Y}_{t+1,T}$, respectively. Then applying Bayes' theorem,

$$f_t(\beta|\mathcal{Y}_T) = \sum_{k=1}^{K} f_t(\beta, s_t = k|\mathcal{Y}_T) \propto \sum_{k=1}^{K} f_t(\beta, s_t = k|\mathcal{Y}_t)f_t(\beta, s_t = k|\mathcal{Y}_{t+1,T})/\pi(\beta, s_t = k).$$

The right hand side is a mixture of different states, hence for the event $[s_t = k]$, we have

$$f_t(\beta, s_t = k|\mathcal{Y}_t)f_t(\beta, s_t = k|\mathcal{Y}_{t+1,T})/\pi(\beta, s_t = k)$$

$$= \Big\{\sum_{i=1}^{t} p^{(k)}_{it}f^{(k)}_{i,t}(\beta)\Big\}\Big\{\tilde{q}_{kk}\sum_{j=t+1}^{T} q^{(k)}_{t+1,j}f^{(k)}_{t+1,j}(\beta) + \Big(\sum_{l\neq k}\tilde{q}_{lk}q^{(l)}_{t+1}\Big)f^{(k)}_{0,0}(\beta)\Big\}\Big/\big(\pi_k f^{(k)}_{0,0}(\beta)\big)$$

$$= \sum_{i=1}^{t} p^{(k)}_{it}\Big(\sum_{l\neq k}\frac{\tilde{q}_{lk}}{\pi_k}q^{(l)}_{t+1}\Big)f^{(k)}_{i,t}(\beta) + \frac{\tilde{q}_{kk}}{\pi_k}\sum_{1\leq i\leq t<j\leq T} p^{(k)}_{it}q^{(k)}_{t+1,j}\frac{f^{(k)}_{i,t}(\beta)f^{(k)}_{t+1,j}(\beta)}{f^{(k)}_{0,0}(\beta)}.$$

Simple algebra shows that

$$f^{(k)}_{i,t}(\beta)f^{(k)}_{t+1,j}(\beta)/f^{(k)}_{0,0}(\beta) = \Big(\psi^{(k)}_{ij}/(\psi^{(k)}_{it}\psi^{(k)}_{t+1,j})\Big)f^{(k)}_{i,j}(\beta).$$

Hence (10) and (11) are proved.

References

Ang, A., & Bekaert, G. (2002a). Short rate non-linearities and regime switches. *Journal of Economic Dynamics and Control, 26*, 1243–1274.

Ang, A., & Bekaert, G. (2002b). Regime switches in interest rates. *Journal of Business & Economic Statistics, 20*, 163–182.

Cai, J. (1994). A Markov model of unconditional variance in ARCH. *Journal of Business & Economic Statistics, 12*, 309–316.

Diebold, F. X., & Rudebusch, G. D. (1996). Measuring business cycles: A modern perspective. *The Review of Economics and Statistics, 78*, 67–77.

Durland, M. J., & McCurdy, T. H. (1994). Duration-dependent transitions in a Markov model of U.S. GNP growth. *Journal of Business & Economic Statistics, 12*, 279–288.

Filardo, A. J., & Gordon, S. F. (1998). Business cycles durations. *Journal of Econometrics, 85*, 99–123.

Gray, S. F. (1996). Modeling the conditional distribution of interest rates as a regime-switching process. *Journal of Financial Economics, 42*, 27–62.

Hamilton, J. D. (1989). A new approach to the economic analysis of nonstationary time series and the business cycle. *Econometrica, 57*, 357–384.

Hamilton, J. D. (1990) Analysis of time series subject to changes in regimes. *Journal of Econometrics, 45*, 39–70.

Hamilton, J. D. (1996). Specification testing in Markov-switching time series models. *Journal of Econometrics, 70*, 127–157.

Hamilton, J. D., & Susmel, R. (1994). Autoregressive conditional heteroscedasticity and changes in regime. *Journal of Econometrics, 64*, 307–333.

Kim, C. J. (1994). Dynamic linear models with Markov-switching. *Journal of Econometrics, 60*, 1–22.

Kim, C. J., Piger, J., & Startz, R. (2008). Estimation of Markov regime-switching regression models with endogenous switching. *Journal Econometrics, 143*, 263–273.

Lai, T. L., & Xing, H. (2011). A simple Bayesian approach to multiple change-points. *Statistica Sinica, 21*, 539–569.

Smith, D. R. (2002). Markov-switching and stochastic volatility diffusion models of short-term interest rates. *Journal of Business & Economic Statistics, 20*, 183–197.

So, M. K. P., Lam, K., & Li, W. K. (1998). A stochastic volatility model with Markov switching. *Journal of Business & Economic Statistics, 16*, 244–253.

Direction Estimation in a General Regression Model with Discrete Predictors

Yuexiao Dong and Zhou Yu

Abstract Consider a general regression model, where the response Y depends on discrete predictors $\mathbf{X}$ only through the index $\boldsymbol{\beta}^T\mathbf{X}$. It is well-known that the ordinary least squares (OLS) estimator can recover the underlying direction $\boldsymbol{\beta}$ exactly if the link function between Y and X is linear. Li and Duan (Ann Stat 17:1009–1052, 1989) showed that the OLS estimator can recover $\boldsymbol{\beta}$ proportionally if the predictors satisfy the linear conditional mean (LCM) condition. For discrete predictors, we demonstrate that the LCM condition generally does not hold. To improve the OLS estimator in the presence of discrete predictors, we model the conditional mean $\mathrm{E}(\mathbf{X} \mid \boldsymbol{\beta}^T\mathbf{X})$ as a polynomial function of $\boldsymbol{\beta}^T\mathbf{X}$ and use the central solution space (CSS) estimator. The superior performances of the CSS estimators are confirmed through numerical studies.

1 Introduction

Consider univariate response $Y \in \mathbb{R}$ and q-dimensional predictor $\mathbf{X} \in \mathbb{R}^q$. For $\boldsymbol{\beta} \in \mathbb{R}^q$, let $\theta = \boldsymbol{\beta}^T\mathbf{X}$ be a linear combination of the predictor $\mathbf{X}$. Suppose the probability distribution function of Y depends on $\mathbf{X}$ only through θ, such that

$$Y \sim F_\theta(Y), \text{ where } \theta = \boldsymbol{\beta}^T\mathbf{X}. \tag{1}$$

Model (1) allows Y to be continuous or discrete, and we will refer to it as the general regression model. Many popular regression models can be formulated under this framework, such as linear regression, single index model, transformation models, and generalized linear regression.

As a special case of the general regression model (1), single index model (SIM) considers $Y = g(\boldsymbol{\beta}^T\mathbf{X}) + \varepsilon$ for continuous response Y and unknown link

Y. Dong (✉)
Department of Statistics, Temple University, Philadelphia, PA 19122, USA
e-mail: ydong@temple.edu

Z. Yu
East China Normal University, Shanghai 200241, China
e-mail: zyu@stat.ecnu.edu.cn

Z. Jin et al. (eds.), *New Developments in Statistical Modeling, Inference and Application*, ICSA Book Series in Statistics, DOI 10.1007/978-3-319-42571-9_4

function $g : \mathbb{R} \mapsto \mathbb{R}$. SIM is a semiparametric model that allows for flexibility through the nonparametric link function and mitigates the curse of dimensionality through the parametric index structure. The estimation problem in SIM involves estimation of the index $\boldsymbol{\beta}$ and the link function $g(\cdot)$ simultaneously. Some classical references include Powell et al. (1989), Härdle et al. (1993), Ichimura (1993), Horowitz and Härdle (1996), Carroll et al. (1997), etc. Cui et al. (2011) considered a more general model, where the response can be continuous or discrete, and the single index appears in both the mean component and the variance component. Since nonparametric smoothing is involved in all the aforementioned methods, theses methods require that the link function $g(\cdot)$ is smooth and at least one predictor is continuous. To avoid nonparametric smoothing, methods based on distance covariance and Hilbert-Schmidt Independence Criterion are proposed, respectively, in Sheng and Yin (2013) and Zhang and Yin (2015).

In this paper, we aim to estimate the index $\theta = \boldsymbol{\beta}^T\mathbf{X}$ in the general regression model (1), where all the predictors are discrete. To the best of our knowledge, Cook and Li (2009) and Sheng and Yin (2013) are the only methods in the literature that allow all the predictors to be discrete. Let $\mathbf{X} = (X_1, \ldots, X_q)^T$. Cook and Li (2009) assumed that the conditional distribution of $X_i \mid Y$ follows a one-parameter exponential family distribution for $i = 1, \ldots, q$, and used the maximum likelihood estimator of the inverse regression model to recover the direction $\boldsymbol{\beta}$ in the original forward regression. On the other hand, Sheng and Yin (2013) argued that $\boldsymbol{\beta}$ can be recovered through maximizing the distance covariance between $\boldsymbol{\eta}^T\mathbf{X}$ and Y over $\boldsymbol{\eta} \in \mathbb{R}^p$. The estimator in Sheng and Yin (2013) is desirable as its asymptotic normality has been established under some technical conditions.

We provide an alternative method for direction recovery with discrete predictors. Denote $\text{var}(\mathbf{X}) = \boldsymbol{\Sigma}$ and assume $\text{E}(\mathbf{X}) = \mathbf{0}$ without loss of generality. The classical ordinary least squares (OLS) estimator from the linear regression model is $\boldsymbol{\beta}_{\text{OLS}} = \boldsymbol{\Sigma}^{-1}\text{E}(\mathbf{X}Y)$. A surprising fact revealed by Li and Duan (1989) is that $\boldsymbol{\beta}_{\text{OLS}}$ is proportional to the true direction $\boldsymbol{\beta}$ in model (1) under the following linear conditional mean (LCM) condition

$$\text{E}(\mathbf{X} \mid \boldsymbol{\beta}^T\mathbf{X}) \text{ is a linear function of } \boldsymbol{\beta}^T\mathbf{X}. \tag{2}$$

For continuous $\mathbf{X}$, it is well-known that if (2) holds for all $\boldsymbol{\beta} \in \mathbb{R}$, then $\mathbf{X}$ has to follow an elliptically-contoured distribution. Variable transformation and elliptical trimming (Cook and Nachtsheim 1994) are thus useful data preprocessing tools for continuous predictors. For discrete predictors, variable transformation and elliptical trimming no longer work, and new direction recovery method is needed when the LCM condition (2) is violated. This motivates us to consider the OLS estimator based on the central solution space (CSS). Although the CSS estimators have been systematically studied in Li and Dong (2009), Dong and Li (2010), and Dong and Yu (2012), we are the first to study CSS estimators in the presence of exclusively discrete predictors.

The rest of the paper is organized as follows. In Sect. 2, we examine the OLS estimator with discrete predictors and examine the role of the LCM condition. In

Sect. 3, we demonstrate that the LCM condition is oftentimes violated with discrete predictors, and introduce the central solution space estimator as an extension of OLS. Numerical studies are performed in Sect. 4 and we conclude the paper with some discussions in Sect. 5.

2 Two Scenarios That OLS Works

We explore the two scenarios when $\boldsymbol{\beta}_{\mathrm{OLS}}$ can be used to recover the true direction $\boldsymbol{\beta}$. In the first scenario, the response Y and the discrete predictor $\mathbf{X}$ have a linear relationship. In the second scenario, the discrete predictor $\mathbf{X}$ satisfies the LCM condition (2). We assume $\mathrm{E}(\mathbf{X}) = \mathbf{0}$ unless specified otherwise.

2.1 OLS with Linear Link Function

In the case with continuous Y, suppose Y and $\mathbf{X}$ follow the linear model $Y = \alpha + \boldsymbol{\beta}^T\mathbf{X} + \varepsilon$, where $\alpha \in \mathbb{R}$, $\boldsymbol{\beta} \in \mathbb{R}^q$, and ε is independent of $\mathbf{X}$. Then obviously we have

$$\boldsymbol{\beta}_{\mathrm{OLS}} = \boldsymbol{\Sigma}^{-1}\mathrm{E}(\mathbf{X}Y) = \alpha\boldsymbol{\Sigma}^{-1}\mathrm{E}(\mathbf{X}) + \boldsymbol{\Sigma}^{-1}\mathrm{E}(\mathbf{X}\mathbf{X}^T)\boldsymbol{\beta} + \boldsymbol{\Sigma}^{-1}\mathrm{E}(\mathbf{X})\mathrm{E}(\varepsilon) = \boldsymbol{\beta},$$

where the last equality holds because $\mathrm{E}(\mathbf{X}) = \mathbf{0}$ and $\mathrm{E}(\mathbf{X}\mathbf{X}^T) = \boldsymbol{\Sigma}$.

In the case with discrete Y, $\boldsymbol{\beta}_{\mathrm{OLS}}$ can be a good estimator of $\boldsymbol{\beta}$ when Y and $\mathbf{X}$ satisfy $Y = \alpha + \boldsymbol{\beta}^T\mathbf{X}$, which will be referred to as the no-error linear model. To fix the idea, consider the following two examples. We will see that the response and the predictors exactly follow the no-error linear model in Example 1, while the no-error linear model is a good approximation in Example 2.

Example 1. Consider the zoo data from the UCI machine learning repository http://archive.ics.uci.edu/ml/datasets/Zoo. This data set contains 101 animals with 16 attributes. Except for the number of legs, all the other attributes (aquatic or not; feathers or not; milk or not; etc.) are binary. The response is the type of the animal, with mammals (41 cases) and birds (20 cases) being the two dominant types. We collapse the other 40 cases into the third category, which includes insects, fish, reptiles, molluscs, and amphibians. The sample OLS estimator has only two coefficients that are significantly different from zero. Not surprisingly, the corresponding attributes are feathers and milk. For this particular data set, all the animals that milk are mammals, and all the animals with feathers are birds.

Example 2. Consider the congressional voting records from the 98th Congress, 2nd session in 1984, which is available at the UCI machine learning repository http://archive.ics.uci.edu/ml/datasets/Congressional+Voting+Records. The data set consists of votes from 435 U.S. House of Representatives Congressmen on 16 subjects, with each vote being one of the three categories: yea, nay, and unknown disposition. The response here is whether the Congressman is democrat or republican. From the sample OLS estimator, we see that the most dominant coefficient corresponds to a bill related to physician fee freeze. It turns out that 245 of 267 democrats voted against this bill, while 163 of 168 republicans voted for the same bill.

2.2 OLS with the LCM Condition

For nonlinear link functions, Li and Duan (1989) showed that $\boldsymbol{\beta}_{\text{OLS}}$ is proportional to the true direction $\boldsymbol{\beta}$ in model (1) under the LCM condition (2). For $\mathbf{a}, \mathbf{b} \in \mathbb{R}^q$, the $\boldsymbol{\Sigma}$-inner product between $\mathbf{a}$ and $\mathbf{b}$ is $\langle \mathbf{a}, \mathbf{b} \rangle_{\boldsymbol{\Sigma}} = \mathbf{a}^T \boldsymbol{\Sigma} \mathbf{b}$. Let $\mathbf{P}_{\boldsymbol{\Sigma}}(\boldsymbol{\beta}) = \boldsymbol{\Sigma}\boldsymbol{\beta}(\boldsymbol{\beta}^T\boldsymbol{\Sigma}\boldsymbol{\beta})^{-1}\boldsymbol{\beta}^T$ be the projection matrix onto the column space of $\boldsymbol{\beta}$ under the $\boldsymbol{\Sigma}$-inner product. The LCM condition (2) then implies that $\mathrm{E}(\mathbf{X} \mid \boldsymbol{\beta}^T\mathbf{X}) = \mathbf{P}_{\boldsymbol{\Sigma}}(\boldsymbol{\beta})\mathbf{X}$. Under model (1), we have

$$\mathrm{E}(\mathbf{X}Y) = \mathrm{E}\{\mathbf{X}\mathrm{E}(Y \mid \mathbf{X})\} = \mathrm{E}\{\mathbf{X}\mathrm{E}(Y \mid \boldsymbol{\beta}^T\mathbf{X})\} = \mathrm{E}\{\mathrm{E}(\mathbf{X} \mid \boldsymbol{\beta}^T\mathbf{X})Y\}. \tag{3}$$

Plug in $\mathrm{E}(\mathbf{X} \mid \boldsymbol{\beta}^T\mathbf{X}) = \mathbf{P}_{\boldsymbol{\Sigma}}(\boldsymbol{\beta})\mathbf{X}$ and pre-multiply $\boldsymbol{\Sigma}^{-1}$, we get

$$\boldsymbol{\beta}_{\text{OLS}} = \boldsymbol{\Sigma}^{-1}\mathrm{E}(\mathbf{X}Y) = \boldsymbol{\Sigma}^{-1}\mathbf{P}_{\boldsymbol{\Sigma}}(\boldsymbol{\beta})\mathrm{E}(\mathbf{X}Y) = \boldsymbol{\beta}(\boldsymbol{\beta}^T\boldsymbol{\Sigma}\boldsymbol{\beta})^{-1}\boldsymbol{\beta}^T\mathrm{E}(\mathbf{X}Y) \propto \boldsymbol{\beta},$$

where "$\propto$" means proportional to.

Remark 1. A related concept is sufficient dimension reduction (SDR) (Cook 1998). SDR aims to find $\mathbf{B} = \{\boldsymbol{\beta}_1, \ldots, \boldsymbol{\beta}_d\} \in \mathbb{R}^{q \times d}$ with the smallest possible column space, such that

$$Y \perp\!\!\!\perp \mathbf{X} \mid \mathbf{B}^T\mathbf{X}, \tag{4}$$

where "$\perp\!\!\!\perp$" means statistical independence. Correspondingly, the smallest column space is called the central space for the regression between Y and $\mathbf{X}$, and is denoted as $\mathcal{S}_{Y|\mathbf{X}}$. (4) implies that Y depends on $\mathbf{X}$ only through $\mathbf{B}^T\mathbf{X}$. Under the general regression model (1), Y is independent of $\mathbf{X}$ given the index $\theta = \boldsymbol{\beta}^T\mathbf{X}$, which guarantees the second equality in (3). Model (1) can thus be viewed as a special case of (4) with the number of indices $d = 1$. Using the SDR terminology, the finding in Li and Duan (1989) becomes that $\boldsymbol{\beta}_{\text{OLS}} \in \mathcal{S}_{Y|\mathbf{X}}$.

Remark 2. Sheng and Yin (2013) proposed direction recovery in model (1) through distance covariance. They require a technical condition that

$$\mathbf{P}_{\boldsymbol{\Sigma}}(\boldsymbol{\beta})\mathbf{X} \perp\!\!\!\perp \mathbf{Q}_{\boldsymbol{\Sigma}}(\boldsymbol{\beta})\mathbf{X}, \tag{5}$$

where $\mathbf{Q}_{\boldsymbol{\Sigma}}(\boldsymbol{\beta}) = \mathbf{I}_q - \mathbf{P}_{\boldsymbol{\Sigma}}(\boldsymbol{\beta})$ with $\mathbf{I}_q$ being the $q \times q$ dimensional identity matrix. Note that $Y \perp\!\!\!\perp \mathbf{Q}_{\boldsymbol{\Sigma}}(\boldsymbol{\beta})\mathbf{X} \mid \mathbf{P}_{\boldsymbol{\Sigma}}(\boldsymbol{\beta})\mathbf{X}$ under model (1). Together with (5), we have

$\{Y, \mathbf{P}_{\boldsymbol{\Sigma}}(\boldsymbol{\beta})\mathbf{X}\} \perp\!\!\!\perp \mathbf{Q}_{\boldsymbol{\Sigma}}(\boldsymbol{\beta})\mathbf{X}$. It follows that

$$\mathrm{E}(\mathbf{X}Y) = \mathrm{E}\{\mathbf{P}_{\boldsymbol{\Sigma}}(\boldsymbol{\beta})\mathbf{X}Y\} + \mathrm{E}\{\mathbf{Q}_{\boldsymbol{\Sigma}}(\boldsymbol{\beta})\mathbf{X}Y\} = \mathrm{E}\{\mathbf{P}_{\boldsymbol{\Sigma}}(\boldsymbol{\beta})\mathbf{X}Y\} = \mathbf{P}_{\boldsymbol{\Sigma}}(\boldsymbol{\beta})\mathrm{E}(\mathbf{X}Y),$$

where the second equality holds because $\mathrm{E}\{\mathbf{Q}_{\boldsymbol{\Sigma}}(\boldsymbol{\beta})\mathbf{X}Y\} = \mathbf{Q}_{\boldsymbol{\Sigma}}(\boldsymbol{\beta})\mathrm{E}(\mathbf{X})\mathrm{E}(Y) = \mathbf{0}$. Under the same technical condition (5) as in Sheng and Yin (2013), we have shown that $\boldsymbol{\beta}_{\mathrm{OLS}} \propto \boldsymbol{\beta}$.

Next we present an example with discrete predictors and demonstrate that $\boldsymbol{\beta}_{\mathrm{OLS}} \propto \boldsymbol{\beta}$ when the LCM condition (2) is satisfied. The square link function is used for the ease of demonstration. Other types of link functions lead to similar results. We do not require $\mathrm{E}(\mathbf{X}) = \mathbf{0}$, and the OLS estimator $\boldsymbol{\beta}_{\mathrm{OLS}} = \boldsymbol{\Sigma}^{-1}\mathrm{E}\{(\mathbf{X} - \mathrm{E}(\mathbf{X}))Y\}$ is used in this example.

Example 3. Consider $\mathbf{X} = (X_1, X_2)^T$, $\boldsymbol{\beta} = (1, 1)^T$, and $Y = (\boldsymbol{\beta}^T\mathbf{X})^2$.

Case i: $X_1 \sim \text{Poisson}(l_1)$, $X_2 \sim \text{Poisson}(l_2)$, and $X_1 \perp\!\!\!\perp X_2$. It is easy to see

$$X_1 \mid (X_1 + X_2 = m) \sim \text{Binomial}\,(m, \rho) \;\text{ with } \rho = l_1/(l_1 + l_2).$$

It follows that $\mathrm{E}(X_1 \mid X_1 + X_2) = \rho(X_1 + X_2)$ is linear in $X_1 + X_2$. Similarly $\mathrm{E}(X_2 \mid X_1 + X_2)$ is linear in $X_1 + X_2$. Together the LCM condition (2) holds. On the other hand, we have

$$\boldsymbol{\Sigma} = \begin{pmatrix} l_1 & 0 \\ 0 & l_2 \end{pmatrix} \text{ and } \mathrm{E}\{(\mathbf{X} - \mathrm{E}(\mathbf{X}))Y\} = \begin{pmatrix} l_1(2l_1 + 2l_2 + 1) \\ l_2(2l_1 + 2l_2 + 1) \end{pmatrix}.$$

It follows that

$$\boldsymbol{\beta}_{\mathrm{OLS}} = \boldsymbol{\Sigma}^{-1}\mathrm{E}\{(\mathbf{X} - \mathrm{E}(\mathbf{X}))Y\} = \begin{pmatrix} 2l_1 + 2l_2 + 1 \\ 2l_1 + 2l_2 + 1 \end{pmatrix} \propto \begin{pmatrix} 1 \\ 1 \end{pmatrix} = \boldsymbol{\beta}.$$

Case ii: $X_1 \sim \text{Binomial}(n_1, p)$, $X_2 \sim \text{Binomial}(n_2, p)$, and $X_1 \perp\!\!\!\perp X_2$. Then

$$X_1 \mid (X_1 + X_2 = m) \sim \text{Hypergeometric}(n_1 + n_2, m, n_1).$$

It is easy to see that the LCM condition is satisfied. We also have

$$\boldsymbol{\Sigma} = \begin{pmatrix} n_1p & 0 \\ 0 & n_2p \end{pmatrix} \text{ and } \mathrm{E}\{(\mathbf{X} - \mathrm{E}(\mathbf{X}))Y\} = \begin{pmatrix} n_1p(1-p)(1 - 2p + 2n_1p + 2n_2p) \\ n_2p(1-p)(1 - 2p + 2n_1p + 2n_2p) \end{pmatrix}.$$

It follows that

$$\boldsymbol{\beta}_{\mathrm{OLS}} = \boldsymbol{\Sigma}^{-1}\mathrm{E}\{(\mathbf{X} - \mathrm{E}(\mathbf{X}))Y\} = \begin{pmatrix} (1-p)(1 - 2p + 2n_1p + 2n_2p) \\ (1-p)(1 - 2p + 2n_1p + 2n_2p) \end{pmatrix} \propto \begin{pmatrix} 1 \\ 1 \end{pmatrix} = \boldsymbol{\beta}.$$

Case iii: $(X_1, X_2, W)^T \sim \text{Multinomial}(n, (p_1, p_2, p_3))$. We have

$$X_1 \mid (X_1 + X_2 = m) \sim \text{Binomial}\,(m, \pi) \;\; \text{with}\; \pi = p_1/(p_1 + p_2).$$

Thus the LCM condition is satisfied. The explicit calculation of $\boldsymbol{\beta}_{\text{OLS}}$ shows that it is proportional to $\boldsymbol{\beta}$, and the details are provided in the Appendix.

3 Central Solution Space with Discrete Predictors

We have seen in Sect. 2 that the LCM condition plays an important role for $\boldsymbol{\beta}_{\text{OLS}}$ to recover $\boldsymbol{\beta}$ in model (1). We will see that the LCM condition is more often than not violated with discrete predictors. Transformation or trimming, which are popular methods for continuous predictors, are not applicable for discrete predictors. This motivates us to consider the central solution space estimator (Li and Dong 2009), which does not require the LCM condition.

3.1 Beyond the LCM Condition

Consider $\mathbf{X} = (X_1, X_2)^T$, $X_1 \sim \text{Binomial}(n_1 = 2, p_1)$, $X_2 \sim \text{Binomial}(n_2 = 3, p_2)$, and $X_1 \perp\!\!\!\perp X_2$. We are interested in $\text{E}(X_1 \mid \boldsymbol{\beta}^T\mathbf{X})$ as a function of $\boldsymbol{\beta}^T\mathbf{X}$ for different combinations of p_1, p_2 and $\boldsymbol{\beta}$. The explicit form of $\text{E}(X_1 \mid \boldsymbol{\beta}^T\mathbf{X})$ may not be easily derived. Instead, we generate $N = 10^6$ random samples and calculate the sample conditional mean $\text{E}_N(X_1 \mid \boldsymbol{\beta}^T\mathbf{X})$ as an approximation of $\text{E}(X_1 \mid \boldsymbol{\beta}^T\mathbf{X})$. Specifically, let $\{\mathbf{X}^{(i)}, i = 1, \ldots, N\}$ be an i.i.d. sample of $\mathbf{X}$, where $\mathbf{X}^{(i)} = (X_1^{(i)}, X_2^{(i)})^T$. Suppose Ω is the support of $\boldsymbol{\beta}^T\mathbf{X}$. For any $\omega \in \Omega$, let $I(\boldsymbol{\beta}^T\mathbf{X} = \omega)$ be the indicator function of $\boldsymbol{\beta}^T\mathbf{X} = \omega$. Then $\text{E}(X_1 \mid \boldsymbol{\beta}^T\mathbf{X} = \omega)$ can be approximated by

$$\text{E}_N(X_1 \mid \boldsymbol{\beta}^T\mathbf{X} = \omega) = \frac{\text{E}_N\{X_1 I(\boldsymbol{\beta}^T\mathbf{X} = \omega)\}}{\text{E}_N\{I(\boldsymbol{\beta}^T\mathbf{X} = \omega)\}} = \frac{\sum_{i=1}^N X_1^{(i)} I(\boldsymbol{\beta}^T\mathbf{X}^{(i)} = \omega)}{\sum_{i=1}^N I(\boldsymbol{\beta}^T\mathbf{X}^{(i)} = \omega)}.$$

We plot $\text{E}_N(X_1 \mid \boldsymbol{\beta}^T\mathbf{X})$ versus $\boldsymbol{\beta}^T\mathbf{X}$ in Fig. 1. The linear, quadratic and cubic fit between $\text{E}_N(X_1 \mid \boldsymbol{\beta}^T\mathbf{X})$ and $\boldsymbol{\beta}^T\mathbf{X}$ are also included. The upper left panel confirms the finding in case ii of Example 3. Namely, $\text{E}(X_1 \mid \boldsymbol{\beta}^T\mathbf{X})$ is a linear function of $\boldsymbol{\beta}^T\mathbf{X}$ and the LCM condition is satisfied when $p_1 = p_2$ and $\boldsymbol{\beta} = (1, 1)^T$. In the first row of Fig. 1, we fix $\boldsymbol{\beta} = (1, 1)^T$ and modify p_1 and p_2. It is clear that $\text{E}(X_1 \mid \boldsymbol{\beta}^T\mathbf{X})$ is a nonlinear function of $\boldsymbol{\beta}^T\mathbf{X}$ when $p_1 \neq p_2$. In the second row of Fig. 1, we fix $p_1 = p_2 = 0.1$ and modify $\boldsymbol{\beta}$. We see that the LCM condition will not hold when $\boldsymbol{\beta}$ is not proportional to $(1, 1)^T$. Similar results hold true for cases i and iii of Example 3, which are not reported here.

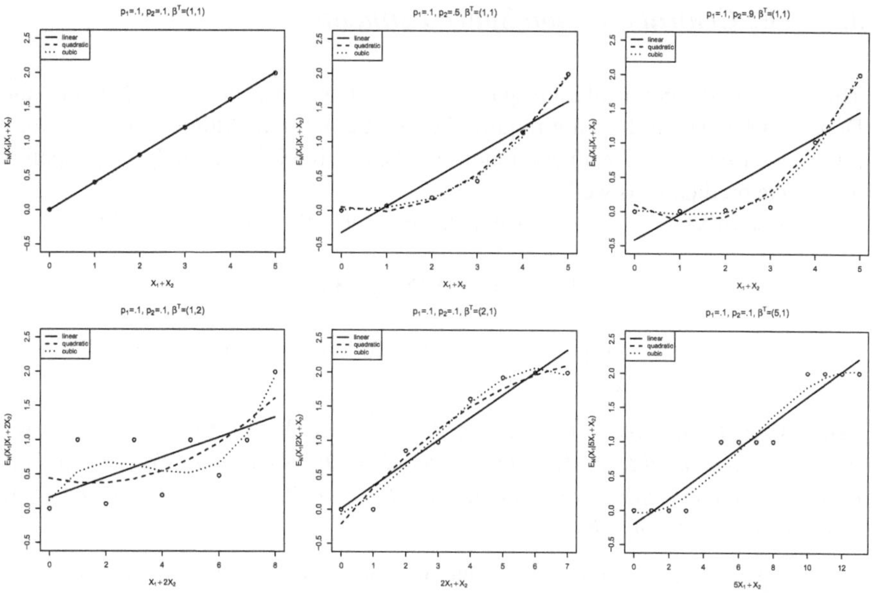

Fig. 1 $E_N(X_1 \mid \boldsymbol{\beta}^T\mathbf{X})$ v.s. $\boldsymbol{\beta}^T\mathbf{X}$. $N = 10^6$, $X_1 \sim$ Binomial $(2, p_1)$, $X_2 \sim$ Binomial $(3, p_2)$, and X_1 independent of X_2

We see from Fig. 1 that the LCM condition could easily be violated with discrete predictors. The next example demonstrates that without the LCM condition, $\boldsymbol{\beta}_{\text{OLS}}$ may not be able to recover $\boldsymbol{\beta}$.

Example 4. Let $\mathbf{X} = (X_1, X_2)^T$, $\boldsymbol{\beta} = (1, 1)^T$, and $Y = (\boldsymbol{\beta}^T\mathbf{X})^3$. Suppose $X_1 \sim$ *Bernoulli*(p_1), $X_2 \sim$ *Bernoulli*(p_2), and $X_1 \perp\!\!\!\perp X_2$. Similar to Fig. 1, one can check that the LCM condition is violated if $p_1 \neq p_2$. On the other hand, we have

$$\boldsymbol{\Sigma} = \begin{pmatrix} p_1 & 0 \\ 0 & p_2 \end{pmatrix} \text{ and } \mathrm{E}\{(\mathbf{X} - \mathrm{E}(\mathbf{X}))Y\} = \begin{pmatrix} p_1 - p_1^2 + 6p_1p_2 - 6p_1^2p_2 \\ p_2 - p_2^2 + 6p_1p_2 - 6p_1p_2^2 \end{pmatrix}.$$

It follows that

$$\boldsymbol{\beta}_{\text{OLS}} = \boldsymbol{\Sigma}^{-1}\mathrm{E}\{(\mathbf{X} - \mathrm{E}(\mathbf{X}))Y\} = \begin{pmatrix} 1 - p_1 + 6p_2 - 6p_1p_2 \\ 1 - p_2 + 6p_1 - 6p_1p_2 \end{pmatrix},$$

which is not proportional to $\boldsymbol{\beta} = (1, 1)^T$ unless $p_1 = p_2$.

3.2 The Central Solution Space Estimator

The OLS-based central solution space (CSS) estimator was first proposed in Li and Dong (2009), which does not require the LCM condition. Although Li and Dong (2009) focused on CSS with continuous predictors, the CSS method can be applied to discrete predictors as well.

Suppose $\mathrm{E}(\mathbf{X}) = \mathbf{0}$. Under model (1), we observe the following equality

$$\mathrm{E}(\mathbf{X}Y) = \mathrm{E}\{\mathrm{E}(\mathbf{X} \mid \boldsymbol{\beta}^T\mathbf{X})Y\}. \tag{6}$$

Denote the solution of Eq. (6) as $\boldsymbol{\beta}_{\mathrm{CSS}}$. The following result is a special case of Theorem 4.1 in Li and Dong (2009).

Proposition 1. *Suppose* $\Pr(\mathrm{E}\{\mathrm{E}(\mathbf{X} \mid \boldsymbol{\eta}^T\mathbf{X})Y\} \neq \mathrm{E}\{\mathrm{E}(\mathbf{X} \mid \boldsymbol{\beta}^T\mathbf{X})Y\}) > 0$ *whenever* $\boldsymbol{\eta}$ *is not proportional to* $\boldsymbol{\beta}$. *Then under model (1), the solution of Eq. (6) is unique up to a scalar multiplication, and satisfies* $\boldsymbol{\beta}_{\mathrm{CSS}} \propto \boldsymbol{\beta}$. *Furthermore, if the LCM condition (2) holds, then* $\boldsymbol{\beta}_{\mathrm{CSS}} \propto \boldsymbol{\beta}_{\mathrm{OLS}}$.

The first part of Proposition 1 states that one can use $\boldsymbol{\beta}_{\mathrm{CSS}}$ to recover $\boldsymbol{\beta}$ without the LCM condition (2). The second part reveals that $\boldsymbol{\beta}_{\mathrm{CSS}}$ coincides with $\boldsymbol{\beta}_{\mathrm{OLS}}$ when the LCM condition is true. Ichimura (1993) provided an example that the parameters in the index $\boldsymbol{\beta}$ are unidentifiable when the predictors are all discrete. Our assumption in Proposition 1 eliminates such pathological situations, and guarantees that the CSS estimator is unique even with exclusively discrete predictors.

For $\mathbf{a} = (a_1, \ldots, a_q)^T \in \mathbb{R}^q$, let $\|\mathbf{a}\| = \sqrt{\sum_{i=1}^q a_i^2}$. To find the solution of Eq. (6), Li and Dong (2009) suggested solving the following optimization problem

$$\text{minimize } L(\boldsymbol{\eta}) \text{ over } \boldsymbol{\eta} \in \mathbb{R}^q, \text{ where } L(\boldsymbol{\eta}) = \|\mathrm{E}\{\mathbf{X}Y - \mathrm{E}(\mathbf{X} \mid \boldsymbol{\eta}^T\mathbf{X})Y\}\|^2. \tag{7}$$

Denote the minimizer of $L(\boldsymbol{\eta})$ as $\boldsymbol{\eta}_0$. As long as all the moments involved exist, Theorem 4.2 in Li and Dong (2009) states that $\boldsymbol{\eta}_0$ is proportional to $\boldsymbol{\beta}_{\mathrm{CSS}}$ under the same condition as in Proposition 1.

The sample level CSS estimator is based on minimizing $L_N(\boldsymbol{\eta})$, the sample objective function of $L(\boldsymbol{\eta})$ in (7). Motivated from the observations in Sect. 3.1, we model $\mathrm{E}(\mathbf{X} \mid \boldsymbol{\eta}^T\mathbf{X})$ as a polynomial function of $\boldsymbol{\eta}^T\mathbf{X}$. As we have seen in Fig. 1, for discrete predictors, using quadratic and cubic functions of $\boldsymbol{\eta}^T\mathbf{X}$ may be more suitable than using linear functions of $\boldsymbol{\eta}^T\mathbf{X}$. For any function $r(\mathbf{X}, Y)$ and an i.i.d. sample $\{(\mathbf{X}^{(i)}, Y^{(i)}), i = 1, \ldots, N\}$, we denote the sample estimator of $\mathrm{E}\{r(\mathbf{X}, Y)\}$ by $\mathrm{E}_N\{r(\mathbf{X}, Y)\} = N^{-1}\sum_{i=1}^N r(\mathbf{X}^{(i)}, Y^{(i)})$. The step-by-step algorithm is as follows.

1. Center $Y^{(i)}$ and $\mathbf{X}^{(i)}$ as $\hat{Y}^{(i)} = Y^{(i)} - \mathrm{E}_N(Y)$, $\hat{\mathbf{X}}^{(i)} = \mathbf{X}^{(i)} - \mathrm{E}_N(\mathbf{X})$.
2. Set $k = 2$ or $k = 3$. Denote $G(\boldsymbol{\eta}^T\hat{\mathbf{X}}^{(i)})$ as $\{1, \boldsymbol{\eta}^T\hat{\mathbf{X}}^{(i)}, \ldots, (\boldsymbol{\eta}^T\hat{\mathbf{X}}^{(i)})^k\}^T$. The sample estimator of $\mathrm{E}(\hat{\mathbf{X}} \mid \boldsymbol{\eta}^T\hat{\mathbf{X}})$ becomes

$$\mathrm{E}_N(\hat{\mathbf{X}} \mid \boldsymbol{\eta}^T\hat{\mathbf{X}}) = \mathrm{E}_N\{\hat{\mathbf{X}}G^T(\boldsymbol{\eta}^T\hat{\mathbf{X}})\}\left(\mathrm{E}_N\{G(\boldsymbol{\eta}^T\hat{\mathbf{X}})G^T(\boldsymbol{\eta}^T\hat{\mathbf{X}})\}\right)^{-1} G(\boldsymbol{\eta}^T\hat{\mathbf{X}}).$$

3. Estimate $\boldsymbol{\beta}$ by solving the following optimization problem

$$\text{minimize } L_N(\boldsymbol{\eta}) \text{ over } \boldsymbol{\eta} \in \mathbb{R}^q, \text{ where } L_N(\boldsymbol{\eta}) = \|\mathrm{E}_N\{\hat{\mathbf{X}}\hat{Y} - \mathrm{E}_N(\hat{\mathbf{X}} \mid \boldsymbol{\eta}^T\hat{\mathbf{X}})\hat{Y}\}\|^2,$$

where the minimizer is denoted as $\hat{\boldsymbol{\beta}}^{(k)}_{\text{CSS}}$.

A Newton-Raphson type estimator can be implemented to find the minimizer in step 3 of the above algorithm. See, for example, Cook and Li (2009), Dong and Yu (2012).

4 Numerical Studies

In this section, we demonstrate the effectiveness of CSS estimator with discrete predictors via simulation studies. For $\mathbf{X} = (X_1, \ldots, X_q)^T$ and $\boldsymbol{\beta} \in \mathbb{R}^q$, consider three settings of $\boldsymbol{\beta}^T\mathbf{X}$ as follows,

Case (i): $\boldsymbol{\beta} = (1, -1, 1, 0, \ldots, 0)^T, X_1 \sim \text{Binomial}(2, 0.1), X_2 \sim \text{Binomial}(3, 0.9),$

$X_3, \ldots, X_q \sim \text{Bernoulli}(0.5)$, and $X_i \perp\!\!\!\perp X_j$ for $i \neq j$.

Case (ii): $\boldsymbol{\beta} = (-1, -1, 3, 0, \ldots, 0)^T, X_1 \sim \text{Poisson}(1), X_2 \sim \text{Poisson}(0.5),$

$X_3, \ldots, X_q \sim \text{Bernoulli}(.5)$, and $X_i \perp\!\!\!\perp X_j$ for $i \neq j$.

Case (iii): $\boldsymbol{\beta}=(1, 0, -1, 0, \ldots, 0)^T, (X_1, X_2, W)^T \sim \text{Multinomial}(4, (0.2, 0.4, 0.4)),$

$X_3, \ldots, X_q \sim \text{Bernoulli}(0.5)$, and $X_i \perp\!\!\!\perp X_j$ for $i \neq j$ except for X_1 and X_2.

For each combination of $\boldsymbol{\beta}$ and $\mathbf{X}$, consider the following models

$$\text{Model I:} \quad Y = 0.2\exp(\boldsymbol{\beta}^T\mathbf{X} + 2) + 0.2\varepsilon,$$

$$\text{Model II:} \quad Y = 0.2(\boldsymbol{\beta}^T\mathbf{X})^3 + 0.2\varepsilon,$$

$$\text{Model III:} \quad Y = \begin{cases} 1 & \text{if} \boldsymbol{\beta}^T\mathbf{X} \geq 0, \\ 0 & \text{if} \boldsymbol{\beta}^T\mathbf{X} < 0. \end{cases}$$

In Model I and II, we have continuous response with error $\varepsilon \sim N(0, 1)$ and $\varepsilon \perp\!\!\!\perp X$. The response in Model III is discrete. All three models are special cases of the general regression model (1). Denote $\boldsymbol{\Sigma}_N$ as the sample covariance matrix of $\mathbf{X}$. Then the classical ordinary least squares estimator is $\hat{\boldsymbol{\beta}}_{\text{OLS}} = \boldsymbol{\Sigma}_N^{-1}\mathrm{E}_N\{(\mathbf{X} - \mathrm{E}_N(\mathbf{X}))Y\}$. Two CSS estimators $\hat{\boldsymbol{\beta}}^{(2)}_{\text{CSS}}$ and $\hat{\boldsymbol{\beta}}^{(3)}_{\text{CSS}}$ are also included for the comparison, where we estimate $\mathrm{E}(\mathbf{X} \mid \boldsymbol{\beta}^T\mathbf{X})$ as a quadratic or a cubic function of $\boldsymbol{\beta}^T\mathbf{X}$. Let $R^2(\hat{\boldsymbol{\beta}}, \boldsymbol{\beta})$ be the squared sample Pearson correlation between $\boldsymbol{\beta}^T\mathbf{X}$ and $\hat{\boldsymbol{\beta}}^T\mathbf{X}$, which will be used to measure the performances of different estimators.

Table 1 Comparison of OLS and CSS estimators based on 100 repetitions

Case	Model	$\widehat{R^2}(\hat{\boldsymbol{\beta}}_{\text{OLS}}, \boldsymbol{\beta})$	$\widehat{R^2}(\hat{\boldsymbol{\beta}}^{(2)}_{\text{CSS}}, \boldsymbol{\beta})$	$\widehat{R^2}(\hat{\boldsymbol{\beta}}^{(3)}_{\text{CSS}}, \boldsymbol{\beta})$
(i)	I	0.9262 (0.0032)	0.9562 (0.0021)	0.9712 (0.0018)
	II	0.9641 (0.0012)	0.9984 (0.0001)	0.9994 (0.0001)
	III	0.8038 (0.0084)	0.7976 (0.0144)	0.8700 (0.0099)
(ii)	I	0.9721 (0.0015)	0.9547 (0.0020)	0.9803 (0.0013)
	II	0.8997 (0.0035)	0.9180 (0.0034)	0.9430 (0.0040)
	III	0.9593 (0.0020)	0.9543 (0.0021)	0.9803 (0.0009)
(iii)	I	0.9602 (0.0018)	0.9855 (0.0020)	0.9977 (0.0004)
	II	0.9389 (0.0023)	0.9647 (0.0025)	0.9880 (0.0008)
	III	0.9102 (0.0029)	0.9846 (0.0009)	0.9794 (0.0015)

We fix predictor dimension $q = 10$, sample size $N = 200$, and report the simulation results in Table 1 based on 100 repetitions. Each entry of Table 1 is formatted as $a(b)$, where a is the average of $\widehat{R^2}(\hat{\boldsymbol{\beta}}, \boldsymbol{\beta})$ across the 100 repetitions, and b is the standard error of the average. We see that $\hat{\boldsymbol{\beta}}^{(2)}_{\text{CSS}}$ outperforms $\hat{\boldsymbol{\beta}}_{\text{OLS}}$ in six out of nine settings, while $\hat{\boldsymbol{\beta}}^{(3)}_{\text{CSS}}$ consistently outperforms $\hat{\boldsymbol{\beta}}_{\text{OLS}}$ in all nine settings. $\hat{\boldsymbol{\beta}}^{(3)}_{\text{CSS}}$ enjoys the best overall performances, as it is better than $\hat{\boldsymbol{\beta}}^{(2)}_{\text{CSS}}$ in all but one setting. This simulation study confirms our intuition in Sect. 3. Namely, when the LCM condition is violated and $\text{E}(\mathbf{X} \mid \boldsymbol{\beta}^T\mathbf{X})$ can not be modeled by linear functions of $\boldsymbol{\beta}^T\mathbf{X}$, the CSS estimators can improve the OLS estimator as long as we can model $\text{E}(\mathbf{X} \mid \boldsymbol{\beta}^T\mathbf{X})$ properly.

5 Discussion

To recover the direction $\boldsymbol{\beta}$ in the general regression model (1) with discrete predictors, we examine the OLS and the CSS-based OLS estimators in this paper. In the case when the link function is linear, or when the predictor distribution satisfies the LCM condition, OLS can recover the true direction up to a multiplicative scalar. If the link function is nonlinear and the LCM condition is not satisfied, OLS is no longer suitable. By relaxing the LCM condition and modeling $\text{E}(\mathbf{X} \mid \boldsymbol{\beta}^T\mathbf{X})$ as polynomial functions of $\boldsymbol{\beta}^T\mathbf{X}$, the CSS-based estimators improve OLS and lead to better accuracy at recovering $\boldsymbol{\beta}$. Our development addresses a gap in the existing CSS literature, which mainly focuses on continuous predictors (Dong and Li 2010; Dong and Yu 2012; Li and Dong 2009). In the case of continuous predictors, Theorem 6.1 in Li and Dong (2009) provides the consistency results of the CSS estimators. From Fig. 1, it is obvious that $\text{E}(\mathbf{X} \mid \boldsymbol{\beta}^T\mathbf{X})$ can not be consistently estimated by polynomial functions of $\boldsymbol{\beta}^T\mathbf{X}$. Finding consistent CSS estimators with discrete predictors is a topic worth future investigation.

Appendix

Proof of $\boldsymbol{\beta}_{\text{OLS}} \propto \boldsymbol{\beta}$ *in Example 3, case iii.* For $(X_1, X_2, W)^T \sim$ Multinomial $(n, (p_1, p_2, p_3))$, it is well-known that $X_i \sim$ Binomial(n, p_i) for $i = 1, 2$, and $\text{cov}(X_1, X_2) = -np_1p_2$. It follows that $\text{E}(X_1X_2) = n(n-1)p_1p_2$. It can be shown that

$$\text{E}(X_1^3) = np_1 + 3n(n-1)p_1^2 + n(n-1)(n-2)p_1^3.$$

Next we denote $k_3 = n - k_1 - k_2$ and calculate $\text{E}(X_1^2X_2)$ as follows

$$\begin{aligned}
\text{E}(X_1^2X_2) &= \sum_{k_1,k_2} k_1^2 k_2 \frac{n!}{k_1!k_2!k_3!} p_1^{k_1} p_2^{k_2} p_3^{k_3} \\
&= n(n-1)p_1p_2 \sum_{k_1,k_2} (k_1 - 1 + 1) \frac{(n-2)!}{(k_1-1)!(k_2-1)!k_3!} p_1^{k_1-1} p_2^{k_2-1} p_3^{k_3} \\
&= n(n-1)(n-2)p_1^2p_2 \sum_{k_1,k_2} \frac{(n-3)!}{(k_1-2)!(k_2-1)!k_3!} p_1^{k_1-2} p_2^{k_2-1} p_3^{k_3} \\
&\quad + n(n-1)p_1p_2 \sum_{k_1,k_2} \frac{(n-2)!}{(k_1-1)!(k_2-1)!k_3!} p_1^{k_1-1} p_2^{k_2-1} p_3^{k_3} \\
&= n(n-1)p_1p_2(1 + np_1 - 2p_1).
\end{aligned}$$

For $Y = (X_1 + X_2)^2$, we thus have

$$\begin{aligned}
&\text{E}\{(X_1 - \text{E}(X_1))Y\} = \text{E}(X_1^3) - \text{E}(X_1)\text{E}(X_1^2) + \text{E}(X_1X_2^2) + \text{E}(X_1X_2^2) \\
&\quad - \text{E}(X_1)\text{E}(X_2^2) + 2\text{E}(X_1^2X_2) - 2\text{E}(X_1)\text{E}(X_1X_2) \\
&= np_1\{1 + (2n-3)p_1 - (2n-2)p_1^2 + p_2(2n - 3 - (2n-2)p_2 - (4n-4)p_1)\}.
\end{aligned}$$

Similarly, $\text{E}\{(X_2 - \text{E}(X_2))Y\}$ is equal to

$$np_2\{1 + (2n-3)p_2 - (2n-2)p_2^2 + p_1(2n - 3 - (2n-2)p_1 - (4n-4)p_2)\}.$$

Recall that $\mathbf{X} = (X_1, X_2)^T$ and $\text{var}(\mathbf{X}) = \boldsymbol{\Sigma}$. Let $|\boldsymbol{\Sigma}|$ be the determinant of $\boldsymbol{\Sigma}$. Since the first row of $\boldsymbol{\Sigma}^{-1}$ is $|\boldsymbol{\Sigma}|^{-1}\{np_2(1-p_2), np_1p_2\}$, the first component of $\boldsymbol{\beta}_{\text{OLS}}$ becomes

$$\begin{aligned}
&|\boldsymbol{\Sigma}|^{-1}[np_2(1-p_2)\text{E}\{(X_1 - \text{E}(X_1))Y\} + np_1p_2\text{E}\{(X_2 - \text{E}(X_2))Y\}] \\
&\quad = |\boldsymbol{\Sigma}|^{-1}n^2p_1p_2\{1 + (2n-3)(p_1+p_2) - (2n-2)(p_1^2 + p_2^2)\}.
\end{aligned}$$

Due to the symmetry between p_1 and p_2 in the expression above, the second component of $\boldsymbol{\beta}_{\mathrm{OLS}}$ is exactly the same as the first component. Thus we have $\boldsymbol{\beta}_{\mathrm{OLS}} \propto (1,1)^T = \boldsymbol{\beta}$. □

Proof of Proposition 1. Assume $\mathrm{E}\{\mathrm{E}(\mathbf{X} \mid \boldsymbol{\eta}^T\mathbf{X})Y\} = \mathrm{E}\{\mathrm{E}(\mathbf{X} \mid \boldsymbol{\beta}^T\mathbf{X})Y\}$ with probability 1 for some $\boldsymbol{\eta}$, such that $\boldsymbol{\eta}$ is not proportional to $\boldsymbol{\beta}$. Then both $\boldsymbol{\eta}$ and $\boldsymbol{\beta}$ will satisfy Eq. (6), which means the solution of (6) is not unique up to a scalar multiplication. Thus under the assumption that $\Pr(\mathrm{E}\{\mathrm{E}(\mathbf{X} \mid \boldsymbol{\eta}^T\mathbf{X})Y\} \neq \mathrm{E}\{\mathrm{E}(\mathbf{X} \mid \boldsymbol{\beta}^T\mathbf{X})Y\}) > 0$ whenever $\boldsymbol{\eta}$ is not proportional to $\boldsymbol{\beta}$, the solution of (6) is unique. Because $\boldsymbol{\beta}$ satisfies (6) and the solution of (6) is unique up to a scalar multiplication, we have $\boldsymbol{\beta}_{\mathrm{CSS}} \propto \boldsymbol{\beta}$. Under the additional LCM condition (2), $\boldsymbol{\beta}_{\mathrm{OLS}}$ is also proportional to $\boldsymbol{\beta}$. Consequently we have $\boldsymbol{\beta}_{\mathrm{CSS}} \propto \boldsymbol{\beta}_{\mathrm{OLS}}$. □

References

Carroll, R. J., Fan, J., Gijbels, I., & Wand, M. P. (1997). Generalized partially linear single-index models. *Journal of the American Statistical Association, 92*, 477–489.

Cook, R. D. (1998). *Regression graphics*. New York: Wiley.

Cook, R. D., & Li, L. (2009). Dimension reduction in regressions with exponential family predictors. *Journal of Computational and Graphical Statistics, 18*, 774–791.

Cook, R. D., & Nachtsheim, C. (1994). Reweighting to achieve elliptically contoured covariates in regression. *Journal of the American Statistical Association, 89*, 592–599.

Cui, X., Härdle, W., & Zhu, L. X. (2011). The EFM approach for single-index models. *The Annals of Statistics, 39*, 1658–1688.

Dong, Y., & Li, B. (2010). Dimension reduction for non-elliptically distributed predictors: Second order methods. *Biometrika, 97*, 279–294.

Dong, Y., & Yu, Z. (2012). Dimension reduction for the conditional *k*th moment via central solution space. *Journal of Multivariate Analysis, 112*, 207–218.

Härdle, W., Hall, P., & Ichimura, H. (1993). Optimal smoothing in single-index models. *The Annals of Statistics, 21*, 157–178.

Horowitz, J. L., & Härdle, W. (1996). Direct semiparametric estimation of single-index models with discrete covariates. *Journal of the American Statistical Association, 91*, 1632–1640.

Ichimura, H. (1993). Semiparametric least square (SLS) and weighted SLS estimation of single-index models. *Journal of Econometrics, 58*, 71–120.

Li, B., & Dong, Y. (2009). Dimension reduction for non-elliptically distributed predictors. *The Annals of Statistics, 37*, 1272–1298.

Li, K. C., & Duan, N. (1989). Regression analysis under link violation. *The Annals of Statistics, 17*, 1009–1052.

Powell, J. L., Stock, J. M., & Stoker, T. M. (1989). Semiparametric estimation of index coefficients. *Econometrica, 57*, 1403–1430.

Sheng, W., & Yin, X. (2013). Direction estimation in single-index models via distance covariance. *Journal of Multivariate Analysis, 122*, 148–161.

Zhang, N., & Yin, X. (2015). Direction estimation in single-index regressions via Hilbert-Schmidt independence criterion. *Statistica Sinica, 25*, 743–758.

Part II
New Developments in Trial Design

Futility Boundary Design Based on Probability of Clinical Success Under New Drug Development Paradigm

Yijie Zhou, Ruji Yao, Bo Yang, and Ramachandran Suresh

Abstract Statistical significance has been the traditional focus of clinical trial design due to the classic requirement for regulatory approval of a new therapy. However, an increasing emphasis is placed on a medical and payer perspective, where the value of a new therapy is generally measured by the magnitude of treatment effect based on point estimates. It is often the case that the magnitude of point estimates to demonstrate sufficient medical value is larger than that to demonstrate statistical significance. Therefore, a new clinical trial design should take into account both statistical significance and the magnitude of point estimates.

In line with the traditional trial design focus being on statistical significance, traditional futility analysis is designed based on power or conditional power to preserve the probability of achieving statistical significance at the end of a trial. With the additional trial objective for a sufficiently large point estimate, we propose an alternative futility analysis design approach where futility boundaries are selected based on the probability of observing a sufficiently large point estimate of treatment effect. We denote such probability as "probability of clinical success". Additionally, we define "relative retention rate" of this probability, and propose one futility boundary selection criteria to be 90 % relative retention rate. Via an illustrative example, we have extensively evaluated the operational characteristics of this approach including the conditional probability of clinical success based on the interim data and the probability of correct and incorrect stopping, all of which can/should be taken in consideration for futility boundary selection.

Y. Zhou (✉)
Data and Statistical Science, AbbVie Inc., North Chicago, IL 60064, USA
e-mail: yijie.zhou@abbvie.com

R. Yao
Merck Research Laboratory, Merck & Co., Inc., Kenilworth, NJ 07033, USA

B. Yang
Biometrics, Global Medicines Development & Affairs, Vertex Pharmaceuticals, Boston, MA 02210, USA

R. Suresh
Global Biometric Sciences, Bristol-Myers Squibb, Plainsboro, NJ 08536, USA

Z. Jin et al. (eds.), *New Developments in Statistical Modeling, Inference and Application*, ICSA Book Series in Statistics, DOI 10.1007/978-3-319-42571-9_5

1 Introduction

1.1 A New Paradigm of Drug Development from Medical and Payer Perspective

To obtain regulatory approval of a new therapy has been the focus of classic drug development, where statistical significance on the primary and/or key secondary efficacy endpoints is required in two replicated confirmatory clinical trials. As a result, demonstrating statistical significance has been viewed as the classic criterion for trial success. More importantly in the clinical trial design stage, substantial emphasis has been placed on statistical testing such as sample size and power calculation, as well as multiplicity control on the family-wise type I error rate across testing multiple hypotheses (e.g., testing of multiple endpoints or multiple doses).

However, direct users of a therapy including (1) physicians and clinicians who are the prescribers of therapies and who represent the medical community and (2) insurance companies and patients who are the payers of therapies, view clinical trial data from a different angle. They pay more attention to point estimates as a representation of efficacy instead of statistical significance or p-values. This perspective from medical community and payers gains increasing importance nowadays. This is because given the availability of existing drugs and competitive landscape of drug development, new therapies need to offer sufficient clinical benefit in order to be viewed valuable by the medical community and thus to reach patients who need them (Man-Son-Hing et al. 2002; The Practice Committee 2008; Dearing et al. 2014; Hoffmann et al. 2014). Point estimates play a critical role here because in the absence of head-to-head comparison within a single trial, it is a common practice that the cross-trial indirect comparison of point estimates measures the relative clinical benefit across different therapies, and the magnitude of point estimates to be viewed as clinically meaningful can be beyond that to demonstrate statistical significance.

Moreover, it is often the case that confirmatory clinical trials are sized large to meet the regulatory safety database requirement and thus are overpowered for efficacy endpoints. With a large sample size, the magnitude of point estimates required to demonstrate statistical significance can be small and therefore the clinical relevance of the point estimates becomes more important.

1.2 A Motivating Example

The example utilizes the clinical trial frame work of an investigational therapy for Crohns' Disease; however, the idea applies to clinical trials in general.

Crohn's Disease is an inflammatory disease that can cause a variety of systemic symptoms including abdominal pain, diarrhea, vomiting, and weight loss, etc. Existing therapies include corticosteroids, immuno-suppressant such as azathioprine and methotrexate, and biologic treatments such as infliximab, adalimumab, certolizumab, and natalizumab. A patient's disease activity is assessed using the Crohn's Disease Activity Index (CDAI) score, with a lower score indicating a lower disease activity. One typical efficacy endpoint in a Crohn's Disease clinical trial is the Binomial proportion of patients achieving a response based on reduction of the CDAI score.

Given the multiple therapies that are currently available, it is determined clinically that a new therapy needs to demonstrate 20 % (0.2) or more increase in response rate when compared with placebo in order to bring additional medical benefit to treating the disease. It is natural to design a clinical trial assuming an underlying placebo-adjusted treatment difference of 20 % in the response rate. The placebo group response rate is assumed at 25 % based on historical data. With a sample size of 100 subjects per group, the trial has approximately 85 % power to reject the null hypothesis when assuming $\Delta = 20\,\%$ and $P_{pbo} = 25\,\%$, with 2-sided α of 0.05 based on a Chi-square test.

With the sample size of 100 subjects per group, the required point estimate of treatment difference to reject the null hypothesis, i.e., to achieve statistical significance with 2-sided p-value < 0.05, is approximately 13 %. However, as stated earlier a difference of 20 % or more is required for this investigational therapy to be competitive with existing therapies. Therefore, success of this clinical trial constitutes a point estimate of 20 % or more for treatment difference at the final analysis, which is beyond merely rejecting the null hypothesis.

1.3 Futility Analysis Under the New Perspective

Futility analysis is commonly used when designing a clinical trial for a new therapy, where the trial can be stopped early due to lack of efficacy. It provides the advantage to limit patient exposure to non-efficacious therapies and more importantly to save time and resource towards identifying better therapies as quickly as possible. Futility analysis is implemented through interim monitoring during trial conduct, and interim monitoring is typically performed by an independent data monitoring committee in order to protect the integrity of trial data. Therefore, a concrete futility stopping criteria, i.e., a futility boundary, needs to be prespecified to facilitate decision making by the data review committee.

Various statistical methods have been developed to derive futility stopping boundaries in clinical trial settings (Snapinn et al. 2006), including group sequential design to specify the beta-spending functions (Pocock 1977; O'Brien and Fleming 1979; Lan and DeMets 1983; Chang et al. 1998; Jennison and Turnbull 2000; DeMets and Ware 1980, 1982; Pampallona and Tsiatis 1994; Pampallona et al. 2001), the use of stochastic curtailment such as conditional power (Lan et al. 1982; Halperin et al. 1982; Lachin 2005), predictive power (Spiegelhalter et al. 1986; Choi et al. 1985; Choi and Pepple 1989) and predictive probabilities (Dmitrienko and Wang 2006; Daimon 2008). However, majority of the existing methods are in line with the classic drug development paradigm which focuses on statistical significance. This is because both power and conditional power are essentially the probability to achieve statistical significance. In another words, the term "*futility*" thus far in literature and statistical research refers only to the situation that it is unlikely to achieve statistical significance if the study would proceed to the end. Under the new paradigm of drug development from medical and payer perspective, the objective of interim monitoring for futility should be shifted accordingly. The term "futility" should be considered in a broader sense as the inability of an investigational therapy to demonstrate sufficient efficacy which includes a non-satisfactory point estimate. Therefore, instead of targeting on the ability to achieve statistical significant at the end of the trial, a futility analysis should be designed to target on the ability to achieve a desired point estimate in addition to the statistical significance at the end of the trial. In the motivating example, a futility analysis should be designed to protect the probability of observing a desired point estimate of 20 % or more treatment difference at the final analysis, rather than the 13 % or more for statistical significance.

The predictive probability approach (Dmitrienko and Wang 2006; Daimon 2008) where the inference is based on the Bayesian posterior distribution also utilizes probability for the decision making on trial success or futility. Under certain parameterization and a non-informative prior, this posterior probability decision criteria is similar or equivalent to the above mentioned probability based on the observed point estimate. However, the proposed cutoff selection for the posterior probability decision criteria is still derived from the hypothesis testing setting and related to the frequentist significant level. As a result, the suggested selection of the futility criteria parameter is also based on the hypothesis testing setting and therefore is not directly applicable when trial success is based on observing a desired point estimate.

In the context of this paper, we consider the "success" of a clinical trial as achieving a desired point estimate in addition to the statistical significance, and propose a futility boundary design based on the probability of "clinical success" (POCS). POCS is defined as the probability of observing certain treatment effect at the end of the trial and thus differs from the concept of "probability of success (POS)" in literature which is typically related to average or expected power (Chuang-Stein 2006; Jiang 2011; Carroll 2013; Ibrahim et al. 2015). As an analogue to the power calculation in the commonly used group sequential design accounting for futility analyses, POCS decreases with the incorporation of futility analyses because additional opportunities are provided to make a false negative decision. However, unlike power where people have a general expectation (e.g., 80 % or 90 % power), the scale of POCS and its decrease can vary largely depending on the desired target value, and thus selecting a futility boundary based on the absolute value of POCS or conditional POCS can be challenging. Therefore, we propose a futility design based on the relative scale of POCS. Specifically, we calculate the POCS with and without a futility analysis and we define the ratio of the two probabilities as "relative retention rate", and propose one futility boundary selection criteria such as greater or equal to 90 % relative retention rate. Under the framework of the motivating example in Sect. 1.2, we have extensively evaluated the operational characteristics of this approach including the conditional probability of "success" based on the interim data and the probability of correct and incorrect stopping, all of which should be taken into consideration when designing a futility boundary. Specifically, the above mentioned operational characteristics are evaluated as a function of potential futility boundary, the underlying true treatment difference, and the timing of the futility analysis.

The article is structured as follows. In Sect. 2, we describe the proposed futility boundary design based on the probability of observing the desired point estimate. Section 3 presents the analysis of the motivating example trial with simulation to evaluate the operational characteristics of the proposed futility boundary design. Discussion in Sect. 4 follows.

2 Futility Analysis Design Based on Probability of Clinical Success

2.1 Probability of Clinical Success (POCS)

We introduce the concept of *probability of clinical success* (POCS) when rejecting the null hypothesis is no longer sufficient for trial success. In the motivating example in Sect. 1.2, the probability of clinical success is the probability of observing a point estimate of 20 % or more treatment difference at the final analysis. In this article, we consider POCS in the following form:

$$\Pr\ (\text{observed treatment difference}\ \geq\ c)\,, \tag{1}$$

where the value c is larger than the value required to reject the null hypothesis, so achieving statistical significance is implied.

Consider testing the treatment difference between two independent means or proportions. Let n_1 and n_2 denote the sample size per group before and after an interim analysis, respectively, and $n = n_1 + n_2$. Let random variables X_1 and X_2 denote the treatment difference before and after the interim analysis, respectively. Note that X_1 and X_2 are independent of each other. The *POCS* defined in Eq. (1) can be written as

$$\text{POCS} = Pr\ (w_1 X_1 + w_2 X_2 \geq c)\,, \tag{2}$$

where w_1 and w_2 are the sample size based weight that $w_1 = n_1/n$ and $w_2 = n_2/n$. POCS accounting for an interim futility analysis, also called *overall POCS*, can then be presented as

$$\text{POCS}_{\text{overall}} = Pr\ (w_1 X_1 + w_2 X_2 \geq c \text{ AND } X_1 > \xi) \tag{3}$$

where ξ is the futility boundary. Let f_1 and f_2 denote the density function for X_1 and X_2 with the corresponding cumulative distribution functions denoted by F_1 and F_2 respectively. The probability in Eq. (3) can be written as

$$\int_{\xi}^{\infty}\left[1-F_2\left(\frac{c-w_1x}{w_2}\right)\right]f_1(x)dx \tag{4}$$

which can be calculated by numerical integration. As an analogue to conditional power, the conditional POCS given the observed data at the interim analysis can be presented as

$$\begin{aligned}\mathrm{POCS}_c &= Pr\left(w_1X_1+w_2X_2\geq c \middle| X_1=x_1\right)\\ &= 1-F_2\left(\frac{c-w_1x_1}{w_2}\right)\end{aligned} \tag{5}$$

When the variables being analyzed are continuous, X_1 and X_2 are differences in means that typically are assumed to follow a normal distribution. Therefore, $f_1(\cdot)$and $f_2(\cdot)$ are the corresponding normal density functions and $F_1(\cdot)$and $F_2(\cdot)$ are the corresponding cumulative normal distribution function $\Phi_1(\cdot)$and $\Phi_2(\cdot)$. In cases that X_1 and X_2 are differences in binomial proportions, the integration can be presented as the summation below. Denote $D_1 = n_1X_1$ and $D_2 = n_2X_2$ which are the difference in the number of cases up to and after an interim analysis, respectively.

$$\mathrm{POCS}_{\mathrm{overall}} = \sum_{k=\xi n_1+1}^{n_1} \Pr(D_2 \geq cn-k)\Pr(D_1=k), \tag{6}$$

where $\Pr(D_2 \geq cn - k)$ is $\mathrm{POCS_c}$ conditioned on $D_1 = k$. Without loss of generality, we assume $k \geq 0$. Therefore

$$\Pr(D_1=k) = \sum_{j=0}^{n_1-k} C_{n_1}^{k+j}{p_1}^{k+j}(1-p_1)^{n_1-(k+j)}C_{n_1}^{j}{p_2}^{j}(1-p_2)^{n_1-j}, \tag{7}$$

where p_1 and p_2 are the Binary probabilities for the two groups, and

$$\Pr(D_2 \geq cn-k) = \sum_{i=cn-k}^{n_2}\Pr(D_2=i) \tag{8}$$

where $\Pr(D_2 = i)$can be calculated similarly as $\Pr(D_1 = k)$.

2.2 Relative Retention of POCS

When the goal of trial design has shifted from simply achieving statistical significance to a more aggressive criterion which is to observe a sufficiently large point estimate, we propose to design a futility analysis accordingly. In analogue with the conventional group sequential design, it is noted that

1. Adding a futility interim analysis will reduce the overall POCS, similarly as reducing the overall power due to the additional opportunities to make a type II error.
2. A high futility boundary is desired to maximize the probability of interim stopping when the trial is less likely to meet the success criteria at the final analysis. Such futility boundary is expected to be higher than that from a conventional group sequential design if the success criterion is more aggressive than achieving statistical significance.
3. The higher the futility boundary, the lower the overall POCS because it is more likely to stop the trial, even if the underlying true treatment effect exists as desired.

Given these observations, we could design a futility analysis based on POCS preservation instead of power or conditional power preservation. To measure the extent of POCS preservation, we define the relative percentage

$$\mathrm{POCS}_{\mathrm{overall}} / \, \mathrm{POCS}, \tag{9}$$

as *relative retention rate*. Using this metric, the futility boundary could be designed as the highest one with at least 90 % relative retention rate when calculating POCS and $\mathrm{POCS}_{\mathrm{overall}}$ under assumed Δ.

2.3 Probability of Interim Stopping

We define a positive (negative) trial based on observing a point estimate for treatment difference of c or more (less than c) at the final analysis. Note that we assume statistical significance is achieved when observing c. As analogues to the probability of interim stopping under H_0 and H_a in the conventional group sequential design, we define the probability of correct (incorrect) interim stopping as the probability that a negative (positive) trial is stopped at the futility interim analysis. In another words,

$$\begin{aligned} \Pr\ (\text{correct stopping}) &= \Pr\left(X_1 \leq \xi \,\middle|\, w_1X_1 + w_2X_2 < c\right) \\ &= \int_{-\infty}^{\xi} F_2\left(\frac{c - w_1x}{w_2}\right) f_1(x)dx / F(c), \end{aligned} \tag{10}$$

and

$$\Pr\ (\text{incorrect stopping}) = \Pr\left(X_1 \leq \xi \,\middle|\, w_1X_1 + w_2X_2 \geq c\right)$$

$$= \int_{-\infty}^{\xi} \left[1 - F_2\left(\frac{c - w_1x}{w_2}\right)\right] f_1(x)dx / \left[1 - F(c)\right], \quad (11)$$

where F is the cumulative distribution for the difference regardless of interim analysis.

For continuous variable, normal density function and normal cumulative functions will be used in Eqs. (10) and (11). For Binomial proportions,

$$\Pr\ (\text{correct stopping}) = \sum_{k=-n_1}^{\xi n} \Pr\left(D_2 < cn - k\right) \Pr\left(D_1 = k\right) / \Pr\left(D < cn\right), \quad (12)$$

$$\Pr\ (\text{incorrect stopping}) = \sum_{k=-n_1}^{\xi n} \Pr\left(D_2 \geq cn - k\right) \Pr\left(D_1 = k\right) / \Pr\left(D \geq cn\right), \quad (13)$$

where D is the difference in the number of cases at final analysis.

3 Analysis of the Motivating Example Trial

In the motivating example in Sect. 1.2, a futility analysis is planned when data of 40 subjects per group are available. It is a common practice to conduct futility analysis when 40 % or 50 % of the information is available (Gould 2005). In general, a futility analysis conducted earlier than that is associated with great uncertainty; on the same token, a futility analysis conducted later than that has limited time and resource saving.

The conventional group sequential futility design is provided in Table 1, where we present 2 scenarios based on overall power preservation at 80 % and sufficient conditional power at 20 %. The corresponding futility boundaries are 7.5 and 8.5 %, respectively. The calculations are conducted in EAST 5.4 using non-binding efficacy and futility boundaries.

As pointed out earlier, such selected futility boundaries are not directly linked to the trial objective of observing a point estimate of 20 % or more.

To help meet the trial success criterion of observing a point estimate of 20 % or more, we design the futility boundaries using the proposed approach based on POCS. With this sample size of 40 per treatment group at the interim futility analysis, one additional subject being a responder corresponds to a 2.5 % incremental in the Binomial proportion of response rate with a group. Therefore, we

Table 1 Conventional futility interim analysis design for a parallel-design two-group clinical trial with Binomial outcome (n = 100 per group, futility analysis n1 = 40 per group, assuming $P_{pbo} = 25\,\%$, $P_{active} - P_{pbo} = 20\,\%$, 2-sided $\alpha = 0.05$, calculation in EAST 5.4 using non-binding efficacy and futility boundaries.)

		Scenario 1: power preservation at 0.80	Scenario 2: conditional power at 0.20 under observed difference
Decision criteria in terms of observed treatment difference		Futile if <7.5 %	Futile if <8.5 %
Conditional power[a]		0.15	0.20
Overall power		0.80	0.78
Probability of futility stopping	Under H_0	0.76	0.79
	Under H_a	0.11	0.14
Probability of passing	Under H_0	0.24	0.21
	Under H_a	0.89	0.86
β spending	At interim	0.11	0.14
	At final analysis	0.09	0.08

[a]Conditional power under observed difference

Table 2 Futility interim analysis design for a parallel-design two-group clinical trial with Binomial outcome based on POCS under H_a (Trial setting: parallel 2-arm trial with Binomial endpoint, n = 100 per group, futility analysis at 40 per group, assuming $P_{pbo} = 25\,\%$)

	POCS = Pr($\delta \geq 20\,\%$)						
	Without futility	With futility					
True effect size	POCS	Futility bound	$POCS_{overall}$	Relative retention rate	$POCS_c$[a]	Pr (correct stopping)	Pr (incorrect stopping)
$\Delta = 20\,\%$	53.2 %	$\delta \leq 7.5\,\%$	51.3 %	96.4 %	2.8 %	12.2 %	1.9 %
		$\delta \leq 10\,\%$[*]	**49.9 %**	**93.6 %**	**8.1 %**	**16.7 %**	**3.4 %**
		$\delta \leq 12.5\,\%$	47.5 %	89.2 %	18.7 %	21.6 %	5.5 %

δ: observed treatment difference
[a]Calculated at observed difference at interim, i.e., assuming Δ is the same as futility bound
[*]: selected futility bound based on criteria "Relative retention rate > 90 %"

consider the distinct potential futility boundaries that are in incremental of 2.5 %. Table 2 presents the POCS without the futility analysis, overall POCS with the futility analysis, the relative retention rate, the conditional POCS, the probability of correct and incorrect stopping for 3 futility boundary candidates: 7.5, 10, and 12.5 %. According to the proposed criteria of selecting the highest futility boundary with at least 90 % relative retention rate, the boundary of 10 % is selected.

Figure 1a plots the overall power and overall POCS under various futility boundaries ranging from 0 to 20 % with incremental change of 2 %. Reference lines are placed at 86 and 53.2 % which correspond to the original power and POCS without futility analysis. It can be seen from the plot that there is a significant power loss as the futility boundary increases; on the contrast, the POCS loss is relatively small.

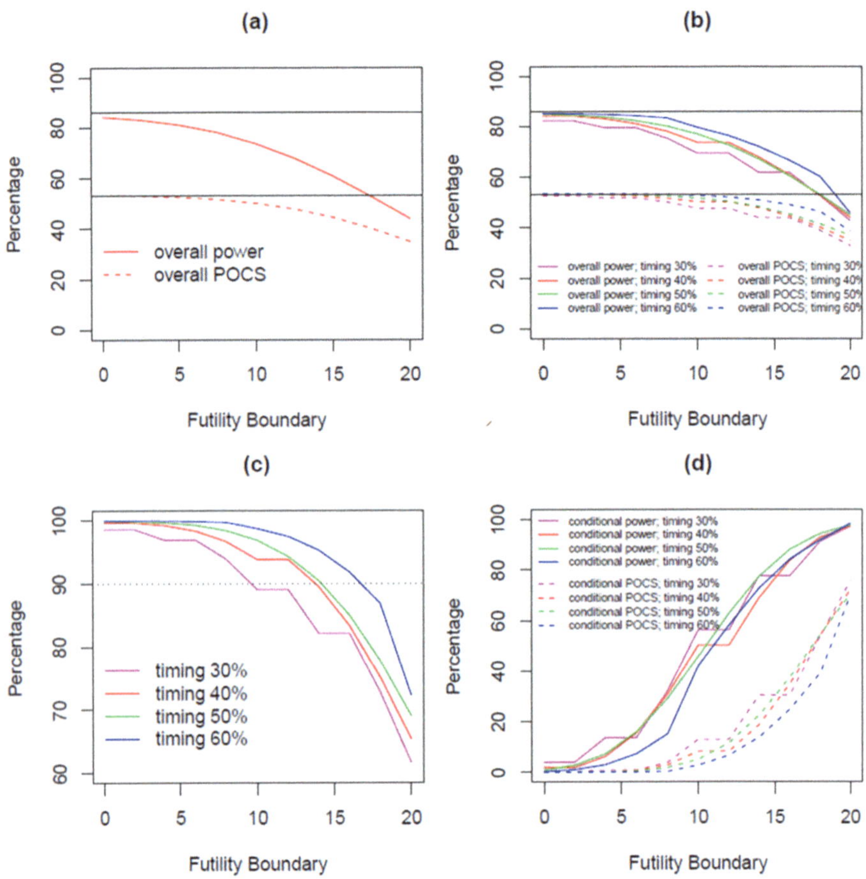

Fig. 1 (**a**) Overall power and overall POCS for futility analysis at timing of 40 % sample size; (**b**) Overall power and overall POCS, (**c**) relative retention rate, (**d**) conditional POCS and conditional power calculated at observed difference at interim, for futility analysis at timing of 30, 40, 50 and 60 % of total sample size. Reference lines for overall power and overall POCS are placed at 86 % and 53.2 %, respectively, which are the original power and POCS without futility analysis. Reference line for relative retention rate is placed at 90 % which is the futility boundary selection criteria. (Trial setting: parallel 2-arm trial with Binomial endpoint, n = 100 per group, assuming $P_{pbo} = 25\,\%$ and $\Delta = 20\,\%$)

We further evaluate the operational characteristics of the proposed futility analysis design for various futility boundaries, and its sensitivity with respect to the timing of the futility analysis as well as to the underlying true treatment difference. Under the assumed true treatment difference of 20 %, Fig. 1b plots the overall power and overall POCS for different futility boundaries and for different timing of the futility analysis at 30%, 40 %, 50 % or 60 % of the sample size, and Fig. 1c plots the corresponding relative retention rate. It can be seen that when the underlying true treatment difference is as desired, conducting a futility analysis at a later timing can lead to higher values in overall power, overall POCS and relative retention rate.

This is not unexpected because a futility analysis at a later timing has a larger sample size and utilizes more information, and therefore has a higher likelihood to make the correct decision. When comparing the two commonly used middle timing at 40 % or 50 % of the sample size, it can be seen that the difference in relative retention rate is relatively small. This result supports the initial timing selection of 40 % for early decision making without a large compromise in the data evidence available for this decision making. Figure 1d plots the conditional POCS in comparison with conditional power calculated under the observed difference at the interim, for different futility boundaries and for different timing of the futility analysis at 30 %, 40 %, 50 % or 60 % of the sample size. As expected, the conditional POCS is much lower than the conditional power, which supports again that futility boundaries derived using conditional power are disconnected with the trial objective based on the desired point estimate.

Figure 2a plots the probability of a positive trial and a negative trial, and probability of correct and incorrect interim stopping when using the 10 % futility boundary, with respect to different scenarios for the underlying true treatment difference. As defined in Sect. 2.3, a positive (negative) trial refers to observing 20 % or more (less than 20 %) treatment difference at the final analysis, and the probability of correct (incorrect) interim stopping refers to the probability that a negative (positive) trial is stopped at the futility interim analysis. Figure 2b further plots these probabilities with respect to different timing of the futility analysis at 30 %, 40 %, 50 % or 60 % of the sample size. It can be seen from Fig. 2a that as expected, the probability of a negative trial decreases (thus the probability of a positive trial increases) as the underlying true treatment difference increases. In addition, the larger the underlying true treatment difference, the lower the probability to stop the trial because the interim analysis data are more likely to exceed the pre-specified futility boundary. By using the futility boundary of 10 %, majority of the negative trials can be stopped at the futility analysis, especially when the underlying true treatment difference is not as large as the desired 20 %. In the meanwhile, the tradeoff in terms of incorrect stopping is very small, because only a negligible portion of the positive trials are stopped at the interim futility analysis. This is observed throughout all scenarios of the underlying true treatment difference that are considered. Figure 2b suggests that when the underlying true treatment difference is around the desired magnitude which is 20 %, an earlier futility interim analysis has slightly higher probability to stop a negative trial. This is because the sampling distribution from a smaller sample size has a wider spread and therefore the left tail probability of less than 10 % futility boundary is larger. However, the probability of incorrectly stopping a positive trial is also increased for an earlier timing, and the magnitude of increase is significant for the early timing at 30 % of the sample size.

Figure 2c further displays the partition of correct and incorrect stopping among the overall futility interim stopping for different scenarios of underlying true treatment difference. It can be seen that the proportion of incorrect stopping increases dramatically for earlier timing of futility interim analysis, which suggests that we should design the futility interim analysis with a comfortable level of data evidence.

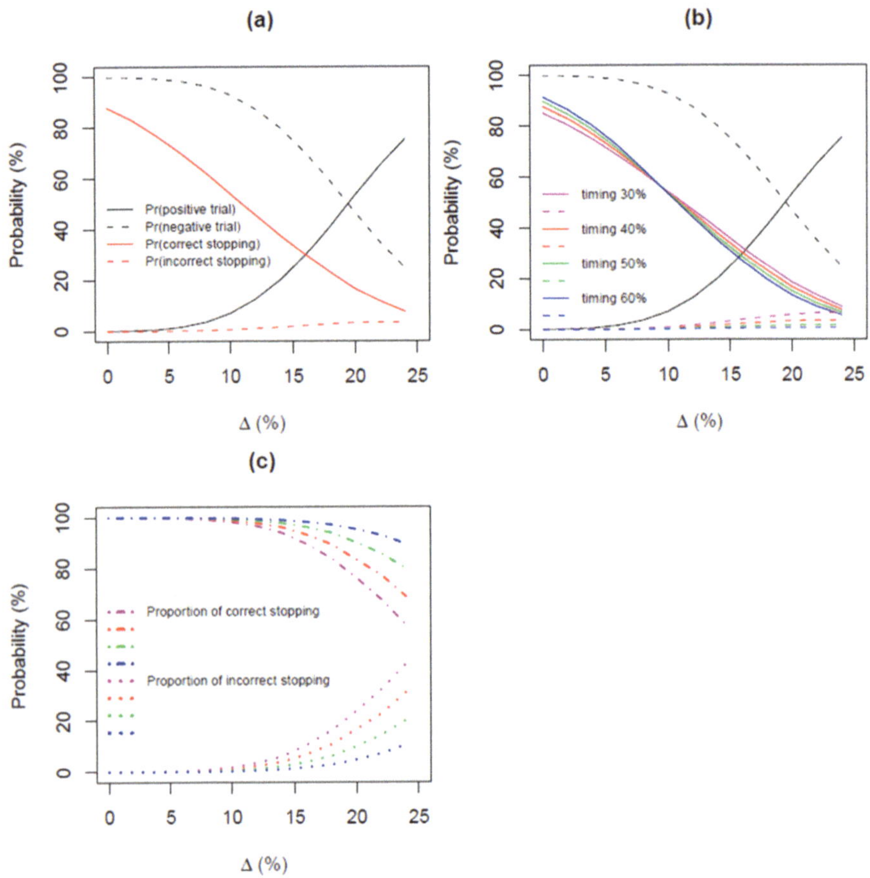

Fig. 2 (**a**) Probability of a positive trial and a negative trial, and probability of correct and incorrect interim stopping with a futility boundary of 10 % at timing of 40 % sample size for different true treatment effect size Δ; (**b**) Probability of correct and incorrect interim stopping, (**c**) Proportion of correct and incorrect stopping out of total futility interim stopping, with a futility boundary of 10 % at timing of 30, 40, 50 and 60 % of total sample size. A positive (negative) trials refers to observing 20 % or more (less than 20 %) treatment difference in the final analysis, and the probability of correct (incorrect) interim stopping refers to the probability that a negative (positive) trial is stopped at the futility interim analysis. (Trial setting: parallel 2-arm trial with Binomial endpoint, n = 100 per group, assuming $P_{pbo} = 25\,\%$)

4 Discussion

When the benefit of a therapy is evaluated though the magnitude of treatment effect, achieving statistical significance is no longer sufficient for a clinical trial to be successful. The conventional futility design to preserve the probability of achieving statistical significance becomes de-linked with the evolved trial success objectives. In this article, we propose an alternative futility analysis design approach based on POCS which directly targets the desired trial success criteria on clinical relevance, i.e., observing a sufficiently large point estimate in addition to statistical significance. Note that power is also a form of POCS where the threshold c equals $z_{1-\alpha/2}{}^*\sqrt{[\mathrm{Var}(w_1X_1 + w_2X_2)]}$. It is worth pointing out that both statistical significance and clinical relevance are important for a clinical trial to be successful (Carroll 2009), and in this article, we consider the scenario that meeting clinical relevance automatically implies meeting statistical significance. If statistical significance is not achieved even with a sufficiently large point estimator, it is likely due to variability. For example, the actual variability is larger than the planned variability, which we won't know at the design stage.

The concept of POCS can also be applied in the drug development program besides within a single trial. The thinking in developing a best-in-class drug can be very different from that in developing a first-in-class drug. In addition to the minimal requirement of statistical significance, there is a target product profile that a best-in-class drug candidate needs to achieve in order to bring additional benefit to the patient, medical community and payers. If statistical significance is achieved but the target product profile is not met in Phase 2, the chance of meeting it in Phase 3 is likely to be low. While making a decision of futility stop during Phase 3, the totality of data including the second trial data in the program should be carefully considered before such futility decision can be made.

We define a quantity *relative retention rate* to measure the degree of POCS preservation, and propose a futility boundary selection criteria based on relative retention rate (e.g., greater or equal to 90 % relative retention rate). Note that when true $\Delta = \mathrm{c}$, POCS = 50 % if it is a symmetrical distribution (e.g., normal distribution), and this probability is independent of sample size. In this situation, $\mathrm{POCS}_{\mathrm{overall}}/\mathrm{POCS} = 90\,\%$ is equivalent to $\mathrm{POCS}_{\mathrm{overall}} = 45\,\%$. Similarly as in group sequential design, conditional POCS, probabilities of correct and incorrect stopping can be evaluated for the proposed futility analysis design approach. Sample size adjustment based on the loss of POCS can also be considered.

It is important to note that relative retention rate is one of several metrics that can be used to design a futility boundary. The futility boundary can also be designed based on probability of correct stopping, probability of incorrect stopping, and conditional POCS, or all these factors above taken into consideration. This is similar to the common practice in a conventional group sequential design that, maintaining a decent overall power after accounting for a futility analysis is one approach to select futility boundary and there are many other metrics that can be used for boundary selection, including conditional power, probability of correct stopping under the null, and probability of incorrect stopping under the alternative, etc.

We use a Crohn's Disease clinical trial as an example to illustrate the proposed futility analysis design, and perform extensive evaluation of the operational characteristics of the proposed design in terms of conditional POCS based on interim data, probability of correct and incorrect stopping, with respect to different underlying true treatment differences and different timing of the futility interim analysis. The results suggest that such proposed futility design has a high chance to correctly stop a trial if the outcome at the final analysis is undesired, and at the same time has a very low chance to incorrectly stop a trial if the outcome at final analysis is satisfactory, which is a negligible tradeoff. While the group sequential futility analysis design is typically evaluated only at $H_0 = 0$, $H_a = \Delta$ and $H_a = \Delta/2$, we propose to evaluate the selected futility boundary over the continuous range between $H_0 = 0$ and the desired magnitude for true treatment difference, because it is also of great interest how the futility stopping boundary performs when treatment effect exists but not as large as desired. Additionally, the results also suggest that the timing of the futility analysis around 40 % of the planned sample size provides sufficient data evidence as well as POCS preservation.

When the trial success criteria are more aggressive than rejecting the null hypothesis, POCS is generally lower than power. Comparing the overall power with overall POCS, we note that a high futility boundary can cause significant amount of power loss, but relatively small POCS loss. Therefore, one should not be concerned about power loss in selecting the futility boundary when achieving statistical significance is not the ultimate goal.

References

Carroll, K. J. (2009). Back to basics: Explaining sample size in outcome trials, are statisticians doing a thorough job? *Pharmaceutical Statistics, 8*, 333–345.

Carroll, K. J. (2013). Decision making from Phase II to Phase III and the probability of success: Reassured by assurance? *Journal of Biopharmaceutical Statistics, 23*, 1188–1200.

Chang, M. N., Hwang, I. K., & Shih, W. J. (1998). Group sequential designs using both type I and type II error probability spending functions. *Communications in Statistics Theory and Methods, 27*, 1323–1339.

Choi, S. C., & Pepple, P. A. (1989). Monitoring clinical trials based on predictive probability of significance. *Biometrics, 45*, 317–323.

Choi, S. C., Smith, P. J., & Becker, D. P. (1985). Early decision in clinical trials when the treatment differences are small. *Controlled Clinical Trials, 6*, 280–288.

Chuang-Stein, C. (2006). Sample size and the probability of a successful trial. *Pharmaceutical Statistics, 5*, 305–309.

Daimon, T. (2008). Predictive checking for Bayesian interim analyses in clinical trials. *Contemporary Clinical Trials, 29*, 740–750.

Dearing, K. R., Sangal, A., & Weiss, G. J. (2014). Maintaining clarity: Review of maintenance therapy in non-small cell lung cancer. *World Journal of Clinical Oncology, 5*, 103–113.

DeMets, D. L., & Ware, J. H. (1980). Group sequential methods for clinical trials with a one-sided hypothesis. *Biometrika, 67*, 651–660.

DeMets, D. L., & Ware, J. H. (1982). Asymmetric group sequential boundaries for monitoring clinical trials. *Biometrika, 69*, 661–663.

Dmitrienko, A., & Wang, M.-D. (2006). Bayesian predictive approach to interim monitoring in clinical trials. *Statistics in Medicine, 25*, 2178–2195.

Gould, L. (2005). Timing of futility analyses for 'proof of concept' trials. *Statistics in Medicine, 24*, 1815–1835.

Halperin, M., Lan, K. K. G., Ware, J., Johnson, N. J., & DeMets, D. L. (1982). An aid to data monitoring in long-term clinical trials. *Controlled Clinical Trials, 3*, 311–323.

Hoffmann, T. C., Thomas, S. T., Ng Hung Shin, P., & Glasziou, P. P. (2014). Cross-sectional analysis of the reporting of continuous outcome measures and clinical significance of results in randomized trials of non-pharmacological interventions. *Trials, 15*(1), 362.

Ibrahim, J. G., Chen, M. H., Lakshminarayanan, M., Liu, G. F., & Heyse, J. F. (2015). Bayesian probability of success for clinical trials using historical data. *Statistics in Medicine, 34*, 249–264.

Jennison, C., & Turnbull, B. W. (2000). *Group sequential methods with applications to clinical trials*. London: Chapman and Hall/CRC.

Jiang, K. (2011). Optimal sample sizes and go/no-go decisions for phase II/III development programs based on probability of success. *Statistics in Biopharmaceutical Research, 3*, 463–475.

Lachin, J. M. (2005). A review of methods for futility stopping based on conditional power. *Statistics in Medicine, 24*, 2747–2764.

Lan, K. K. G., & DeMets, D. L. (1983). Discrete sequential boundaries for clinical trials. *Biometrika, 70*, 659–663.

Lan, K. K. G., Simon, R., & Halperin, M. (1982). Stochastically curtailed tests in long-term clinical trials. *Communications in Statistics Part C Sequential Analysis, 1*, 207–219.

Man-Son-Hing, M., Laupacis, A., O'Rourke, K., Molnar, F.J., Mahon, J., Chan, K.B.Y., and Wells, G. (2002). Determination of the clinical importance of study results: A review. *Journal of General Internal Medicine, 17*, 469–476.

O'Brien, P. C., & Fleming, T. R. (1979). A multiple testing procedure for clinical trials. *Biometrics, 35*, 549–556.

Pampallona, S., & Tsiatis, A. A. (1994). Group sequential designs for one-sided and two-sided hypothesis testing with provision for early stopping in favor of the null hypothesis. *Journal of Statistical Planning and Inference, 42*, 19–35.

Pampallona, S., Tsiatis, A. A., & Kim, K. (2001). Interim monitoring of group sequential trials using spending functions for the type I and type II error probabilities. *Drug Information Journal, 35*, 1113–1121.

Pocock, S. J. (1977). Group sequential methods in the design and analysis of clinical trials. *Biometrika, 64*, 191–199.

Snapinn, S., Chen, M. G., Jiang, Q., & Koutsoukos, T. (2006). Assessment of futility in clinical trials. *Pharmaceutical Statistics, 5*, 273–281.

Spiegelhalter, D. J., Freedman, L. S., & Blackburn, P. R. (1986). Monitoring clinical trials: Conditional or predictive power? *Controlled Clinical Trials, 7*, 8–17.

The Practice Committee of the American Society for Reproductive Medicine. Interpretation of clinical trial results. *Fertil Steril®, 90*, S114–S120 (2008) doi:10.1016/j.fertnstert.2008.08.037.

Bayesian Modeling of Time Response and Dose Response for Predictive Interim Analysis of a Clinical Trial

Ming-Dauh Wang, Dominique A. Williams, Elisa V. Gomez, and Jyoti N. Rayamajhi

Abstract Bayesian approach has been increasingly applied to various aspects of design and analysis of clinical trials. We present one application concerning an interim futility analysis of a trial. Longitudinal data were collected for a range of the studied doses. Bayesian analysis was first conducted to predict observations at the end of treatment for patients not yet followed through treatment, based on all interim observed data. The predicted data in combination with observed data at the end of treatment were then analyzed using a Bayesian normal dynamic linear model for dose response inference. Summary of the Bayesian analysis was used to aid an interim futility decision.

1 Introduction

Clinical trials conducted for drug development in the exploratory stage, commonly Phase 1 or 2, are often designed to optimize the learning of response curves in relation to time and dose. Consequently, one dose or two of the experimental drug can be selected for further confirmatory testing. Better quantification of the response curves in the former would more clearly inform dose selection as well as dosing frequency for the latter. Patient exposure to the experimental drug of an exploratory trial is typically short with respect to its stabilized effect on the target biomarker or clinical endpoint after long-term use. Thus the study would often be longitudinal to enhance estimation of the time response curve and prediction of the long-term effect. Meanwhile, the focus would still be primarily on the end of treatment duration as it tends to most closely resemble the long-term repeated use of the drug than interim time points, and dose response learned at the end of treatment would normally drive dose selection for subsequent trials.

M.-D. Wang (✉) • D.A. Williams • E.V. Gomez • J.N. Rayamajhi
Global Statistical Sciences, Eli Lilly and Company, Indianapolis, IN 46285, USA
e-mail: wang_ming-dauh@lilly.com

Z. Jin et al. (eds.), *New Developments in Statistical Modeling, Inference and Application*, ICSA Book Series in Statistics, DOI 10.1007/978-3-319-42571-9_6

Modeling of time and dose responses can be approached through well-defined mean response functions if shapes of the curves are sure to reasonably explain the relationships. For example, Emax models and their variations have been widely validated to be useful in early phase drug development (Fu and Manner, 2010; Thomas et al., 2014). Nevertheless, in cases where time or dose response is not confidently known, other less shape-specific models can be applied. Among such, models that utilize the Markov property for the description of dependence across doses or time points seem a flexible choice. A class of such models are called Normal Dynamic Linear Models (NDLMs) (Bornkamp et al., 2007; Krams et al., 2003; Smith et al., 2006; West and Harrison, 1997).

Interim analysis is frequently conducted for exploratory as well as confirmatory trials for both economical and ethical reasons. In the case of interim futility analysis in an exploratory trial where time and dose responses are yet being learned, certainty of the learning for interim decisions could be low given partially observed data of the already relatively small trial at the interim look. Thus interim analysis approaches that account for not only the interim observed data but also future observables could increase the probability of correct interim decisions. A Bayesian predictive approach to interim analysis of such like was proposed by Dmitrienko and Wang (2006), where formulas for the normal and binary cases are provided. The approach can be generalized for application in more complex cases through Bayesian simulation.

Taking the Bayesian predictive approach, the first step of an interim analysis is to predict observations not yet available at later time points, especially at the end of treatment duration. So the emphasis is first on the longitudinal dimension of drug response. The predicted observables along with the interim observed data are then analyzed to illuminate dose response at the end of treatment duration for interim decision. The first step is about prediction, where patients still ongoing in the trial, but have not progressed to the primary time point would have their yet unobserved measurements predicted given all available longitudinal data from all subjects. Afterwards, dose response inference for the time point of interest is made with both the observed and predicted data, and posterior probabilities of hypotheses on parameters of interest are computed for use in the interim decision.

We specify and discuss the time and dose response models employed for the Bayesian predictive interim futility analysis of a Phase 2 clinical trial in Sect. 2. Section 3 contains simulations performed to assess operating characteristics of the applied approach prior to the interim analysis. The actual interim analysis for the futility decision is presented in Sect. 4. We conclude with discussion in Sect. 5.

2 Bayesian Predictive Interim Analysis

A generalized application of the Bayesian predictive approach to interim analysis proposed by Dmitrienko and Wang (2006) is illustrated through its implementation in a Phase 2 clinical trial.

2.1 A Phase 2 Clinical Trial

A Phase 2 clinical trial was conducted for an experimental drug, with a continuous measure for the primary efficacy assessment. The primary endpoint of the trial was percent change from baseline to the end of the treatment period in the primary efficacy measure. Still yet exploratory, three doses of the drug were studied to understand the response in relation to dose, along with a placebo group as the control. Power calculation was performed for detecting a meaningful difference in the primary endpoint between the active doses and placebo, which was performed through Bayesian simulation. One particular aspect of the sample size determination was that it was addressed by probability of study success (PrSS or POS) (Chuang-Stein, 2006; Wang, 2015; Wang and Li, 2013) rather than the conventional frequentist approach. Resulted from the Bayesian sample size calculation, about 100 patients were planned to be enrolled to each of the three active doses and placebo, with approximately 80 to reach the end of treatment. In addition to the primary endpoint at the end of treatment, for the purpose of eliciting longitudinal properties of response to treatment, as well as for providing intermediate data to enhance interim prediction of response at the primary time point, another measurement of the primary efficacy measure was taken at an earlier time point. Due to the consideration of cost, there was only one interim measurement.

The dose response relationship of the primary endpoint was still highly uncertain when the trial was designed. For this reason, a planned interim analysis was embedded in the design for allowance of a futility stopping. If the interim efficacy signal was convincingly weak at all active doses, it would be wise to suspend the trial and reassess further development of the drug. On the other hand, if promising efficacy was demonstrated earlier at the interim, the trial would still continue for gathering more information to better design subsequent trials. To be consistent in the manner of assessing study success, the interim analysis was centered around calculating probabilities of hypotheses of parameters that had been looked at for the same size determination of the trial, which are to be presently defined. Since the interim analysis was not intended for claiming efficacy earlier, inflation of type-I error was not of concern. Our current emphasis is on the interim analysis of the trial, thus the design of the trial will not be further elaborated.

2.2 Modeling of Time Response and Dose Response

To specify the models, denote the primary endpoint of subject i at dose d and time t as $Y_{i,d,t}$, $d = 1, 2, 3, 4$, $t = 1, 2$, where $d = 1$ is for placebo and $d = 2, 3, 4$ are for the low, middle, and high doses of the tested drug; $t = 1$ is for the time point of the interim measurement of the primary efficacy measure and $t = 2$ is for the primary time point at the end of treatment. Although the notation as well as the models to be defined are for the specific trial here considered, they can be extended to cases with more time points or doses. Observations at the primary time point were first predicted for patients that were still in the trial but had not progressed to the end of treatment. The predicted values along with the observed at the primary time point were then analyzed through a dose response model. To note, only patients with an interim or a final observation were included in the analysis.

2.2.1 Modeling Time Response for Prediction

For the goal of predicting the data yet unobserved at the primary time point, using all available interim data, the following simple regression model was first used:

$$Y_{i,d,2}|y_{i,d,1} \sim \alpha_D + \beta_D y_{i,d,1} + N(0, \lambda_D^2), D = 1, 2,$$

where $D = 1$ for placebo is to distinguish from $D = 2$ for the active doses. It indicated the state of belief that time dependence of the response is different between placebo and the active doses, and the trend is consistent among the active doses. If more suitable for other situations, the consistency assumption can be relaxed to allow for incongruent coefficients across active doses. Also, covariates deemed relevant can be added to the model. Priors of the regression coefficients and random errors $\alpha_D, \beta_D, \lambda_D^2, D = 1, 2$ were assigned common for placebo and the active doses as the following Normal (*N*) and Inverse Gamma (*IG*) distributions:

$$\alpha_D \sim N(\mu_\alpha, \sigma_\alpha^2),$$
$$\beta_D \sim N(\mu_\beta, \sigma_\beta^2),$$
$$\lambda_D^2 \sim IG\left(\frac{\lambda_n}{2} \cdot \frac{\lambda_\mu^2 \lambda_n}{2}\right).$$

The values of the prior parameters actually used for analysis were: $\mu_\alpha = 0$, $\sigma_\alpha = 10$, $\mu_\beta = 0$, $\sigma_\beta = 10$, $\lambda_\mu = 5$, and $\lambda_n = 1$, which together represented a vague knowledge about the parameters at the time of the interim analysis.

In addition, the following more general mixed model repeated measures (MMRM) model was employed:

$$Y_{i,d,t} \sim s_i + \alpha_{d,t} + N(0, \lambda_D^2),$$

where s_i is the random subject effect, $\alpha_{t,d}$ is the fixed effect at dose d and time t, and λ_D^2 is the variance of observation random error. Again, relevant covariates can be incorporated. Prior distributions of the model parameters were designated as

$$s_i \sim N(0, \sigma_s^2),$$
$$\alpha_{d,t} \sim N(\mu_{d,t}, \sigma_{d,t}^2),$$

$$\lambda_D^2 \sim IG\left(\frac{\lambda_n}{2}.\frac{\lambda_\mu^2 \lambda_n}{2}\right).$$

Making the priors diffuse, the values of the prior parameters actually used for the interim analysis were: $\sigma_s = 10$, $\mu_{d,t} = 0$, $\sigma_{d,t} = 10$, $\lambda_\mu = 5$, and $\lambda_n = 1$.

Our simulations and interim analysis showed that the regression and MMRM models resulted in similar results. Thus in the subsequent simulations and analysis sections, we only present results by the MMRM model. The MMRM model indeed simultaneously models time and dose effects, and it is not response shape driven, so is generally flexible. But to more specifically focus on the end time point of interest, we chose an NDLM model for dose response estimation to be next developed.

As the primary objective of the first step, prediction of the unobserved data at t=2 was through the Bayesian predictive paradigm. In general, if θ denotes the model parameters, Y_o the observed data, and Y_u the unobserved, then prediction of Y_u is by

$$f(y_u|y_o) \propto \int f(y_u|\theta)f(\theta|y_o)d\pi(\theta),$$

where f signifies a density or likelihood function and $\pi(\theta)$ is the given prior density. In the case now presented, Y_o consists of all data observed at $t = 1$ and 2, and Y_u designates the data yet to be observed at $t = 2$. Such Bayesian predictive inference is according to the likelihood principle (Wang and Li, 2013).

2.2.2 Modeling Dose Response for Interim Decision

With aggregation of the observed data at the time of the interim analysis and the predicted values of unobserved data from the preceding time response modeling step, dose response relationship at the primary time point was modeled, adjusting for certain covariates. This was performed through the following NDLM model adjusted for the baseline value of the primary measure and age:

$$Y_{i,d,2} \sim N(\theta_d + \beta_b x_{i,0} + \beta_{age} y_{i,0}, \sigma^2), d = 1, 2, 3, 4,$$
$$\theta_d \sim N(\theta_{d-1} + \xi_{d-1}, \tau_{d-1}^2), d = 2, 3, 4,$$

where θ_d is the mean response of dose group $d = 1, 2, 3, 4$, $x_{i,0}$ and $y_{i,0}$ are the baseline values for the primary measure and age respectively, β_b and β_{age} are the coefficients for $x_{i,0}$ and $y_{i,0}$, σ^2 is the variance of the response, ξ_d is the slope parameter that allows movement from dose $d-1$ to dose $d, d = 2, 3, 4$, and $\tau_d^2, d = 2, 3, 4$ permit variability around relations between the mean responses. Note that we did not define ξ_d's recursively as in Smith et al. (2006), and thus to avoid over smoothing. We further define

$$\tau_{d-1}^2 = \tau^2(\nu_d - \nu_{d-1}),$$

where ν_d is the actual dosage of dose d, with $\nu_1 = 0$ for placebo. It indicated that the more distant apart between 2 neighboring doses, the more uncertain of their relation. The difference of dosages can be replaced by a function of the dosages to generalize the application.

Our NDLM analysis was Bayesian, with the following prior distributions for the model parameters:

$$\begin{aligned}
\beta_b &\sim N(\mu_{\beta_b}, \sigma^2_{\beta_b}),\\
\beta_{age} &\sim N(\mu_{\beta_{age}}, \sigma^2_{\beta_{age}}),\\
\sigma^2 &\sim IG\left(\frac{\sigma_n}{2}, \frac{\sigma^2_\mu \sigma_n}{2}\right),\\
\theta_1 &\sim N(\mu_{01}, \nu^2_{01}),\\
\xi_d &\sim N(\mu_{d0}, \sigma^2_{d0}), d = 1, 2, 3,\\
\tau^2 &\sim IG\left(\frac{\tau_n}{2}. \frac{\tau_n \tau^2_\mu}{2}\right).
\end{aligned}$$

The actual assigned values of the parameters in the prior distributions were $\mu_{\beta_b} = 0$, $\sigma_{\beta_b} = 100$, $\mu_{\beta_{age}} = 0$, $\sigma_{\beta_{age}} = 100$, $\sigma_\mu = 12$, $\sigma_n = 1$, $\mu_{01} = 0$, $\nu_{01} = 20$, $\mu_{d0} = 0$, $\sigma_{d0} = 20$, $\tau_\mu = 8$, and $\tau_n = 1$, which again expressed the lack of knowledge of the parameters at the time of the interim analysis.

2.3 Interim Futility Decision Rule

The interim futility decision rule was defined so that a decision to abort the trial early was deemed reasonable in the standard of exploratory drug development. By the proposed Bayesian predictive approach, our interest was in testing hypotheses directly on the parameters than by a statistical test (Wang, 2015; Wang and Li, 2013). Our application compared the three active doses respectively with placebo and checked if a greater response in the primary endpoint than placebo by a given margin was demonstrated. It was expressed in terms of probabilities as

$$P_d = Pr\left(\theta_d - \theta_1 > \delta\right), d = 2, 3, 4.$$

The maximum of these probabilities among the doses is denoted as

$$P_m = Max\left\{P_d, d = 2, 3, 4\right\}.$$

If none of the active doses showed a probability greater than a pre-specified threshold probability η, i.e. if $P_m < \eta$, the trial would be regarded futile. To take into account the correlations among the doses in making interim decisions, the following probability was also looked at:

$$P_a = Pr\left((\theta_2 - \theta_1 < \delta) \; or \; (\theta_3 - \theta_1 < \delta) \; or \; (\theta_4 - \theta_1 < \delta)\right),$$

which was then again compared to η.

The principle for the choice of η is that for an exploratory purpose, η is not set too high, so as to avoid attrition of a potential efficacious drug candidate with a high probability. Reflecting this principle, $\eta = 0.2$ was suggested (Dmitrienko and Wang, 2006).

3 Simulations Prior to Interim Analysis

To adequately prepare for the interim analysis, simulations were performed to illuminate likely outcomes under different scenarios. Three of the scenarios are summarized in Table 1, representing the more promising (scenario 1), neutral (scenario 2), and futile (scenario 3) cases, respectively. The main purpose was to make sure the approach would inform a clear-cut interim futility stopping for cases with all drug doses inefficacious and suggest unambiguous continuation of the trial for cases with some active doses clearly superior to placebo. The within-subject correlation between the two time points was considered. All patients were assumed having progressed to the first time point, and a percentage were yet without an observation at the end time point. In each scenario, the number of patients in each treatment group was set at 25 to reflect the timing of the actual interim analysis, and the standard deviation of the primary end point was estimated to be 6.7 % across treatment groups. For example, in the first scenario, the mean responses with the doses are 0, 0.25, 0.75, and 1.75 % at the first time point, and are 0, 0.5, 0.75, and 3.5 % at the end time point; within-subject correlation coefficient between the two time points is 0.6; only 50 % of patients have values observed at the end time point.

Table 1 Scenarios for pre-trial simulations

		Mean of primary endpoint (%)			
Scenario	Time point	Placebo	Low dose	Med dose	High dose
1	1	0	0.25	0.75	1.75
	2	0	0.50	1.50	3.50
2	1	0	0.25	0.25	0.75
	2	0	0.50	0.50	1.75
3	1	0.10	0.10	0.10	0.10
	2	0.25	0.25	0.25	0.25

Within-subject correlation coefficient between time points: 0.6
Percentage of patients with observation at Time=2: 50 %

Table 2 Summary of Bayesian analysis of simulated trials

Scenario	Primary endpoint (%) Mean of posterior means of simulated trials			
	Placebo	Low dose	Med dose	High dose
1	−0.03	0.55	1.51	3.46
2	0.02	0.53	0.51	1.73
3	0.27	0.25	0.25	0.25

For each scenario, $N = 1000$ trials (which was assessed as adequate) were simulated, and the proposed Bayesian predictive approach was applied to analyze the simulated trials. The simulations and analysis were conducted in R and the R package BRrugs for Markov Chain Monte Carlo (MCMC). MCMC properties, including convergence and auto-correlations, were monitored to ensure adequacy of the MCMC simulations. To compare the estimated effects with the assumed in the scenarios, Table 2 summarizes the means of posterior means of treatment effects at the end time point over the simulated trials for the scenarios, where the exhibited estimation accuracy by comparison with the numbers in Table 1 shows the adequacy of the proposed approach.

For each simulated trial, its predictive probabilities of showing superiority of the drug, individually by $P_i, i = 2, 3, 4$ and collectively by P_a and P_m, were calculated. To proffer more comprehensive information for internal development decisions on an exploratory trial, it is beneficial to look at a set of values of δ than to fix at one. With this in mind, a few values of the superiority margin δ, namely $0.5, 1.5, 2.5\,\%$, were explored. An interim futility stopping would be recommended by predictive probabilities that are less than the pre-specified threshold $\eta = 0.2$. Within each scenario, the percentage of the simulated trials that were labeled for futility stopping was the estimated predictive probability of stopping a trial at the interim for futility. The predictive probabilities of futility stopping for the scenarios are summarized in the upper panel of Table 3, with the collective probability P_a or P_m driving the interim decision.

The simulation results show that the probability of falsely stopping the trial is low for scenario 1 (promising case) across the different superiority margins, and that the probability of falsely continuing the trial is low for scenario 3 (futile case) as long as the rule for stopping is not set too loose by using a very low superiority margin as $\delta = 0.5$. The summary assured us on the appropriateness of applying the proposed Bayesian predictive approach to the interim futility analysis. It was also observed that the two collective probabilities P_a and P_m were generally very close.

To demonstrate the benefit of incorporating the predicted data in the interim analysis, the same Bayesian analysis was repeated on only interim observed data without prediction. The results are summarized in the lower panel of Table 3 as compared against the predictive analysis in the upper panel. The comparison indicates higher probabilities of correct decisions by the predictive approach than without prediction. For instance, for scenario 2 with $\delta = 2.5$, all active doses are below expectation by assumption; for which the predictive approach renders a probability of $P_a = 0.6$ for futility stopping, whereas the probability is only 0.38 if estimated without prediction.

Table 3 Summary of simulations

		Probability of futility: $Pr(P < \eta), \eta = 0.2$				
Scenario	δ	$P = P_2$	$P = P_3$	$P = P_4$	$P = P_a$	$P = P_m$
With predicted observations at Time 2						
1	2.5	0.95	0.63	0.07	0.07	0.07
	1.5	0.71	0.25	<0.01	<0.01	<0.01
	0.5	0.30	0.03	<0.01	<0.01	<0.01
2	2.5	0.95	0.95	0.64	0.60	0.62
	1.5	0.70	0.73	0.22	0.17	0.19
	0.5	0.31	0.31	0.04	0.02	0.03
3	2.5	0.98	0.99	0.99	0.96	0.96
	1.5	0.86	0.86	0.86	0.69	0.71
	0.5	0.52	0.52	0.50	0.24	0.26
Without predicted observations at Time 2						
1	2.5	0.85	0.50	0.04	0.04	0.03
	1.5	0.56	0.15	<0.01	<0.01	<0.01
	0.5	0.21	0.02	<0.01	<0.01	<0.01
2	2.5	0.85	0.88	0.47	0.38	0.43
	1.5	0.56	0.58	0.15	0.08	0.12
	0.5	0.21	0.20	0.02	0.01	0.01
3	2.5	0.95	0.95	0.94	0.84	0.87
	1.5	0.75	0.76	0.74	0.45	0.52
	0.5	0.38	0.39	0.38	0.10	0.15

4 Actual Interim Analysis

The interim futility analysis was conducted when about a third of the number of patients planned to enroll had observations at the intended end time point, with results summarized in the upper panel of Table 4. Compared to $\eta = 0.2$, the predictive probabilities seem overwhelmingly pointing to futility, except for the low superiority margin $\delta = 0.5$. A further look into the data showed one patient on placebo responded extremely well, the best among all. As an exploration, this observation was regarded an outlier and removed, and the results of re-analysis are summarized in the lower panel of Table 4. It did show improved results toward the benefit of the drug, but it would still suggest stopping for futility if the decision rule is set with a higher superiority margin as $\delta = 2.5$.

It was also found that the observed variability of the primary endpoint was much higher than what was assumed in the design stage. This discrepancy could be attributed to the lack of information about treatment of the disease state for which the drug was developed. There was yet no approved or even experimental drug for this disease, and thus there was no reliable data available about the intended endpoint. Also, the ascertained endpoint as a biomarker was yet highly exploratory

Table 4 Summary of interim analysis

With the outlier						
	Treatment					
Primary endpoint (Δ)	Placebo	Low dose	Med dose	High dose		
Posterior mean	1.80	0.59	1.13	1.58	p_a	p_m
$Pr(\Delta_{Trt} - \Delta_{Pbo} > 2.5)$		< 0.01	< 0.01	0.02	0.02	0.03
$Pr(\Delta_{Trt} - \Delta_{Pbo} > 1.5)$		0.03	0.05	0.10	0.10	0.15
$Pr(\Delta_{Trt} - \Delta_{Pbo} > 0.5)$		0.12	0.18	0.30	0.30	0.40
Without the outlier						
	Treatment					
Primary endpoint (Δ)	Placebo	Low dose	Med dose	High dose		
Posterior mean	1.07	0.73	1.08	1.58	p_a	p_m
$Pr(\Delta_{Trt} - \Delta_{Pbo} > 2.5)$		0.02	0.02	0.07	0.07	0.09
$Pr(\Delta_{Trt} - \Delta_{Pbo} > 1.5)$		0.10	0.12	0.22	0.22	0.31
$Pr(\Delta_{Trt} - \Delta_{Pbo} > 0.5)$		0.28	0.35	0.50	0.50	0.63

Δ percent change from baseline

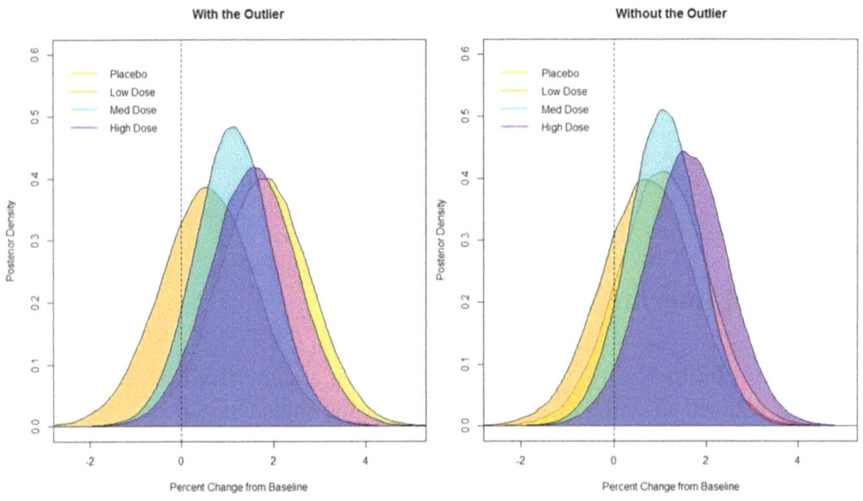

Fig. 1 Posterior distributions of treatment effects at interim analysis

in its correlations with potential clinical endpoints to be next pursued in more confirmatory trials. For the stated reasons and benefits of collecting more data for further elicitation, the trial was continued to the planned end.

To provide a more informative decision making kit, the posterior distributions of the individual treatment effects were plotted alongside one another with different colors for more catching visual comparisons, see Fig. 1. This type of plots have shown to be useful to decision makers, especially non-statisticians.

5 Analysis of Final Data

Given the decision to complete the trial, there was the opportunity to analyze the final data. The analysis results are summarized in Table 5. Differentiation between the active doses and placebo was more clearly demonstrated, which was encouraging for continuing development of the drug.

Posterior distributions of treatment effects are depicted in Fig. 2 for aid in further planning.

Table 5 Summary of final analysis

	Treatment					
Primary endpoint (Δ)	Placebo	Low dose	Med dose	High dose		
Posterior mean	0.13	0.69	1.00	1.32	p_a	p_m
$Pr(\Delta_{Trt} - \Delta_{Pbo} > 2.5)$		< 0.01	< 0.01	0.03	0.03	0.03
$Pr(\Delta_{Trt} - \Delta_{Pbo} > 1.5)$		0.08	0.17	0.32	0.32	0.40
$Pr(\Delta_{Trt} - \Delta_{Pbo} > 0.5)$		0.54	0.71	0.85	0.85	0.92

Δ percent change from baseline

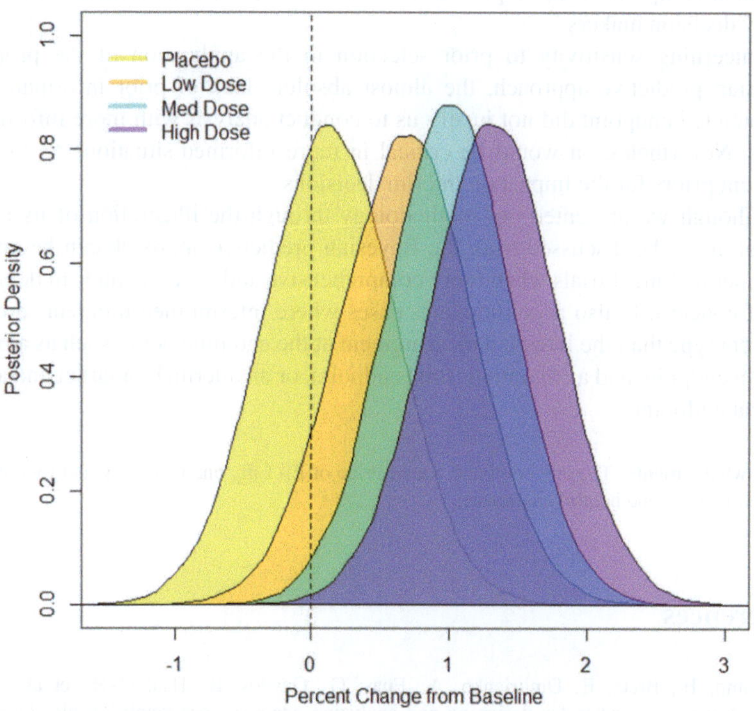

Fig. 2 Posterior distributions of treatment effects at final analysis

6 Discussion

We conducted Bayesian modeling of time response and dose response for the interim futility analysis of a clinical trial. A simulation based generalization of the Bayesian predictive approach proposed by Dmitrienko and Wang (2006) was applied. Prediction of observations not yet seen at the interim analysis was first made for the time point of interest by a Bayesian regression or MMRM model. The predicted values were then incorporated in the modeling of dose response at the time point of interest by a Bayesian NDLM model. Pre-interim simulations showed that this Bayesian predictive approach adequately estimated the assumed dose responses. High predictive probabilities of making correct futility decisions for different scenarios were evidenced. It also demonstrated increased probabilities of making correct decisions than inference without prediction.

For the actual interim analysis, even border-line futility was manifested, the estimated predictive probabilities along with other considerations as given contributed to a no-stop decision. Bayesian analysis of the completed trial revealed more encouraging results, which retrospectively confirmed the interim no-stop decision. The graphical presentation of posterior distributions of the Bayesian analysis for treatment comparisons as employed was found useful for communication with and use by decision makers.

Concerning sensitivity to prior selection in the application of the proposed Bayesian predictive approach, the almost absolute lack of prior information on the intended endpoint did not justify us to conduct analysis with more informative priors. Nevertheless, it would be critical in more informed situations to compare different priors for the impact on interim decisions.

Although we presented our methodology through the illustration of its implementation in the discussed trial, the Bayesian predictive approach can be applied for general clinical trials when more comprehensive and accurate interim decisions are of concern. It also accommodates cases where interim measurements are of a different type than the intended measurement at the end time point, such as a binary interim endpoint and a continuous final endpoint, or an interim biomarker and a final clinical endpoint.

Acknowledgements The authors thank Karen Price of Eli Lilly and Company and two referees for their reviews and helpful comments.

References

Bornkamp, B., Bretz, F., Dmitrienko, A., Enas, G., Gaydos, B., Hsu, C.-H., et al. (2007). Innovative approaches for designing and analyzing adaptive dose-ranging trials. *Journal of Biopharmaceutical Statistics, 17*, 965–995.

Chuang-Stein, C. (2006). Sample size and the probability of a successful trial. *Pharmaceutical Statistics, 5*, 305–309.

Dmitrienko, A., & Wang, M.-D. (2006). Bayesian predictive approach to interim monitoring in clinical trials. *Statistics in Medicine, 25*, 2178–2195.

Fu, H., & Manner, D. (2010). Bayesian adaptive dose-finding studies with delayed responses. *Journal of Biopharmaceutical Statistics, 20*, 1055–1070.

Krams, M., Lees, K. R., Hacke, W., Grieve, A. P., Orgogozo, J. M., & Ford, G. A. for the ASTIN Study investigators (2003). ASTIN: An adaptive dose-response study of UK- 279,276 in acute ischemic stroke. *Stroke, 34*, 2543–2548.

Smith, M. K., Jones, I., Morris, M. F., Grieve, A. P., & Tan K. (2006). Implementation of a Bayesian adaptive design in a proof of concept study. *Pharmaceutical Statistics, 5*, 39–50.

Thomas, N., Sweeney, K., & Somayaji, V. (2014). Meta-analysis of clinical dose response in a large drug development portfolio. *Statistics in Biopharmaceutical Research, 6*, 302–317.

Wang, M.-D. (2015). Applications of probability of study success in clinical drug development. In: Z. Chen, A. Liu, Y. Qu, L. Tang, N. Ting, & Y. Tsong (Eds.). *Applied Statistics in Biomedicine and Clinical Trial Designs: Selected Papers from 2013 ICSA/ISBS Joint Statistical Meetings* (pp. 185–196). Berlin: Springer.

Wang, M.-D., & Li, G. Y. (2013). Bayesian interim inference of probability of clinical trial success. In: M. Hu, Y. Liu, & J. Lin (Eds.) *Topics in Applied Statistics: 2012 Symposium of International Chinese Statistical Association - Springer Proceedings in Mathematics and Statistics* (Vol. 55, pp. 137–147). New York: Springer.

West, M., & Harrison, P. J. (1997). *Bayesian forecasting and dynamic models* (2nd ed.). New York: Springer.

An ROC Approach to Evaluate Interim Go/No-Go Decision-Making Quality with Application to Futility Stopping in the Clinical Trial Designs

Deli Wang, Lu Cui, Lanju Zhang, and Bo Yang

Abstract Interim analyses can be planned to make Go/No-Go decisions in late phase clinical trials and decision quality is an issue of interest because of the timing of interim analysis is often selected based on empirical experience and thresholds for interim Go/No-Go decisions are determined arbitrarily. There is no systematic research to investigate interrelationship among three commonly used statistical methods for interim decision-making, namely conditional power, predictive power, and predicted confidence interval methods. We used a receiver operating characteristic (ROC) approach to evaluate decision-making quality of these methods and they are proved to be equivalent analytically and verified by simulations. To achieve the pre-specified sensitivity and specificity for Go/No-Go decision-making at interim, the required minimum sample size for interim analysis and the threshold for each of three statistical methods can be systematically determined based on the target design parameters of the clinical trials. The application of the obtained results is given for continuous outcome measures.

1 Introduction

Interim analysis is traditionally used to monitor the safety and efficacy of an experimental drug in phase II and III clinical trials. The purpose of the interim analysis is to use the accumulated data in the mid-course of the trial to capture

---

D. Wang (✉)
Global Pharmaceutical Research and Development, AbbVie Inc., North Chicago, IL 60064-6075, USA
e-mail: deli.wang@abbvie.com

L. Cui • L. Zhang
Data and Statistical Science, AbbVie Inc., North Chicago, IL, USA

B. Yang
Biometrics, Global Medicines Development & Affairs, Vertex Pharmaceutical, 50 Northern Ave, Boston, MA 02210, USA

Z. Jin et al. (eds.), *New Developments in Statistical Modeling, Inference and Application*, ICSA Book Series in Statistics, DOI 10.1007/978-3-319-42571-9_7

signals of potential undue harm or unexpected efficacy of the experimental drug early so that a decision regarding whether the trial should be continued can be made. The role of interim analysis is further broadened to include possibility to stop a study (Lachin, 2005) if the trial does not have potential to demonstrate the drug efficacy at the end of the study given data observed at interim. In the adaptive design setting, the information based on the analysis of interim data may be used to make various decisions on potential modification of trial parameters or designs. For example, an interim analysis can be used under the adaptive seamless phase II/III design to evaluate the performance of individual doses in a phase II dose ranging phase with the discontinuation of inefficacious doses followed by the confirmation phase to demonstrate the efficacy of a chosen dose.

Various interim decision-making methods have been developed. For example, the group sequential method (Lan and DeMets, 1983; O'Brien and Fleming, 1979; Peto et al., 1976; Pocock, 1977; Wang and Tsiatis, 1987) is often used for the interim analysis intended to stop the trial early for safety or efficacy. Mazumdar and Liu (2003) extended group sequential design method to use standardized AUC (area under the curve) difference statistic in the comparative clinical trials in diagnostic medicine. Futility analysis approaches in clinical trial interim monitoring have also been widely investigated in the literature (DeMets, 2006; Dobbins, 2013; Friedlin et al., 2010; Lachin, 2009; Lan and Wittes, 1988; Zhang and Clarke, 2010). Conditional power (CP), predictive probability (PP), and predictive confidence interval (PCI) methods are commonly used for the interim futility analysis and dose selection with potential dropping off inefficacious doses. The conditional power is the probability that the final trial result would be statistically significant, given the data observed at interim and a specific assumption about the pattern of the data to be observed in the remainder of the study. If the conditional power calculated at interim is less than a pre-specified threshold, the trial will be stopped for futility, otherwise, continue as is. Lachin (2005) provided a systematic review of methods for futility stopping based on the conditional power which can be calculated based on the null hypothesis, the current trend in the data at interim, or under the original design. The conditional power considers only the interim estimate of the primary efficacy measurement but ignores the potential variability of the estimate at interim. On the other hand, the predictive power method (Spiegelhalter et al., 1986) takes the variability of estimates of interest into consideration for decision-making at interim. It is the average conditional power over the entire posterior distribution of the true parameter of interest based on the observed interim data. Evans et al. (2007) proposed to use the predicted confidence interval calculated at interim for decision-making. They defined the minimum clinical meaningful difference as the pre-specified threshold and compared it to the upper bound of the predicted confidence interval for interim decisions.

Interrelationship between conditional power and predictive power has been reviewed (Gallo et al., 2014; Lan et al., 2009) recently in interim futility analysis. However, there is no systematic research to compare conditional power, predictive power, and predicted confidence interval methods and their decision-making quality, performance, and their interconnected relationship. Timing of interim analysis is often selected based on empirical experience and thresholds for interim Go/No-Go decisions are determined arbitrarily. Some researchers used a pre-specified threshold $1 - \gamma$, where γ is the futility index (ranging from 0.8 to 1) (Halperin et al., 1982; Jennison et al., 1990; Lan et al., 1987; Tan, 2008), for conditional power in futility analysis. Methods to determine the timing and thresholds for interim analysis are not clearly defined. ROC curves (Green and Swets, 1966) are widely used to measure the discriminative capability of medical tests and other decision-making procedures (Obuchowski, 2003; Pepe, 2003; Zweig and Campbell, 1993). Chuang-Stein et al. (2011) applied the concept of sensitivity and specificity to Go/No-Go decision-making in drug development. Interim decision quality of different methods were not investigated in the paper by Chuang-Stein et al. (2011). The present research is to investigate the performance and the relationship of three commonly used methods for interim decision-making and also to define a way to determine the timing and threshold for interim analysis via a Receiver Operating Characteristics (ROC) based approach.

In this paper, we assume that the outcome follows a normal distribution. The presentation will be organized as the following. Section 2 will introduce the sensitivity and specificity of a decision-making method relevant to the true desired and undesired treatment effects space. Borrowing the concept of evaluation of diagnostic testing method, an ROC curve associated with each method is derived and relationship among three methods is also demonstrated in Sect. 2. Simulation results will be presented in Sect. 3 to assess the performance characteristics based on the calculated sensitivity, specificity, positive and negative predictive values under assumed ranges of desired treatment effects (usually the target minimum treatment effects) as well as an undesired treatment effect. Utilization of the ROC approach to systematically determining the timing of interim analysis and the threshold for each statistical method and application of the proposed method to the design optimization are presented in Sect. 4 and finally conclusions and discussions follow.

2 ROC Curves for Interim Go/No-Go Decisions for CP, PP, and PCI Methods

An ROC curve can be constructed based on the sensitivity and the specificity of a diagnostic test which uses a cutoff to declare a disease or an abnormal physical condition. Analogy between clinical trials and diagnostic tests was discussed two decades ago by Pater and Willan (1984). Chuang-Stein et al. (2011) applied the concept of sensitivity and specificity in the hypothesis testing setting for Go/No-Go decisions in different stages of drug development; for example, developing a compound from Phase I to Phase II or moving from Phase II to Phase III development. The sensitivity and specificity of the statistical method for interim Go/No-Go decision-making can be viewed as the probabilities that a positive or negative result based on the statistical method matches the underlying truth. In clinical trials with interim analysis, a positive (negative) result often leads to a Go (No-Go) decision, the sensitivity (specificity) can also be interpreted as the probability of a Go (No-Go) decision while the underlying condition in truth is desirable/favorable (undesirable/unfavorable). In the following, we will substantialize the aforementioned concepts and show relevant applications in characterization of the decision-making quality based on CP, PP, and PCI methods.

Let μ be the true treatment difference (a larger treatment effect is more desirable, i.e., $\mu \geq 0$) of the normally distributed endpoint between a treatment arm and a placebo arm in a clinical trial and σ be the common standard deviation across two arms which is assumed to be known for simplicity. One interim futility analysis is planned with stopping for futility only. Let $N = n + m$ be the total number of subjects per arm in the clinical trial. The interim analysis is performed when n subjects per arm are available for the analysis and additional m subjects per arm will be enrolled if a Go decision is made at the interim, and $t = \frac{n}{N}$ is the information fraction under the assumption that subjects are equally allocated between two arms in the interim analysis. Denote $\bar{X}_n$ and $\bar{X}_m$ as the mean treatment difference between two arms from the first $2n$ subjects at the interim and the last $2m$ subjects after the interim, respectively. Denote C as the critical value for the final test statistics, $C = Z_{1-\alpha/2}$ where $Z_{1-\alpha/2}$ is the $(1-\alpha/2) \times 100\,\%$ percentile of the standard normal distribution, α is the significance level. Let Z_n denote the interim Z-statistics based on information from the first $2n$ subjects and Z_N denote the final Z- statistics based on information from all $2N$ subjects at the end of the trial.

For the treatment difference parameter $\mu \in R$, define the undesired treatment effect space as $R_0 = [0, \mu_0]$ and the desired treatment effect space as $R_1 = [\mu_1, +\infty)$, where μ_0 and μ_1 ($\mu_0 \leq \mu_1$) are two thresholds of the treatment effect difference between two arms which can be pre-specified in the design stage based on clinical, commercial or other considerations of a clinical trial. We assume a larger treatment effect is more desirable and the target favorable treatment effect is $\mu \geq \mu_1$ or $\mu \in R_1$ and the unfavorable treatment effect is $\mu \leq \mu_0$ or $\mu \in R_0$. An interim decision is often made based on whether or not a test statistics can pass a pre-determined threshold. A Go decision can be made if it is believed that the true treatment difference falls in the desired space R_1 given the observed interim data. A No-Go decision can be made if it is believed that the true treatment difference falls in the undesired space R_0 given the observed interim data. We name $S_w(u_w, \mu_1)$ as the sensitivity for Method $w = cp, pp, pci$, which is defined as the probability of a correct interim Go decision at threshold u_w based on an interim test statistics given the underlying true treatment difference is from the desired treatment space R_1 (e.g. $\mu_1 \in R_1$). We name $S_w(u_w, \mu_0)$ as the specificity, which is defined as the probability of a correct interim No-Go decision at threshold u_w based on an interim test statistics given the underlying true treatment difference is from the undesired treatment space R_0 (e.g. $\mu_0 \in R_0$). The threshold u_w in $S_w(u_w, \mu_1)$ and $S_w(u_w, \mu_0)$ is the method specific cutoff value for the interim decision-making. Hence, $S_w(u_w, \mu_1)$ and $1 - S_w(u_w, \mu_0)$, $-\infty < u_w < +\infty$, define a curve with respective to u_w.

We still name it the ROC curve since the curve describes the receiving operating characteristics of a statistical decision method. This research focuses on evaluation of the interim decision-making quality of three commonly used statistical methods, namely the conditional power, the predictive power, and the predicted confidence interval methods. The ROC curves for the interim Go and No-Go decisions and functional forms of the three methods for sensitivity and specificity are derived in the following subsections.

2.1 Conditional Power ROC

The conditional power is the conditional probability of a statistically significant result at the end of a clinical trial given the current data observed at interim and a specific assumption of the treatment effect of remaining data in the study. The assumption could be the current observed treatment effect will be the same in the remaining part of the trial after the interim, or the original design effect holds for the remaining data, or the treatment effect is similar to the null hypothesis (Lachin, 2005). Following a commonly used assumption, we assume the trend of the treatment effect observed at interim continues, i.e. $\mu = \bar{X}_n$. With some algebra (see section "Conditional Power Derivation in Sect. 2.1" in Appendix), the conditional power based on Z-test at interim time t can be obtained as

$$\begin{aligned}\mathrm{CP}_t &= P\left(Z_N \geq C \mid \bar{X}_n\right)\\ &= \Phi\left(-C\sqrt{\frac{N}{m}} + \frac{N}{\sqrt{m}}\frac{\bar{X}_n}{\sigma}\right),\end{aligned} \tag{1}$$

where Φ is the standard normal distribution function. A Go/No-Go decision is made based on the conditional power projected at the end of the trial with additional m subjects per arm enrolled based on the interim data. Suppose a Go decision will be made at interim t if the conditional power calculated in Eq. (1) is greater than or equal to a threshold $\varsigma (0 < \varsigma < 1)$, i.e., $\mathrm{CP}_t \geq \varsigma$. The decision function for CP based on the interim data is defined as

$$D = \begin{cases} 1 \text{ if } \mathrm{CP}_t \geq \varsigma; \\ 0 \text{ otherwise,} \end{cases}$$

equivalently, D=1 when $-C\sqrt{\frac{N}{m}} + \frac{N}{\sqrt{m}}\frac{\bar{X}_n}{\sigma} \geq u$, D=0 otherwise, where $\Phi(u) = \varsigma$. After some algebra (see section "Conditional Power Derivation in Sect. 2.1" in Appendix), the probability of a Go decision based on CP_t with the treatment effect difference of μ is

$$\mathrm{Prob(D=1)} = P\left(-C\sqrt{\frac{N}{m}} + \frac{N}{\sqrt{m}}\frac{\bar{X}_n}{\sigma} \geq u\right) = 1 - \Phi\left(C\sqrt{\frac{n}{N}} - \frac{\sqrt{n}\mu}{\sigma} + \frac{\sqrt{mn}}{N}u\right). \tag{2}$$

The probability of a No-Go decision with the treatment effect difference of μ is 1-Prob(D=1), i.e.,

$$\text{Prob}(\text{D}=0) = \Phi\left(C\sqrt{\frac{n}{N}} - \frac{\sqrt{n}\mu}{\sigma} + \frac{\sqrt{mn}}{N}u\right). \tag{3}$$

The sensitivity for CP at interim t is the probability of a correct interim Go decision (D= 1) based on a conditional power criterion ($\text{CP}_t \geq \varsigma$) calculated from the observed interim data under the target treatment effect $\mu = \mu_1 \in R_1$. The specificity for CP at interim t is the probability of a correct No-Go decision (D=0) based on a conditional power criterion ($\text{CP}_t < \varsigma$) calculated from the observed interim data under the undesired treatment effect $\mu = \mu_0 \in R_0$. Replacing μ with μ_1 and μ_0 in Eqs. (2) and (3), respectively, the sensitivity and the specificity for CP at interim time t at cutoff u are obtained as the following

$$S_{cp}(u, \mu_1) = 1 - \Phi\left(C\sqrt{\frac{n}{N}} - \frac{\sqrt{n}\mu_1}{\sigma} + \frac{\sqrt{mn}}{N}u\right), \tag{4}$$

$$S_{cp}(u, \mu_0) = \Phi\left(C\sqrt{\frac{n}{N}} - \frac{\sqrt{n}\mu_0}{\sigma} + \frac{\sqrt{mn}}{N}u\right). \tag{5}$$

Accordingly, the ROC curve for the interim Go and No-Go decision based on CP can be constructed by varing u in $-\infty < u < +\infty$.

2.2 *Predictive Power ROC*

The predictive power (Spiegelhalter et al., 1986) uses weighted average of conditional power values to consider the variability of the estimate of μ at interim. Suppose the prior distribution of the true treatment difference μ is $g(\mu)$ and its posterior probability density function is $g(\mu \mid \bar{X}_n)$, then the predictive power at interim time t is

$$\text{PP}_t = \int \text{CP}_t(\mu) g(\mu \mid \bar{X}_n) d\mu.$$

Suppose the mean treatment difference of the remaining m subjects after the interim is $\bar{X}_m \sim N(\mu, \sigma^2/m)$. As suggested by Lan et al. (2009) based on a fiducial argument (Spiegelhalter et al., 1986) and assume a non-informative prior distribution $g(\mu) = 1$, the posterior probability density is $g(\mu \mid \bar{X}_n) = N(\bar{X}_n, \sigma^2/n)$ given the interim data (Tan, 2008). Condition on the interim data, the marginal distribution of $\bar{X}_m$ is normally distributed with mean and variance (see section "Predictive Power Derivation in Sect. 2.2" in Appendix) as the following,

$$\begin{aligned} E(\bar{X}_m) &= E(E(\bar{X}_m|\mu)) = E(\mu) = \bar{X}_n, \\ Var(\bar{X}_m) &= \sigma^2(1/n + 1/m). \end{aligned}$$

Then the predictive power is given by

$$\mathrm{PP}_t = \int \mathrm{CP}_t(\mu) g(\mu \mid \bar{X}_n) d\mu = 1 - \Phi\left[\sqrt{\frac{n}{m}}\left(C - \frac{\bar{X}_n\sqrt{N}}{\sigma}\right)\right], \tag{6}$$

where $\bar{X}_n$ are the mean treatment difference between two arms at the interim. It can be shown that $\frac{\sqrt{n}\bar{X}_n}{\sigma} = Z_n + \frac{\sqrt{n}\mu}{\sigma}$ where $Z_n = \frac{\sqrt{n}(\bar{X}_n - \mu)}{\sigma}$. Then Eq. (6) can be re-written as the following,

$$\mathrm{PP}_t = \Phi\left(-C\sqrt{\frac{n}{m}} + Z_n\sqrt{\frac{N}{m}} + \sqrt{\frac{Nn}{m}}\frac{\mu}{\sigma}\right). \tag{7}$$

Similar to the argument for the conditional power method, suppose a Go decision (D=1) is made at interim t if the predictive power calculated in Eq. (7) is greater than or equal to a threshold $\varsigma (0 < \varsigma < 1)$, i.e., $\mathrm{PP}_t \geq \varsigma$, then the decision function for PP based on the interim data is given by

$$D = \begin{cases} 1 \text{ if } \mathrm{PP}_t \geq \varsigma; \\ 0 \text{ otherwise,} \end{cases}$$

which is equivalent to D=1 when $-C\sqrt{\frac{n}{m}} + Z_n\sqrt{\frac{N}{m}} + \sqrt{\frac{Nn}{m}}\frac{\mu}{\sigma} \geq u$, D=0 otherwise, where $\Phi(u) = \varsigma$. After some algebra (see section "Predictive Power Derivation in Sect. 2.2" in Appendix), the probability of a Go decision based on PP_t with the treatment effect difference of μ is

$$\mathrm{Prob(D = 1)} = P\left(-C\sqrt{\frac{n}{m}} + Z_n\sqrt{\frac{N}{m}} + \sqrt{\frac{Nn}{m}}\frac{\mu}{\sigma} \geq u\right). \tag{8}$$

Similar to the argument for the conditional power method, the sensitivity and the specificity at interim time t at cutoff u for PP will be

$$S_{pp}(u, \mu_1) = 1 - \Phi\left(C\sqrt{\frac{n}{N}} - \frac{\sqrt{n}\mu_1}{\sigma} + \sqrt{\frac{m}{N}}u\right), \tag{9}$$

$$S_{pp}(u, \mu_0) = \Phi\left(C\sqrt{\frac{n}{N}} - \frac{\sqrt{n}\mu_0}{\sigma} + \sqrt{\frac{m}{N}}u\right). \tag{10}$$

Accordingly, the ROC curve for the interim Go and No-Go decision based on PP can be constructed by varing u in $-\infty < u < +\infty$.

2.3 Predicted Confidence Interval ROC

Proposed by Evans et al. (2007), the predicted confidence interval (PCI) is the confidence interval predicted for a future time point (e.g., the end of the study) conditional on data observed at interim, or based on some assumptions for the future data yet to be collected. These assumptions could be the trend of the observed data continues, or the future data is the same as the null hypothesis, or the future data is the same as the alternative hypothesis, or the best/worst scenarios (Evans et al., 2007). The predicted confidence interval at the interim can be expressed as

$$\frac{n\bar{X}_n + m\bar{X}_m}{N} \pm C\frac{\sigma}{\sqrt{N}}.$$

where $\bar{X}_m$ is the simulated group mean difference assuming the current trend observed at interim continues, i.e. $\bar{X}_m \sim N(\bar{X}_n, \sigma^2/m)$. Let CPCI_t be the conditional probability of the upper bound of PCI less than or equal to a threshold d at interim time t given interim data. It is the proportion of PCIs whose upper bounds are less than or equal to threshold d given observed interim data. Simulations can be conducted to obtain CPCI_t using the observed interim data. The theoretical CPCI_t can be obtained as the following (see section "Predicted Confidence Interval Derivation in Sect. 2.3" in Appendix),

$$\begin{aligned}\text{CPCI}_t &= P\left(\frac{n\bar{X}_n + m\bar{X}_m}{N} + \frac{C\sigma}{\sqrt{N}} \le d \mid \bar{X}_n\right)\\ &= \Phi\left(-C\sqrt{\frac{N}{m}} + \frac{Nd}{\sigma\sqrt{m}} - \frac{N\bar{X}_n}{\sigma\sqrt{m}}\right). \end{aligned} \quad (11)$$

A Go decision (D=1) is made at interim t when CPCI_t in Eq. (11) is less than or equal to ς where $0 < \varsigma < 1$, i.e., $\text{CPCI}_t \le \varsigma$. In other words, the smaller the CPCI_t the lower the chance that the PCI upper bound will be less than or equal to d, a Go decision should be made. Otherwise, a No-Go decision should be made. Similar to the argument for the conditional power method, the decision function for PCI based on the interim data is

$$D = \begin{cases} 1 \text{ if } \text{CPCI}_t \le \varsigma; \\ 0 \text{ otherwise,} \end{cases}$$

which is equivalent to D=1 when $-C\sqrt{\frac{N}{m}} + \frac{Nd}{\sigma\sqrt{m}} - \frac{N\bar{X}_n}{\sigma\sqrt{m}} \le u$, D=0 otherwise, where $\Phi(u) = \varsigma$. After some algebra (see section "Predicted Confidence Interval Derivation in Sect. 2.3" in Appendix), the probability of a Go decision (D=1) at interim with the treatment effect difference of μ for PCI can be obtained as the following,

$$\text{Prob(D} = 1) = P\left(-C\sqrt{\frac{N}{m}} + \frac{Nd}{\sigma\sqrt{m}} - \frac{N\bar{X}_n}{\sigma\sqrt{m}} \le u\right)$$
$$= \Phi\left(C\sqrt{\frac{n}{N}} - \frac{(d-\mu)\sqrt{n}}{\sigma} + u\frac{\sqrt{mn}}{N}\right). \quad (12)$$

Similar to the argument for the conditional power method, the sensitivity and the specificity at interim time t at cutoff u, an upper bound threshold d for the PCI method are

$$S_{pci}(u, \mu_1) = \Phi\left(C\sqrt{\frac{n}{N}} - \frac{(d-\mu_1)\sqrt{n}}{\sigma} + \frac{\sqrt{mn}}{N}u\right), \quad (13)$$

$$S_{pci}(u, \mu_0) = 1 - \Phi\left(C\sqrt{\frac{n}{N}} - \frac{(d-\mu_0)\sqrt{n}}{\sigma} + \frac{\sqrt{mn}}{N}u\right). \quad (14)$$

Accordingly, the ROC curve for the interim Go and No-Go decision based on PCI can be constructed by varing u in $-\infty < u < +\infty$.

2.4 Equivalent Conversion of CP, PP, and PCI Methods

It is known that an ROC curve for diagnostic testing is invariant under monotonic transformation of a decision function. For the same reason, the ROC curves defined in Sects. 2.1–2.3 should be identical. In the following, a unified expression is derived, and the conversion formula of cutoff points of different decision methods are derived. ROC curves for CP, PP, and PCI methods have been constructed using the sensitivity and 1-specificity. Considering the conditional power method, let $y = S_{cp}(u, \mu_1)$ and $x = 1 - S_{cp}(u, \mu_0)$, then from Eq. (5),

$$\frac{\sqrt{mn}}{N}u = -C\sqrt{\frac{n}{N}} + \frac{\sqrt{n}\mu_0}{\sigma} - \Phi^{-1}(x) \quad (15)$$

Substituting $\frac{\sqrt{mn}}{N}u$ from Eq. (15) into Eq. (4) and we obtain

$$y = S_{cp}(u, \mu_1) = \Phi\left[\Phi^{-1}(x) + \frac{\sqrt{n}(\mu_1 - \mu_0)}{\sigma}\right]. \quad (16)$$

Equation (16) is a non-parametric expression of an ROC curve based on the conditional power method. It can be shown that the same non-parametric expression of ROC curve can be obtained for the predictive power method and the predicted confidence interval method. Identical ROC curves for the three methods imply equivalence of CP, PP, and PCI in terms of decision-making at interim and they

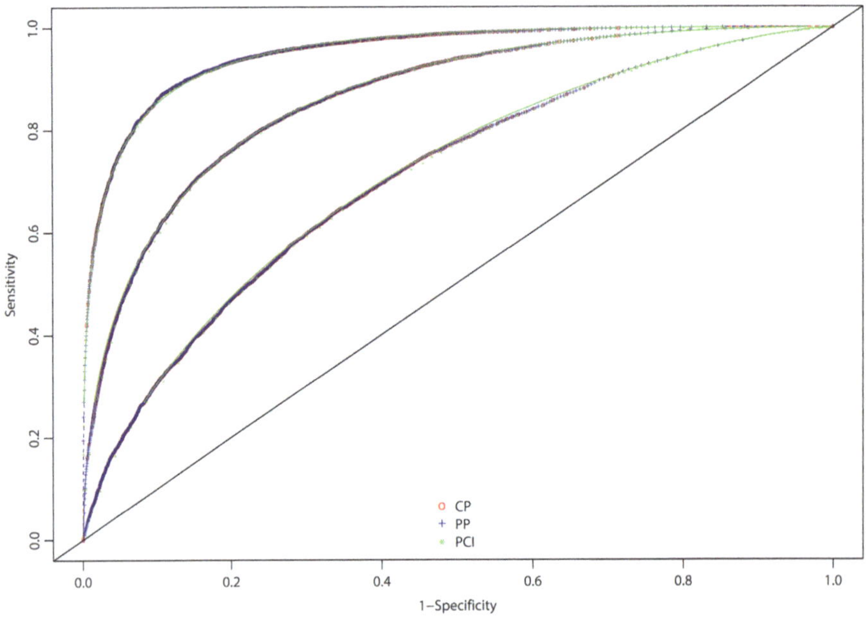

Fig. 1 Simulated ROC curves (points) match theoretical ROC curves for CP, PP, and PCI methods. CP stands for the conditional power method, PP stands for the predictive power method, and PCI stands for the predicted confidence interval method. The simulation (10,000 runs) used a total sample size of N = 60 per arm and the interim sample size was n = 30 per arm. Effect sizes 0.7, 0.5, and 0.3 were assumed as desired effect sizes (μ_1) for three ROC curves from the *top* to the *bottom*. The undesired effect size (μ_0) was 0.1 for all three curves and the common standard deviation was assumed to be 1 in the simulation

are unified by the ROC criteria. Our simulation results presented in Fig. 1 showed the consistency between theoretical ROC curves and simulated ROC curves, which indicates equivalence of the three methods for interim decision-making. For each scenario in Fig. 1, the simulated ROC curves for CP, PP, and PCI are well overlapped with their theoretical ROC curves.

Although three statistical methods are equivalent in terms of overall quality of interim decision-making but thresholds vary among the three methods for the same quality of interim decision-making in terms of the sensitivity and the specificity. The formula for conversion of thresholds between each pair of the three methods can be derived. Let u_{cp}, u_{pp}, and u_{pci} be thresholds for CP, PP, and PCI methods to have the same decision-quality in terms of the sensitivity and the specificity at interim, respectively. After some algebra, the conversion formula of three thresholds are

$$u_{pp} = u_{cp}\sqrt{\frac{n}{N}},$$

Table 1 Optimal thresholds which maximize accuracy of decision-making at interim for the three methods (CP, PP, and PCI) under different desired effect sizes

μ_1	Method	Threshold	Accuracy	μ_1	Method	Threshold	Accuracy
0.7	CP	0.628	0.877	0.3	CP	0.111	0.651
	PP	0.591	0.877		PP	0.194	0.651
	PCI	0.031	0.877		PCI	0.373	0.651
0.6	CP	0.476	0.834	0.2	CP	0.054	0.577
	PP	0.483	0.834		PP	0.127	0.577
	PCI	0.069	0.834		PCI	0.525	0.577
0.5	CP	0.327	0.781	0.1	CP	0.023	0.500
	PP	0.376	0.781		PP	0.079	0.500
	PCI	0.136	0.781		PCI	0.674	0.500
0.4	CP	0.202	0.719	0.0 [a]	CP	0.003	0.500
	PP	0.277	0.719		PP	0.025	0.500
	PCI	0.238	0.719		PCI	0.890	0.500

Note: *CP* the conditional power method; *PP* the predictive power method; *PCI* the predicted confidence interval method where $d = 0.516$ is chosen so that a sample size of 60/arm (N) has 80 % power with a two-sided $\alpha = 0.05$ test

[a] $\mu_0 = 0$, otherwise $\mu_0 = 0.1$. The interim analysis is performed at n = 30 subjects/arm

$$u_{pci} = -2C\sqrt{\frac{N}{m}} + \frac{dN}{\sqrt{m}\sigma} - u_{cp},$$

$$u_{pci} = -2C\sqrt{\frac{N}{m}} + \frac{dN}{\sqrt{m}\sigma} - u_{pp}\sqrt{\frac{N}{n}}.$$

Numerical examples of this mapping can be found in Table 1.

3 Performance Characteristics of ROC Curves

3.1 Factors Associated with the Discriminative Capacity of ROC Curves

As shown in Eq. (16) in Sect. 2.4, the three methods for interim decision-making are equivalent as demonstrated based on ROC criteria. Given a specificity, factors determining the shape of an ROC curve are the interim sample size (n) and the standardized treatment difference between a desired effect and an undesired effect ($\frac{\mu_1-\mu_0}{\sigma}$). Figure 2 presents how the shape of ROC curve changes when the sample sizes increases at interim given a desired effect size is 0.6 and an undesired effect size is 0.1 (Fig. 2a). The area under the ROC curve (AUC), which is the overall measure of decision quality and is the probability of a statistical test to discriminate

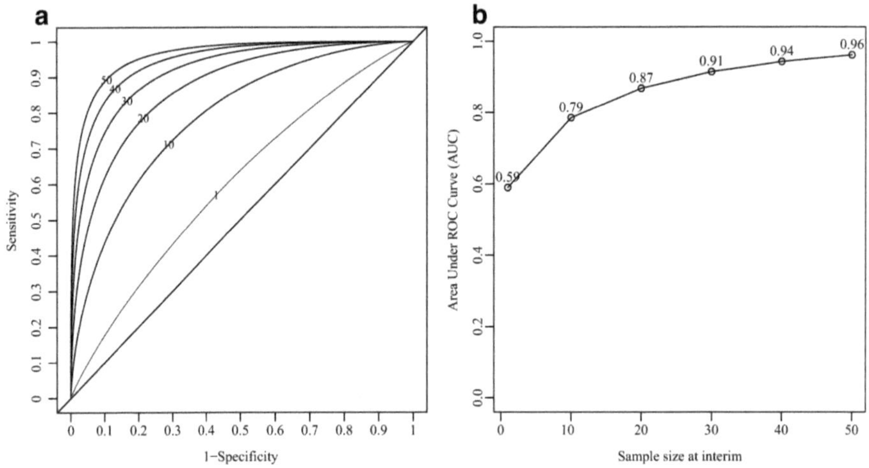

Fig. 2 Conditional power ROC curves at different sample sizes at interim analysis (n = 1, 10, 20, 30, 40, and 50) for a desired effect size of 0.6 and an undesired effect size of 0.1 (**a**). The number on each curve is the assumed sample size/arm associated with that ROC curve at interim. The area under ROC curve in **a** increases along with the increase of the sample size (**b**)

the true positive and the true negative, increases monotonically along with the sample size increases at interim (Fig. 2b). This indicates that the decision quality at interim will be better if more subjects are included in the interim analysis. However, the increase of the AUC is steeper for early cumulative subjects than those accumulated in the later stage of a trial. For example in Fig. 2b, the first 10 subjects/arm contribute 33 % increase of the AUC relative to the AUC with one subject/arm available for interim analysis. About 47 % increase of the AUC is achieved when 20 subjects/arm are available at interim analysis. However, the AUC increase is less than 5 % every 10 subjects/arm increase after 30 subjects/arm are available at interim. Both the sample size at interim and the difference of effect sizes contribute to quality of interim decision-making in terms of AUC. If the sample size is fixed, the larger the difference between the desired and the undesired treatment effects the higher the AUC.

3.2 Performance Comparisons Among the Three Methods by Simulation

One way to evaluate performance of the three methods on the interim decision-making quality is to assess overall accuracy, defined as the average of the sensitivity and the specificity. There are many methods available in the literature to identify optimal points on ROC curves, including minimizing the Euclidean distance method and Youden index (Fluss et al., 2005; Hajian-Tilaki, 2013; Perkins and Schisterman, 2006). We used the method which minimizes the Euclidean distance from the point (x=0,y=1) on the upper left hand corner of the ROC space to any point on the ROC curve to find the optimal point. Suppose the optimal point on the ROC curve described by Eq. (16) has coordinate (x_0, y_0), then $y_0 = h(x_0)$ where $h(x_0)$ is the function of the ROC curve specified by Eq. (16). The approach to identify the optimal point (x_0, y_0) is to minimize the Euclidean distance between Point $(0, 1)$ and a point (x_0, y_0) on the ROC curve defined by Eq. (16), i.e., to minimize $\sqrt{x^2 + (h(x) - 1)^2}$ to obtain (x_0, y_0), where (x, y) is any data point on the ROC curve.

Simulations were conducted to validate the theoretical findings and to compare performance of the three methods in terms of quality of decision-making at interim. We used the following settings to simulate late phase clinical trials with two arms: the total sample size for each arm was 60 which had 80 % power to detect an effect size of 0.516 or had 90 % power to detect 0.6 effect size using a two-sided t-test at the 5 % significance level. The interim analysis was conducted when a half of subjects (30/arm) were available for the analysis. An optimal threshold for each method (CP, PP, or PCI) was identified from theoretical ROC curves and are presented in Table 1 under various desired treatment effect sizes. Performance of optimal thresholds and other thresholds (0.3, 0.4, and 0.5 in the probability scale) for interim decision-making was compared. Besides the probability threshold, an upper bound threshold d in PCI is also required in the simulation. A clinical meaningful threshold is often chosen as d at the design stage. We used a constant (e.g., 0.516) in the simulations using R software (R Development Core Team, 2011). Decision quality was evaluated using the following parameters: sensitivity, specificity, positive predictive value (PPV), negative predictive value (NPV), and overall power. PPV and NPV are commonly used to assess ability of a test to correctly predict the underlying truth using the test result. PPV is the probability to correctly predict the positive truth given the test is positive. NPV is the probability to correctly predict the negative truth given the test is negative.

Performance comparisons among the three methods are presented in Table 2 ($d = 0.516$ in PCI). As expected, all comparative parameters decreased for all three methods when the desired treatment effect decreased at the optimal thresholds. For example, the sensitivity decreased from ∼88 % at $\mu_1 = 0.7$ to ∼50 % at $\mu_1 = 0.1$ which was the undesired effect size or $\mu_1 = 0$ at the null. For other thresholds used at interim decision-making, CP and PP behaved similarly with slightly different numerical values for each comparative parameter but PCI performed differently comparing to CP and PP methods. PCI had a higher sensitivity than CP and PP methods at each desired effect size and the sensitivity decreased when the assumed μ_1 decreased. The specificity for PCI was smaller than CP and PP at each μ_1 level. PCI had a slightly higher NPV and overall power but a slightly lower PPV than CP and PP at each μ_1 level. The type I error rate was well controlled for all three methods at different thresholds except a minor inflation for optimal thresholds. In summary, if optimal thresholds were used for interim decision-making, the three methods performed similarly in terms of decision quality parameters across different desired treatment effect sizes. This result is consistent with our theoretical findings

Table 2 Comparisons of the three methods (CP, PP, and PCI) in terms of the sensitivity, the specificity, the positive predictive value (PPV), the negative predictive value (NPV), and the overall power under different desired effect sizes at various thresholds for decision-making at interim

	Sensitivity			Specificity			PPV			NPV			Power		
Threshold	CP	PP	PCI	CP	PP	PCI	CP	PP	PCI	CP	PP	PCI	CP	PP	PCI
$\mu_1 = 0.7, \mu_0 = 0.1, d = 0.516$															
0.3	0.943	0.954	0.967	0.772	0.738	0.685	0.806	0.784	0.754	0.932	0.941	0.954	0.928	0.937	0.947
0.4	0.928	0.934	0.975	0.810	0.796	0.634	0.830	0.821	0.727	0.918	0.924	0.963	0.915	0.921	0.953
0.5	0.907	0.907	0.983	0.840	0.840	0.586	0.850	0.850	0.704	0.900	0.900	0.971	0.896	0.896	0.959
Opt[a]	0.877	0.877	0.881	0.875	0.875	0.866	0.876	0.876	0.868	0.877	0.877	0.879	0.870	0.870	0.874
$\mu_1 = 0.6, \mu_0 = 0.1, d = 0.516$															
0.3	0.878	0.899	0.923	0.769	0.733	0.686	0.792	0.771	0.746	0.863	0.879	0.900	0.834	0.851	0.868
0.4	0.852	0.860	0.941	0.808	0.792	0.635	0.816	0.806	0.720	0.845	0.850	0.915	0.813	0.821	0.878
0.5	0.822	0.822	0.953	0.840	0.840	0.587	0.837	0.837	0.697	0.825	0.825	0.925	0.789	0.789	0.886
Opt	0.829	0.829	0.823	0.832	0.832	0.832	0.831	0.831	0.831	0.829	0.829	0.824	0.793	0.793	0.789
$\mu_1 = 0.5, \mu_0 = 0.1, d = 0.516$															
0.3	0.795	0.825	0.860	0.767	0.732	0.679	0.773	0.755	0.728	0.789	0.807	0.829	0.698	0.715	0.733
0.4	0.756	0.771	0.887	0.805	0.791	0.628	0.795	0.787	0.705	0.767	0.776	0.847	0.674	0.683	0.748
0.5	0.713	0.713	0.909	0.836	0.836	0.580	0.813	0.813	0.684	0.744	0.744	0.865	0.645	0.645	0.757
Opt	0.783	0.783	0.782	0.778	0.778	0.777	0.779	0.779	0.779	0.782	0.782	0.781	0.691	0.691	0.691
$\mu_1 = 0.4, \mu_0 = 0.1, d = 0.516$															
0.3	0.660	0.697	0.748	0.764	0.731	0.676	0.736	0.721	0.698	0.692	0.707	0.729	0.505	0.522	0.542
0.4	0.611	0.631	0.788	0.808	0.791	0.630	0.761	0.751	0.680	0.675	0.682	0.749	0.481	0.491	0.556
0.5	0.560	0.560	0.823	0.841	0.841	0.583	0.779	0.779	0.663	0.656	0.656	0.767	0.452	0.452	0.566
Opt	0.713	0.713	0.711	0.714	0.714	0.715	0.714	0.714	0.714	0.714	0.714	0.712	0.528	0.528	0.527

$\mu_1 = 0.3, \mu_0 = 0.1, d = 0.516$															
0.3	0.510	0.554	0.616	0.774	0.742	0.693	0.694	0.682	0.667	0.613	0.625	0.643	0.307	0.319	0.333
0.4	0.454	0.475	0.667	0.815	0.800	0.643	0.711	0.704	0.652	0.599	0.604	0.659	0.287	0.295	0.344
0.5	0.406	0.406	0.710	0.847	0.847	0.594	0.726	0.726	0.636	0.588	0.588	0.672	0.270	0.270	0.353
Opt	0.651	0.651	0.654	0.658	0.658	0.658	0.656	0.656	0.657	0.653	0.653	0.656	0.341	0.341	0.341
$\mu_1 = 0.2, \mu_0 = 0.1, d = 0.516$															
0.3	0.357	0.397	0.453	0.772	0.742	0.688	0.611	0.606	0.592	0.546	0.552	0.557	0.155	0.161	0.169
0.4	0.307	0.327	0.510	0.811	0.796	0.641	0.619	0.616	0.587	0.539	0.542	0.567	0.144	0.148	0.177
0.5	0.266	0.266	0.559	0.847	0.847	0.591	0.635	0.635	0.578	0.536	0.536	0.573	0.134	0.134	0.181
Opt	0.567	0.567	0.568	0.581	0.581	0.582	0.575	0.575	0.576	0.573	0.573	0.574	0.182	0.182	0.181
$\mu_1 = 0.1, \mu_0 = 0.1, d = 0.516$															
0.3	0.220	0.255	0.309	0.773	0.738	0.688	0.492	0.493	0.498	0.498	0.498	0.499	0.057	0.061	0.065
0.4	0.184	0.198	0.357	0.813	0.798	0.640	0.497	0.495	0.498	0.499	0.499	0.499	0.053	0.055	0.068
0.5	0.155	0.155	0.404	0.845	0.845	0.592	0.500	0.500	0.498	0.500	0.500	0.499	0.049	0.049	0.070
Opt	0.493	0.493	0.493	0.507	0.507	0.506	0.500	0.500	0.500	0.500	0.500	0.500	0.072	0.072	0.073
$\mu_1 = 0.0, \mu_0 = 0.0, d = 0.516$															
0.3	0.132	0.158	0.194	0.864	0.839	0.802	0.492	0.495	0.495	0.499	0.499	0.499	0.020	0.021	0.022
0.4	0.107	0.116	0.234	0.890	0.881	0.766	0.493	0.493	0.500	0.499	0.499	0.500	0.018	0.019	0.024
0.5	0.088	0.088	0.279	0.911	0.911	0.725	0.497	0.497	0.504	0.500	0.500	0.501	0.017	0.017	0.025
Opt	0.498	0.498	0.493	0.510	0.510	0.517	0.505	0.505	0.505	0.504	0.504	0.505	0.026	0.026	0.027

The $d = 0.516$ in the PCI method

[a] Optimal thresholds were estimated from theoretical formula for each method so that accuracy of decision-making is maximized in each scenario. These values are presented in Table 1. N=60 subjects/arm and interim analysis was conducted at n=30 subjects/arm

that CP, PP, and PCI are equivalent in decision-making quality if appropriate thresholds are chosen for each method.

In practice, the true treatment effect is often unknown and is estimated from previous studies for the similar therapy and the estimated treatment effect is used to design a clinical trial. Suppose a treatment effect size is 0.5, a trial is designed to have 60 subjects/arm to detected this treatment effect with 80 % power using one-sided test at 0.025 level. If the observed treatment effect is also 0.5, then an optimal threshold 0.327 for conditional power has both 78 % sensitivity and specificity for interim Go/No-Go decision making. If the observed treatment effect size is 0.7, then this threshold has 94 % sensitivity and 78 % specificity for interim decision-making. If the observed treatment effect size is 0.3, then this threshold has 50 % sensitivity and 78 % specificity for interim decision-making. Therefore, the assumed true treatment effect is critical for determining criteria which controls interim decision quality.

4 Applications to Design Optimization in Late Phase Clinical Trials

4.1 Timing and Threshold of Interim Analysis Based on ROC Criteria

In late phase clinical trials with interim analyses, one common question is how to determine the time when the interim analysis should be conducted for interim Go/No-Go decisions. The proposed ROC based approach provides an answer to this question. If the sensitivity and the specificity for interim decision-making is pre-specified at the design stage of a trial, then timing of the interim analysis and associated threshold can be determined from the ROC curve. For example, Eqs. (15) and (16) can be used to determine the timing and threshold of interim analysis for the conditional power method. We used the conditional power method to illustrate the details of the application and results are presented in Table 3. For example, at a given total sample size N=60/arm, if the pre-specified sensitivity and specificity both are 85 %, then the interim analysis should be performed when at least 24 subjects per arm are available for the analysis using the conditional power threshold 0.617 for the desired true treatment effect size of 0.7. If the true treatment effect size is 0.5, then the minimum required sample size is 54 subjects per arm for the interim analysis with threshold 0.164. If the true effect size is 0.4, then the current total sample size 60/arm cannot achieve both 85 % sensitivity and 85 % specificity for interim decision-making. In stead, 95 subjects/arm is the minimum required sample size for the same interim decision quality.

Table 3 Sample sizes required under different desired treatment effect sizes to achieve the pre-specified sensitivity and specificity using the conditional power

Pre-specified			μ_1					
Sensitivity	Specificity	Threshold	0.7	0.6	0.5	0.4	0.3	0.2
0.90	0.90	n[a]	37	52	59	59	59	59
		$\Phi(u)$[b]	0.644	0.452	0.0	0.0	0.0	0.0
		n^{*}[c]	37	52	82	146	328	1314
	0.85	n	30	43	59	59	59	59
		$\Phi(u)$	0.532	0.362	0.0	0.0	0.0	0.0
		n^*	30	43	67	119	269	1075
	0.80	n	25	36	56	59	59	59
		$\Phi(u)$	0.443	0.302	0.014	0.0	0.0	0.0
		n^*	25	36	56	100	225	902
0.85	0.90	n	30	43	59	59	59	59
		$\Phi(u)$	0.716	0.576	0.0	0.0	0.0	0.0
		n^*	30	43	67	119	269	1075
	0.85	n	24	34	54	59	59	59
		$\Phi(u)$	0.617	0.474	0.164	0.0	0.0	0.0
		n^*	24	34	54	95	215	859
	0.80	n	20	28	44	59	59	59
		$\Phi(u)$	0.529	0.400	0.202	0.0	0.0	0.0
		n^*	20	28	44	78	176	705
0.80	0.90	n	25	36	56	59	59	59
		$\Phi(u)$	0.773	0.648	0.358	0.0	0.0	0.0
		n^*	25	36	56	100	225	902
	0.85	n	20	28	44	59	59	59
		$\Phi(u)$	0.688	0.554	0.347	0.0	0.0	0.0
		n^*	20	28	44	78	176	705
	0.80	n	16	23	35	59	59	59
		$\Phi(u)$	0.606	0.478	0.310	0.0	0.0	0.0
		n^*	16	23	35	63	142	567

[a] The smallest sample size for the interim analysis with the total sample size of 60/arm
[b] Optimal threshold for interim decision-making with N=60/arm using conditional power
[c] The sample size/arm required to achieve the pre-specified sensitivity and specificity

4.2 *Designs with Global Optimization*

Satisfying both high sensitivity and high specificity for a clinical trial design could be difficult in practice as described in the last subsection. An alternative approach is only to use the sensitivity and the overall power to search an optimal design with the minimum average sample size under the undesired treatment effect. In late phase clinical trials, the overall sample size (N/arm), the sample size at interim (n/arm), and the threshold (u) for Go/No-Go decision at interim analysis are typically pre-specified in the protocol so that the type I error rate is well controlled and the desired power can be achieved. Motivated by Simon's two-stage design in Phase II clinical trials with binary outcomes (Simon, 1989), we propose to use the ROC based approach to optimize a design with interim futility analysis for a continuous endpoint by minimizing the average sample size while maintaining the overall power of the trial. The goal of the proposed design is to minimize the average sample size (ASS) if the underlying treatment effect is undesired while the overall power is reserved. The average sample size under the undesired treatment effect μ_0 is defined as

$$ASS_{\mu_0} = n + (1 - x)(N - n),$$

where x is the specificity defined by any of three methods. Let y be the sensitivity defined by any of three methods, and

$$1 - x = \Phi\left[\Phi^{-1}(y) - \frac{\sqrt{n}(\mu_1 - \mu_0))}{\sigma}\right].$$

To optimize the design, a global search in parameter space for $\{N, n, u, y\}$ needs to be conducted to identify a quadruple $\{N^*, n^*, u^*, y^*\}$ so that ASS_{μ_0} is minimized and the target overall power is still achieved and the type I error rate is controlled. The following procedure can be utilized to find the quadruple $\{N^*, n^*, u^*, y^*\}$ numerically.

1. Determine μ_1 and μ_0 and the maximum sample size N_{max} (based on the resource and time-line considerations);
2. Determine the target power at μ_1 (i.e., $1-\beta$) and the type I error rate α. Calculate the sample size N_0 for the target power based on a fixed sample size design without interim analysis;
3. Choose a sensitivity at μ_1 or y where $1 - \beta < y < 1$;
4. For each N from N_0 to N_{max}, find n in the range of (1,N-1) such that the power of the trial at μ_1 is at least $1 - \beta$ with the minimized ASS_{μ_0} at threshold u under μ_0;
5. Repeat Steps 3 to 4 until a quadruple $\{N^*, n^*, u^*, y^*\}$ minimizing ASS_{μ_0} is identified.

This search procedure is named a global search procedure in parameter space for $\{N, n, u, y\}$ so that the global optimal design can be found. Now, instead of varying N in Step 4, a simplified approach is to determine N upfront using the target power and the sensitivity. Specifically, calculate N^* to target an inflated power $(1 - \beta)/y$ so that the final overall power is no less than the target power. The final n^* and u^* minimizing ASS_{μ_0} are identified as described in Step 4. This simplified search procedure eliminates the search dimension for N in the global search procedure.

One important calculation of the global search procedure is to determine the power in Step 4 for a given quadruple $\{N, n, u, y\}$. Considering equivalence of CP, PP, and PCI methods as shown in Sect. 2.4, we choose CP to demonstrate how the power is calculated in Step 4 in the global search procedure. The overall power is the probability to reject the null hypothesis at the end of a trial with a Go decision at interim. Under the desired treatment effect $\mu = \mu_1$, it is calculated as

$$
\begin{aligned}
1-\beta &= P\left(\frac{\bar{X}_N\sqrt{N}}{\sigma} > C, \bar{X}_n > (u + C\sqrt{\frac{N}{m}})\frac{\sqrt{m}\sigma}{N} \mid \mu = \mu_1\right) \\
&= P\left(\frac{\bar{X}_N - \mu_1}{\sigma/\sqrt{N}} > C - \frac{\mu_1}{\sigma/\sqrt{N}}, \frac{\bar{X}_n - \mu_1}{\sigma/\sqrt{n}} > (u + C\sqrt{\frac{N}{m}})\frac{\sqrt{m}\sigma}{N\sigma/\sqrt{n}} - \frac{\mu_1}{\sigma/\sqrt{n}}\right) \\
&= P\left(Z_N > C - \frac{\mu_1}{\sigma/\sqrt{N}}, Z_n > \frac{u\sqrt{mn}}{N} + C\sqrt{\frac{n}{N}} - \frac{\mu_1\sqrt{n}}{\sigma}\right) \\
&= \int_k^\infty\int_h^\infty g(Z_N, Z_n)\, dz_N dz_n,
\end{aligned}
$$

where $k = C - \frac{\mu_1}{\sigma/\sqrt{N}}$, $h = \frac{u\sqrt{mn}}{N} + C\sqrt{\frac{n}{N}} - \frac{\mu_1\sqrt{n}}{\sigma}$, $g(Z_N, Z_n)$ is the density function of a bivariate normal distribution with mean $\boldsymbol{\mu} = \binom{0}{0}$ and variance covariance matrix $\Sigma = \begin{pmatrix} 1 & \rho \\ \rho & 1 \end{pmatrix}$ with $\rho = \sqrt{\frac{n}{N}}$ for the correlation coefficient between Z_N and Z_n.

An illustration example of this application using the conditional power method is presented in Table 4 for the desired effect size of 0.6 and the undesired treatment effect size of 0.1. Thresholds for PP and PCI were calculated from the CP thresholds using the conversion formula described in Sect. 2.4. With a slightly larger initial sample size, both search procedures led to optimal stopping rules for futility which significantly reduced average sample size by 23–30 % as compared to corresponding fixed sample size designs. The global search procedure had a marginal efficiency than the simplified procedure but both procedures generated designs with similar decision quality at interim.

4.3 An Example

The global optimization procedure based on the proposed method can be easily applied in real clinical trial designs. We used a published phase III clinical trial data as an example to show how to design a trial using the proposed method. Burmester et al. (2013) conducted a study to test if tofacitinib (CP-690,550) was safe and effective in moderate-to-severe rheumatoid arthritis patients taking methotrexate who had an inadequate response to tumor necrosis factor inhibitor treatment. The trial was a 6 month, randomized, double-blind and parallel-group phase 3 study. A total of 399 subjects were equally randomized to receive twice a day treatment with tofacitinib 5 mg, tofacitinib 10 mg or placebo (133 subjects/arm). At Month 3, placebo subjects were equally randomized again to two tofacitinib dose groups. One of the co-primary efficacy endpoints was the change from baseline in

Table 4 Optimal designs for the desired effect size 0.6 and the undesired effect size 0.1 with one interim analysis based on the conditional power

Search	Traditional		N^*	n^*	$\Phi(u^*)$					ASS_{μ_0}	Overall
method	Target power	N/arm	per arm	per arm	CP	PP	PCI[a]	Sensitivity*	Specificity	per arm	power
Global	0.90	60	68	28	0.12	0.23	0.73	0.94	0.62	43.04	0.90
	0.85	51	59	23	0.14	0.25	0.59	0.91	0.64	36.01	0.85
	0.80	45	52	20	0.16	0.27	0.46	0.88	0.66	30.95	0.80
Simplified	0.90	60	76	28	0.15	0.26	0.78	0.94	0.62	46.05	0.91
	0.85	51	62	22	0.086	0.21	0.74	0.93	0.64	39.10	0.87
	0.80	45	61	19	0.18	0.30	0.57	0.88	0.64	34.00	0.83

N^*, n^*, u^* and sensitivity*(=y^*) are components of the quadruple minimizing ASS_{μ_0}
CP conditional power, *PP* predictive power, *PCI* predicted confidence interval
[a] d=0.6 is used in the PCI method

DAS28-4(ESR) at Month 3. This sample size has 90 % power to detect an effect size of 0.4 for a pairwise comparison (treatment vs. placebo) at the 5 % significance level using a two-sided test.

Suppose we want to design a new late phase clinical trial where two treatment arms (a high dose and a low dose) and a placebo arm are included with an allocation ratio of 1:1:1 among three arms. We assume the patient population is similar to one described by Burmester et al. (2013). One interim analysis is planned for futility analysis. We assume the desired effect size $\mu_1 = 0.4$ and the undesired effect size is $\mu_0 = 0.1$, the target power is 90 %, and the significant threshold C for the test is 1.96 under the normal distribution. An optimal design using the proposed method is found that 146 subjects are needed for each arm, an interim analysis could be performed when at least 64 subjects/arm are available for the analysis, the conditional power threshold 0.085 can be used for futility analysis to drop undesired dose arm(s). This design has 95 % chance to make a Go decision and 52 % chance to make a No-Go decision for futility at interim for each dose arm. The average sample size is 103.29 subjects/arm under the undesired effect size of 0.1 and the target power 90 % is reserved for this design. The proposed design has a smaller average sample size than the single stage design if the treatment effect falls in the space of undesired treatment effect. If the undesired treatment effect size is the same as the null hypothesis, i.e. $\mu_0 = 0$,then the optimal design is: 164 subjects/arm are needed, the required minimum interim sample size is 57/ arm, and the conditional power threshold is 0.15 for the interim futility decision-making. The average sample size under the space of undesired treatment effect (the null hypothesis) is 84.26 subjects/arm. This design has 93 % chance to make a Go decision and 74 % chance to make a No-Go decision for futility at interim.

5 Conclusions and Discussions

Interim data monitoring has been used for interim Go/No-Go decision-making in late stage clinical trials. Various interim analysis methods have been used, including conditional power, predictive power and predicted confidence interval. However, the thresholds used for these methods are arbitrary and time (in terms of the sample size) for interim analysis are often chosen based on experience. In addition, although some have discussed the relationship between conditional power and predictive power (Gallo et al., 2014; Lan et al., 2009) , there is no systematic approach to evaluate the performance and relationship among these three methods. In this paper, we propose to use an ROC approach for evaluation of overall decision quality of different interim analysis methods. With this approach, three interim monitoring methods have been shown to be equivalent, leading to the same ROC curve for the same clinical trial. This approach also provides a systematic way of determining the sample size for interim analysis. It was shown that the AUC increased as the interim sample size increased, implying that the interim decision-making quality increased. However, the AUC increase diminished as the interim sample size became larger.

This provides guidance to choose an appropriate interim analysis sample size. For example, one can choose an interim sample size such that the AUC increase does not exceed 5 %. This approach also provides a way of selecting an interim analysis threshold with desired sensitivity and specificity. An ROC curve is furbished once the interim analysis sample size is determined. Then one can choose an interim analysis threshold that meets a target sensitivity and/or specificity. This threshold can then be translated into a cutoff point for conditional power, predictive power, or predicted confidence interval, based on one's preference.

In addition to the application in interim monitoring, this ROC approach can also be integrated into an optimal two-stage design. With obtained expressions of sensitivity and specificity, the global search can be easily conducted and an optimal two-stage design similar to Simon's two-stage design (Simon, 1989) but for continuous outcome (Wason and Mander, 2012) can be obtained. The design with the optimally chosen futility rule minimizes the average sample size while the underlying treatment effect is small. This futility rule can be easily explained to clinicians in terms of conditional power, predictive power or predicted confidence interval which is associated with the sensitivity and the specificity of the interim decision.

This research mainly focuses on the normally distributed endpoint with the equal sample size per arm in clinical trials. It can be easily extended to designs with a unequal sample size per arm. The proposed method can also be extended to the binary endpoint using a normal approximation. Assuming that the underlying treatment response rates for the treatment and placebo arms are P_e and $P_c(P_c > P_e)$, the probabilities of Go/No-Go decisions can be obtained by replacing μ and σ with $P_c - P_e$ and $\sigma = \sqrt{P_c(1-P_c) + P_e(1-P_e)}$ in equations in Sect. 2, respectively. Due to the poor coverage probability for Wald type confidence intervals for the binary endpoint (Agresti and Caffo, 2000; Brown et al., 2001; Newcombe, 1998), especially for scenarios that the sample size is small and the proportion is closed to 0 or 1, the arcsine square root transformation of binomial proportions should be used to calculate predicted confidence intervals to improve the coverage probability of Wald type predicted confidence intervals. The proposed ROC approach can also be extended to the time-to-event endpoint using the normal approximation.

Acknowledgements Disclosure: The design, research, and analysis were supported by AbbVie. AbbVie participated in the interpretation of data, writing, and approval of this manuscript. All authors are employees of AbbVie, Inc.

Appendix

Conditional Power Derivation in Sect. 2.1

As shown in Eq. (1),

$$
\begin{aligned}
\mathrm{CP}_t &= P\left(Z_N \geq C \mid \bar{X}_n\right) \\
&= P\left(\frac{\bar{X}\sqrt{N}}{\sigma} \geq C \mid \bar{X}_n\right) \\
&= P\left(m\bar{X}_m + n\bar{X}_n \geq C\sqrt{N}\sigma \mid \bar{X}_n\right) \\
&= P\left(\bar{X}_m \geq (C\sqrt{N}\sigma - n\bar{X}_n)/m\right) \\
&= P\left[\frac{(\bar{X}_m - \mu)\sqrt{m}}{\sigma} \geq \frac{(C\sqrt{N}\sigma - n\bar{X}_n)\sqrt{m}}{m\sigma} - \frac{\mu\sqrt{m}}{\sigma} \mid \bar{X}_n\right] \\
&= P\left[Z_m \geq \frac{(C\sqrt{N}\sigma - n\bar{X}_n)\sqrt{m}}{m\sigma} - \frac{\mu\sqrt{m}}{\sigma} \mid \bar{X}_n\right].
\end{aligned}
$$

By plugging in $\mu = \bar{X}_n$ under the assumption that the current trend of treatment effect at interim continues, the conditional power is

$$
\mathrm{CP}_t = \Phi\left(-C\sqrt{\frac{N}{m}} + \frac{N}{\sqrt{m}}\frac{\bar{X}_n}{\sigma}\right).
$$

Then Eq. (1) is obtained.

Predictive Power Derivation in Sect. 2.2

$$
\begin{aligned}
Var(\bar{X}_m) &= Var(E(\bar{X}_m|\mu)) + E(Var(\bar{X}_m|\mu)) \\
&= Var(\mu) + E(\sigma^2/m) \\
&= \sigma^2(1/n + 1/m)
\end{aligned}
$$

The predictive power in Eq. (6) is given by

$$
\begin{aligned}
\mathrm{PP}_t &= \int \mathrm{CP}_t(\mu) g(\mu \mid \bar{X}_n) d\mu \\
&= \int P\left(\bar{X}_m \geq (C\sqrt{N}\sigma - n\bar{X}_n)/m \mid \bar{X}_n\right) g(\mu \mid \bar{X}_n) d\mu.
\end{aligned}
$$

Assuming a non-informative prior distribution $g(\mu) = 1$, the posterior probability density is $g(\mu \mid \bar{X}_n) = N(\bar{X}_n, \sigma^2/n)$ given the interim data (Tan, 2008). Condition on the interim data, the marginal distribution of $\bar{X}_m$ is normally distributed with mean $\bar{X}_n$ and variance derived above, then the predictive power at interim time t is

$$\begin{aligned}
\mathrm{PP}_t &= P\left(\frac{\bar{X}_m - \bar{X}_n}{\sigma\sqrt{1/n + 1/m}} \geq \frac{C\sqrt{N}\sigma/m - n\bar{X}_n/m - \bar{X}_n}{\sigma\sqrt{1/n + 1/m}}\right) \\
&= 1 - \Phi\left(\frac{C\sqrt{N}\sigma - N\bar{X}_n}{m\sigma\sqrt{\frac{N}{nm}}}\right) \\
&= 1 - \Phi\left[\sqrt{\frac{n}{m}}\left(C - \frac{\bar{X}_n\sqrt{N}}{\sigma}\right)\right]
\end{aligned}$$

Predicted Confidence Interval Derivation in Sect. 2.3

Assuming $\bar{X}_m$ is the predicted group mean difference given the current trend observed at interim continues in the second half of a trial after the interim, i.e. $\bar{X}_m \sim N(\bar{X}_n, \sigma^2/m)$. Then the probability of the predicted confidence interval upper bound is less than or equal to a threshold d is

$$\begin{aligned}
\mathrm{CPCI}_t &= P\left(\frac{n\bar{X}_n + m\bar{X}_m}{N} + C\frac{\sigma}{\sqrt{N}} \leq d \mid \bar{X}_n\right) \\
&= P\left(\frac{(\bar{X}_m - \mu)\sqrt{m}}{\sigma} \leq \frac{dN}{\sigma\sqrt{m}} - C\sqrt{\frac{N}{m}} - \frac{n\bar{X}_n}{\sqrt{m}\sigma} - \frac{\bar{X}_n\sqrt{m}}{\sigma}\right) \\
&= P\left(Z_m \leq \frac{dN}{\sigma\sqrt{m}} - C\sqrt{\frac{N}{m}} - \frac{N\bar{X}_n}{\sqrt{m}\sigma}\right) \\
&= \Phi\left(-C\sqrt{\frac{N}{m}} + \frac{N(d - \bar{X}_n)}{\sigma\sqrt{m}}\right).
\end{aligned}$$

A Go decision (D=1) is made at interim if $\mathrm{CPCI}_t \leq \varsigma = \Phi(u)$, expressed in the mathematical equation in the following,

$$D = 1\left(-C\sqrt{\frac{N}{m}} + \frac{N(d - \bar{X}_n)}{\sigma\sqrt{m}} \leq u\right).$$

Then the probability of a Go decision at interim is,

$$
\begin{aligned}
E(D) &= P\left(-C\sqrt{\frac{N}{m}} + \frac{N(d-\bar{X}_n)}{\sigma\sqrt{m}} \le u\right) \\
&= P\left(\frac{N\bar{X}_n}{\sigma\sqrt{m}} \ge -C\sqrt{\frac{N}{m}} + \frac{Nd}{\sigma\sqrt{m}} - u\right) \\
&= P\left(\frac{(\bar{X}_n-\mu)\sqrt{n}}{\sigma} \ge -C\sqrt{\frac{n}{N}} + \frac{\sqrt{n}(d-\mu)}{\sigma} - u\frac{\sqrt{mn}}{N}\right) \\
&= P\left(Z_n \ge -C\sqrt{\frac{n}{N}} + \frac{\sqrt{n}(d-\mu)}{\sigma} - u\frac{\sqrt{mn}}{N}\right) \\
&= \Phi\left(C\sqrt{\frac{n}{N}} - \frac{\sqrt{n}(d-\mu)}{\sigma} + u\frac{\sqrt{mn}}{N}\right).
\end{aligned}
$$

Then Eqs. (13) and (14) in Sect. 2.3 are obtained for $S_{pci}(u, \mu_1)$ and $S_{pci}(u, \mu_0)$, respectively.

References

Agresti, A., & Caffo, B. (2000). Simple and effective confidence intervals for proportions and differences of proportions results from adding two successes and two failures. *The American Statistician, 54*, 280–288.

Brown, L. D., Cai, T. T., & DasGupta, A. (2001). Interval estimation for a binomial proportion. *Statistical Science, 16*, 101–117.

Burmester, G. R., Blanco, R., Charles-Schoeman, C., Wollenhaupt, J., Zerbini, C., Benda, B., et al. (2013). Tofacitinib (cp-690,550) in combination with methotrexate in patients with active rheumatoid arthritis with an inadequate response to tumour necrosis factor inhibitors: a randomised phase 3 trial. *The Lancet, 381*, 451–460.

Chuang-Stein, C., Kirby, S., French, J., Kowalski, K., Marshall, S., Smith, M. K., et al. (2011). A quantitative approach for making go/no-go decisions in drug development. *Drug Information Journal, 45*, 187–202.

DeMets, D. L. (2006). Futility approaches to interim monitoring by data monitoring committees. *Clinical Trials, 3*, 522–529.

Dobbins, T. W. (2013). The type II error probability of a group sequential test of efficacy and futility, and considerations for power and sample size. *Journal of Biopharmaceutical Statisticis, 23*, 378–393.

Evans, S. R., Li, L. L., & Wei, L. J. (2007). Data monitoring in clinical trials using prediction. *Drug Information Journal, 41*, 733–742.

Fluss, R., Faraggi, D., & Reiser, B. (2005). Estimation of youden index and its associated cutoff point. *Biomedical Journal, 47*, 458–472.

Friedlin, B., Korn, E. L., & Gray, R. (2010). A general inefficacy interim monitoring rule for randomized clinical trials. *Clinical Trials, 7*, 197–208.

Gallo, P., Mao, L., & Shih, V. H. (2014). Alternative views on setting clinical trial futility criteria. *Journal of Biopharmaceutical Statisticis, 24*, 976–993.

Green, D. M. & Swets, J. A. (Eds.). (1966). *Signal detection theory and psychophysics*. New York, NY: Wiley.

Hajian-Tilaki, K. (2013). Receiver operating characteristics (ROC) curve analysis for medical diagnostic test evaluation. *Caspian Journal of Internal Medicine, 4*, 627–635.

Halperin, M., Lan, K. K. G., Ware, J. H., Johnson, N. J., & DeMets, D. L. (1982). An aid to data monitoring in long-term clinical trials. *Controlled Clinical Trials, 3*, 311–323.

Jennison, C., & Turnbull, B. W. (1990). Statistical approaches to interim monitoring of medical trials: a review and commentary. *Statistical Science, 5*, 299–317.

Lachin, J. M. (2005). A review of methods for futility stopping based on conditional power. *Statistics in Medicine, 24*, 2747–2764.

Lachin, J. M. (2009). Futility interim monitoring with control of type i and type ii error probabilities using the interim z-value or confidence limit. *Clinical Trial, 6*, 565–573.

Lan, K. K. G., & DeMets, D. L. (1983). Discrete sequential boundiaries for clinical trials. *Biometrika, 70*, 659–663.

Lan, K. K. G., Hu, P., & Proschan, M. A. (2009). A conditional power approach to the evaluation of predictive power. *Statistics in Biopharmaceutical Research, 1*, 131–136.

Lan, K. K. G., Simon, R., & Halperin, M. (1987). Stochastically curtailed tests in long-term clinical trials. *Communications in Statistics, C1*, 207–219.

Lan, K. K. G., & Wittes, J. (1988). The b-value: A tool for monitoring clinical trial. *Biometrics, 44*, 579–585.

Mazumdar, M., & Liu, A. (2003). Group sequential design for comparative diagnostic accuracy studies. *Statistics in Medicine, 22*, 727–739.

Newcombe, R. G. (1998). Interval estimation for the difference between independent proportions: Comparison of eleven methods. *Statistics in Medicine, 17*, 873–890.

O'Brien, P. C., & Fleming, T. R. (1979). A multiple testing procedure for clinical trials. *Biometrics, 35*, 549–556.

Obuchowski, N. A. (2003). Receiver operating characteristic curves and their use in radiology. *Radiology, 229*, 3–8.

Pater, J. L., & Willan, A. R. (1984). Clinical trials as diagnostic tests. *Controlled Clinical Trials, 5*, 107–113.

Pepe, M. S. (Ed.) (2003). *The statistical evaluation of medical tests for classification and prediction*. New York, NY: Oxford.

Perkins, N. J., & Schisterman, E. F. (2006). The inconsistency of optimal cut-points obtained using two criteria based on receiver operating characteristics curve. *American Journal of Epidemiology, 163*, 670–675.

Peto, R., Pike, M. C., Armitrage, P., Breslow, N. E., Cox, D. R., Howard, S. V., et al. (1976). Design and analysis of randomized clinical trials requiring prolonged observation of each patient. I. introduction and design. *British Journal of Cancer, 34*, 585–612.

Pocock, S. J. (1977). Group sequential methods in the design and analysis of clinical trials. *Biometrika, 64*, 191–199.

R Development Core Team (2011). *R: A language and environment for statistical computing*. Vienna: R Foundation for Statistical Computing. ISBN:3-900051-07-0.

Simon, R. (1989). Optimal two-stage designs for phase II clinical trials. *Controlled Clinical Trials, 10*, 1–10.

Spiegelhalter, D. J., Freedman, L. S., & Blackburn, P. R. (1986). Monitoring clinical trials: conditional or predictive power ? *Controlled Clinical Trials, 7*, 8–17.

Tan, M. T. (2008). Conditional power in clinical trial monitoring. *Wiley encyclopedia of clinical trials* (pp. 1–7). http://onlinelibrary.wiley.com/. doi:10.1002/9780471462422.eoct448/full

Wang, S. K., & Tsiatis, A. A. (1987). Approximately optimal one-parameter boundaries for group sequential trials. *Biometrics, 43*, 193–199.

Wason, J. M. S., & Mander, A. P. (2012). Minimizing the maximum expected sample size in two-stage phase II clinical trials with continuous outcomes. *Journal of Biopharmaceutical Statistics, 22*, 836–852.

Zhang, Y., & Clarke, W. R. (2010). A flexible futility monitoring method with time-varying conditional power boundary. *Clinical Trials, 7*, 209–218.

Zweig, M. H., & Campbell, G. (1993). Receiver-operating characteristic (ROC) plots: A fundamental evaluation tool in clinical medicine. *Clinical Chemistry, 39*, 561–577.

Part III
Novel Applications and Implementation

Recent Advancements in Geovisualization, with a Case Study on Chinese Religions

Jürgen Symanzik, Shuming Bao, XiaoTian Dai, Miao Shui, and Bing She

Abstract Producing high-quality, map-based displays for economic, medical, educational, or any other kind of statistical data with geographic covariates has always been challenging. Either it was necessary to have access to high-end software or one had to do a lot of detailed programming. Recently, R software for linked micromap (LM) plots has been enhanced to handle any available shapefiles from Geographic Information Systems (GIS). Also, enhancements have been made that allow for a fast overlay of various statistical graphs on Google maps. In this article, we provide an overview of the necessary steps to produce such graphs in R, starting with GIS-based data and shapefiles and ending with the resulting graphs in R. We will use data from a study on Chinese religions and society (provided by the China Data Center at the University of Michigan) as a case study for these graphical methods.

1 Introduction

Geographic visualization, short geovisualization, plays an important role in exploring and mining information from today's huge collections of data with a geographic, that is, spatial context (MacEachren et al., 2004, 1999). Naturally, maps and, even more, interactive maps are an essential tool to extract, visualize, and comprehend complex spatial information (Andrienko and Andrienko, 1999; Andrienko et al., 2001; Roth, 2013). Geovisualization is closely related to exploratory spatial data analysis (ESDA), discussed in detail in Anselin (1994), Bivand (2010), and Symanzik (2014). In fact, Bivand (2010) indicates that *"geovisualization is not separate from exploratory spatial data analysis, but rather constitutes the backbone of ESDA, joining up the large range of techniques proposed for examining spatial data in a shared and easily comprehended visualization framework."*

J. Symanzik (✉) • X. Dai
Department of Mathematics and Statistics, Utah State University, Logan, UT, USA
e-mail: symanzik@math.usu.edu; xiaotian.dai@aggiemail.usu.edu

S. Bao • M. Shui • B. She
China Data Center, University of Michigan, Ann Arbor, MI, USA
e-mail: sbao@umich.edu; shuimiao0915@163.com; bingshe@umich.edu

Z. Jin et al. (eds.), *New Developments in Statistical Modeling, Inference and Application*, ICSA Book Series in Statistics, DOI 10.1007/978-3-319-42571-9_8

In this article, we will discuss advances in geovisualization that make use of two types of maps, that is, linked micromap (LM) plots and overlays on Google maps. The data of interest are Chinese religions at the provincial level, introduced in Sect. 2. In Sect. 3, we discuss LM plots and demonstrate how those can be used for the effective visualization and exploration of the Chinese religions data. In the following Sect. 4, we describe how LM plots can be created interactively in the online *Religion Explorer* software. We briefly describe in Sect. 5 how Google maps can be used as an alternative way to visualize the Chinese religions data. This article is concluded by a brief discussion and outlook in Sect. 6.

2 Religion in China

Religion has a considerable impact on the cultural, social, and economic development of a country. According to Lai (2003), China has experienced a major revival of religious faith and practice since 1979. Based on official statistics, there were about 144 million believers in China in 2003. According to unofficial sources, this number was about 200 million. Apparently, most of the data on this subject are not publicly available or are simply unknown.

The China Data Center (CDC) at the University of Michigan in Ann Arbor, MI, is an international center designed to advance the study and understanding of China (http://chinadatacenter.org/). A primary goal of the CDC is the integration of historical, social, and natural science data in a GIS, where spatial and temporal references are maintained through a relational database. The main data used in this article were derived from the 2004 Economic Census of China provided by the National Bureau of Statistics of the People's Republic of China. This data set includes rough estimates of religious sites and organizations. It consists of 72,968 officially registered religious organizations. The data fields are site name, site address, contact information, year of establishment, ownership type, employee scale, revenue range, primary activities classification, GB (Guo Biao—National Standard) codes for province, city, county and township, province name, city name, county name and township name, zip code, latitude and longitude (Zhu et al., 2014).

Buddhism, Protestantism, Catholicism, Islam, and Daoism (sometimes called "Taoism") are the five big officially recognized religions in China (Hackett et al., 2011; Lai, 2003, Appendix C, p. 99). Zhu et al. (2014) combined Protestantism and Catholicism to Christianity and classified the data to five religious types, based on the name, characteristics, and primary activities of those religious sites and organizations. The five types are Buddhism, Christianity, Daoism, Islam, and "Administration". Administration means administrative organizations like Bureau of Religious Affairs, Religious Authority, Anti-cult Association, religious associations, and so on.

Table 1 Reproduction of Table 1 from Zhu et al. (2014), showing the number of religious sites and organizations for Administration, Buddhism, Daoism, Islam, and Christianity, by province in 2004

ProvinceID	Province	Administration	Buddhism	Daoism	Islam	Christianity	Total
11	Beijing	0	2	0	22	5	29
12	Tianjin	1	6	0	30	25	62
13	Hebei	0	98	31	246	399	774
14	Shanxi	3	280	25	29	411	748
15	Neimenggu	4	109	2	126	304	545
21	Liaoning	2	312	47	89	821	1271
22	Jilin	0	71	8	56	745	880
23	Heilongjiang	1	100	9	64	473	647
31	Shanghai	1	73	21	7	175	277
32	Jiangsu	7	415	62	35	1039	1558
33	Zhejiang	2	2956	1868	10	2830	7666
34	Anhui	3	675	40	98	2132	2948
35	Fujian	10	2745	1030	6	1804	5595
36	Jiangxi	9	1133	288	5	633	2068
37	Shandong	5	14	7	122	306	454
41	Henan	10	187	128	444	1988	2757
42	Hubei	9	756	205	31	198	1199
43	Hunan	5	763	178	36	160	1142
44	Guangdong	10	617	81	3	440	1151
45	Guangxi	1	61	0	14	101	177
46	Hainan	0	2	0	0	5	7
50	Chongqing	1	102	11	3	88	205
51	Sichuan	9	1412	124	116	196	1857
52	Guizhou	1	178	15	80	158	432
53	Yunnan	1	701	102	525	682	2011
54	Xizang	7	1320	0	2	1	1330
61	Shaanxi	2	186	131	69	464	852
62	Gansu	6	530	400	3680	202	4818
63	Qinghai	1	627	42	1266	16	1952
64	Ningxia	0	211	68	3416	22	3717
65	Xinjiang	8	47	1	23,678	105	23,839

Variables related to religions at the provincial level are listed in Table 1. ProvinceID represents the administrative code of a province, and Province is the English name of the 31 provinces from mainland China. "Total" is the total number of all religious sites and organizations within a province, based on available data for 2004.

3 Linked Micromap Plots

Linked micromap plots were introduced about 20 years ago (Carr and Pierson, 1996; Olsen et al., 1996) to overcome some of the limitations of choropleth maps. Rather than focusing on a single detailed geographic map, there are multiple small maps (micromaps) in a LM plot. Areas in these small maps are linked via color to the names of these areas and to one or more statistical panels. The statistical panels may contain any type of statistical plot, such as dotplots with or without confidence intervals or error bars, boxplots, bar charts, line charts or time series plots, scatterplots, and others. With the inclusion of informative statistical plots, information loss that frequently occurs in choropleth maps is no longer a problem in LM plots. A detailed discussion of LM plots can be found in Symanzik and Carr (2008) and Carr and Pickle (2010) and a motivational example with a hypothetical LM plot can be found in Gebreab et al. (2008).

Computer code to construct LM plots has been made available since their introduction in 1996, as summarized in Symanzik and Carr (2008, Sect. 1.5). Numerous developments of code for the production of LM plots in the statistical computing environment R (R Core Team, 2014) followed, as summarized in Symanzik and Carr (2013). However, Payton et al. (2012) observed: "*Producing LMplots [...] has typically been somewhat difficult, and therefore LMplots have seen limited use.*" This changed recently due to the introduction of the two R packages *micromap* (Payton et al., 2015; Payton and Olsen, 2015) and *micromapST* (Carr and Pearson Jr., 2015; Pickle et al., 2015). *micromapST* is focused on LM plots for the United States and *micromap* can be used for any geographic regions, as long as the necessary geographic boundary information (ideally from GIS shapefiles) is available.

3.1 Preparation of Shapefiles

Despite the fact that the newly introduced R packages for micromaps considerably simplify the construction of LM plots, there remains a major practical problem. Many GIS shapefiles are not immediately suitable for use in LM plots. This can be due to the relatively small geographic areas that are almost invisible in a small map as used in LM plots. Similarly, regions that are far away from the main area of interest result in a large unoccupied area in the center of the maps and, furthermore, reduce the size of all areas. Examples for the United States are Washington, D.C. (which is almost invisible in a small map) and Alaska and Hawaii (which are far away from the main area of interest). For LM plots for the United States, this problem was resolved long ago by manually resizing and shifting such areas.

Recently, Symanzik et al. (2014) developed R code that allows to resize and shift problematic areas from arbitrary shapefiles. This R code was further refined and enhanced to facilitate the adjustment of a shapefile from China for use in

LM plots. In the first step, the shapefile was thinned. Thinning, in the context of spatial polygons that represent the outlines of the geographic regions in a shapefile, means that points from the boundaries of a polygon are removed, thus simplifying the boundary and speeding up the drawing of the polygon. Moreover, polygons that describe an area below a particular threshold are removed entirely. The *thinnedSpatialPoly* function from the *maptools* (Bivand and Lewin-Koh, 2014) R package provides an implementation for the thinning of spatial polygons, based on the Douglas–Peucker algorithm (Douglas and Peucker, 1973). This step simplified many of the borders and numerous small islands in the South China Sea that were hardly visible in the maps were removed, thus enlarging all other areas.

In the second step, six small provinces, several of them composed of a single city, had to be enlarged. These were the provinces Beijing, Tianjin, Shanghai, Ningxia, Chongqing, and Hainan. The enlargement of each small province took place in such a way that one of its boundaries was shifted into one of its neighboring provinces (usually the largest one), thus making the small province relatively bigger while reducing the bigger province a bit in size. This step was based on further generalized and enhanced R code that was originally developed for Symanzik et al. (2014).

Overall, these steps required some careful visual reassessment of the resulting new boundaries to guarantee that individual provinces and their relative locations are still recognizable. Too much thinning and/or enlarging one (or multiple) of the provinces by too much might have resulted in a distorted map. No province had to be shifted to produce a map of China suitable for use in LM plots. Figure 1 (left) shows the raw version of the map at the provincial level, Fig. 1 (center) shows the version after thinning and removal of small islands, and Fig. 1 (right) shows the final version after the enlargement of six provinces.

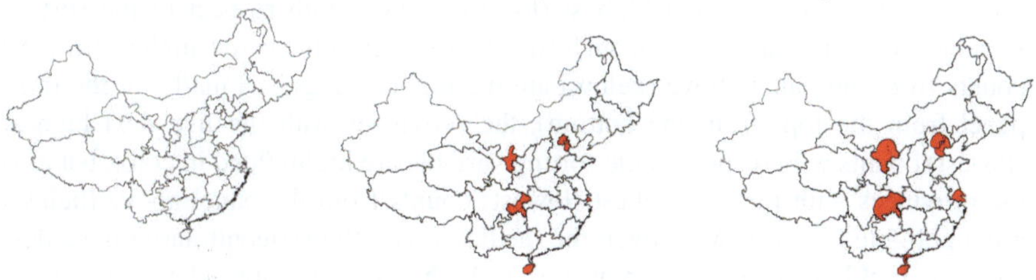

Fig. 1 Provinces from mainland China: Raw version (*left*), after thinning and removal of small islands (*center*), and after enlargement of six small provinces (*right*). The enlarged provinces are shown in *red* before enlargement (*center*) and after enlargement (*right*)

3.2 LM Plots of Chinese Religions

Researchers interested in Chinese religions might have the following questions with respect to the data set shown in Table 1:

1. For the provinces with the highest numbers of religious sites and organizations related to Christianity, how widely is Buddhism represented in those provinces?
2. Is there any association between the number of religious sites and organizations related to Buddhism and Daoism? If so, is this a positive or negative association? Are there regional differences?
3. Is there an outlier, i.e., a province that has an unusually large number of religious sites and organizations related to one of the main religions? How big is this number? And is this also a spatial outlier?

Questions like these cannot be answered easily through a tabular representation as in Table 1. However, answers to these questions (and to many other similar questions) can be easily obtained through LM plots. Figures 2, 3, and 4 show three LM plots that are based on the same data from Table 1. For each of the four religions (Christianity, Buddhism, Daoism, and Islam), the data panel displays a dot plot that shows the number of religious sites and organizations related to one of these religions. Administration and Total have been omitted from these figures.

Different ways exist (see Carr and Pickle, 2010, pp. 64–67, for details) how to highlight additional regions in each of the small maps, beyond the regions that belong to the current perceptual group of the data. In Figs. 2, 3, and 4, two-ended cumulative maps are used. Here, this means that in the top (bottom) panel, only the provinces with the five highest (lowest) counts with respect to the sorting variable are highlighted in color. In the second panel from the top (from the bottom), the provinces with the five next highest (lowest) counts with respect to the sorting variable are highlighted in color, but also the provinces with the five highest (lowest) counts from the panel above (below) are highlighted in gray. Finally, in the third panel from the top (from the bottom), the provinces with the five next highest (lowest) counts with respect to the sorting variable are highlighted in color, but also the provinces with the ten highest (lowest) counts from the panel above (below) are highlighted in gray. Moreover, the median (here, the sixteenth largest/smallest value) is highlighted in a different gray in both adjacent maps. These two-ended cumulative maps make it easy to assess whether there is a general pattern with respect to provinces that have values above and below the median.

In Fig. 2, the provinces and data rows are sorted with respect to decreasing numbers of religious sites and organizations related to Christianity. This allows to answer question 1 from above. Zhejiang and Fujian, which had the largest and fourth largest numbers of religious sites and organizations related to Christianity, also had the largest and second largest numbers of religious sites and organizations related to Buddhism. In Anhui and Henan, ranked second and third with respect to Christianity, Buddhism was much less present. In addition, this figure also shows that for some provinces where Christianity is only rarely present, in particular

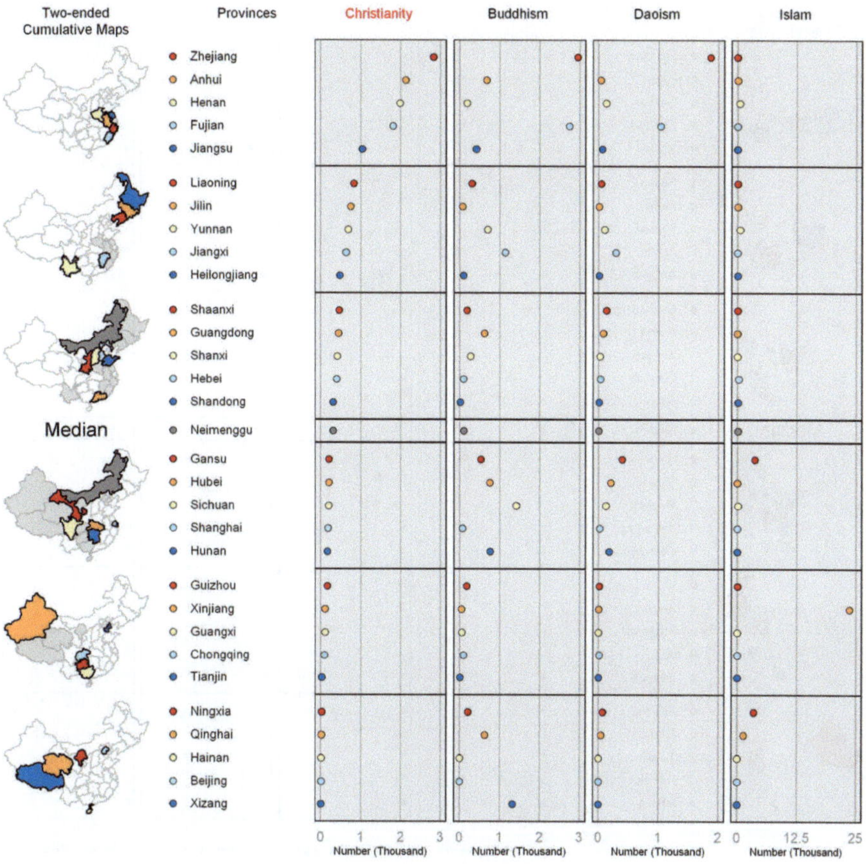

Fig. 2 LM plot of Chinese religions, sorted according to Christianity

Sichuan and Xizang, Buddhism is far more present. In fact, as the next figure will show, these two provinces are ranked third and fourth, respectively, with respect to the number of religious sites and organizations related to Buddhism. When looking at the small maps, it becomes apparent that Christianity was most present in the coastal regions of China in the southeast, reaching as far north as Heilongjiang and as far west as Yunnan. Christianity was less present in the western and central provinces of China.

In Fig. 3, the provinces and data rows are sorted with respect to decreasing numbers of religious sites and organizations related to Buddhism. This allows to answer question 2 from above. It can be seen that the data columns for Buddhism and Daoism run almost parallel to each other, with two exceptions. As discussed in Gebreab et al. (2008), such a pattern is a strong indicator of a strong positive linear association between the numbers of religious sites and organizations related to Buddhism and Daoism. The exceptions are Xizang, where Daoism was far less

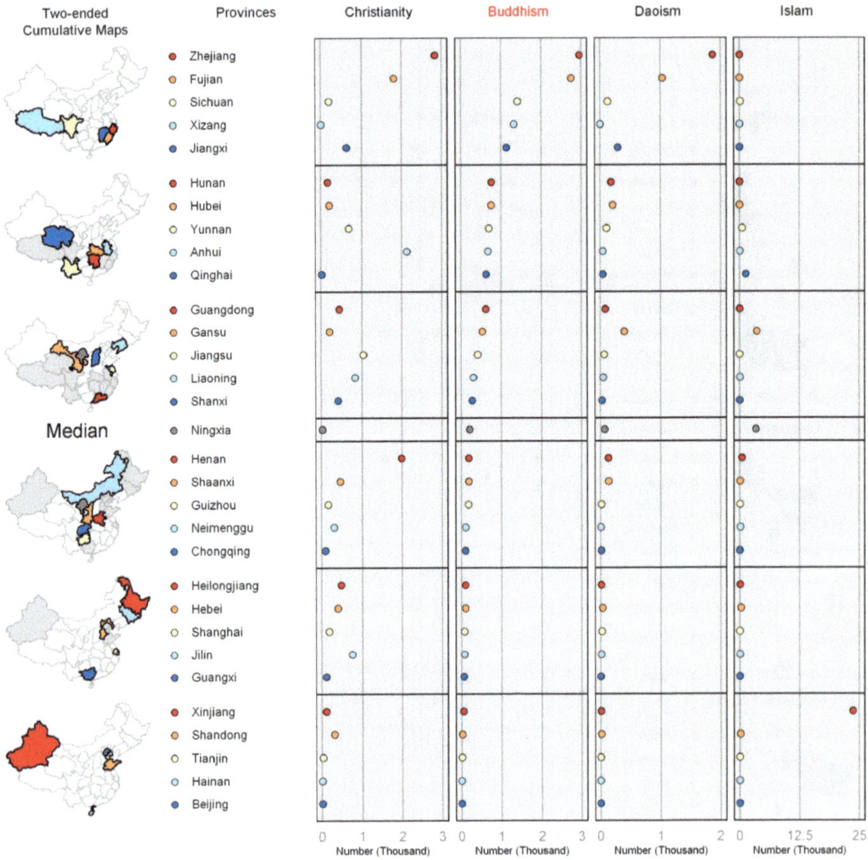

Fig. 3 LM plot of Chinese religions, sorted according to Buddhism

present than the overall relationship with Buddhism would suggest and Gansu, where Daoism was far more present than the overall relationship with Buddhism would suggest. Geographically, the small maps reveal that Buddhism was most present in the southern provinces of China, ranging from Zhejiang in the east to Xizang in the west.

In Fig. 4, the provinces and data rows are sorted with respect to decreasing numbers of religious sites and organizations related to Islam. This allows to answer question 3 from above. A careful look at Table 1 may reveal that the number of 23,678 religious sites and organizations related to Islam in Xinjiang is unusually large. In fact, this number is about eight times bigger then the next highest number of 2956 religious sites and organizations related to Buddhism in Zhejiang. So, this number could be an outlier overall. However, when looking at this province and its neighboring provinces in the maps, it becomes apparent that this is not an overall outlier and not even a spatial outlier. Islam was most present in the western

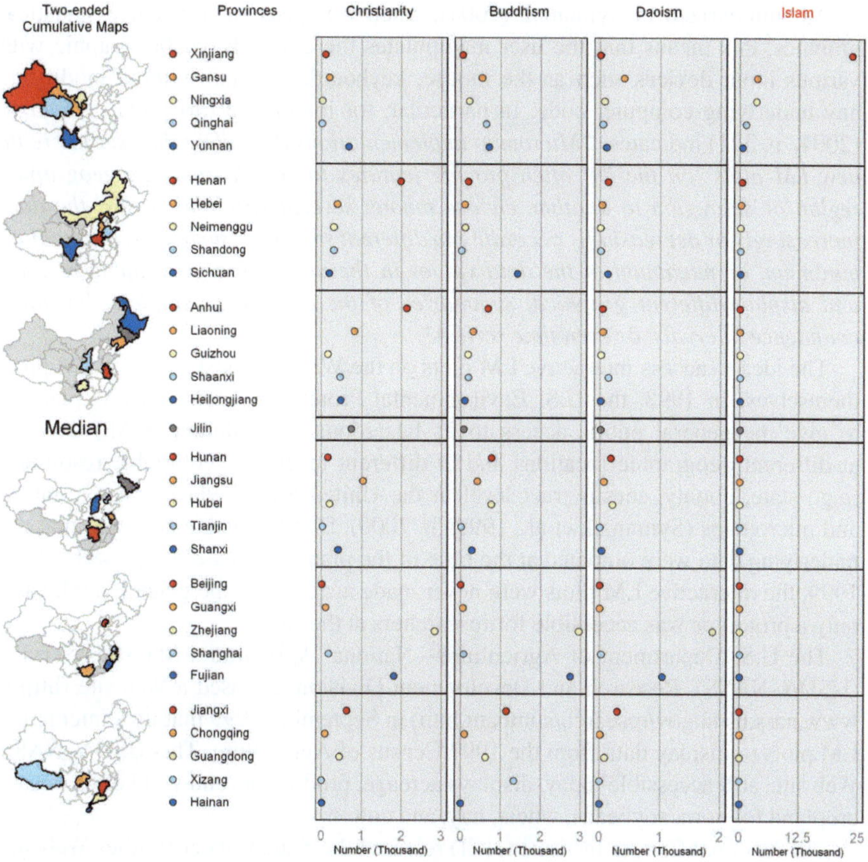

Fig. 4 LM plot of Chinese religions, sorted according to Islam

and northern provinces of China. This is easily explainable by the fact that China is bordered by predominantly Islamic countries to the west, including Pakistan, Afghanistan, Tajikistan, Kyrgyzstan, and Kazakhstan.

4 Interactive LM Plots and *Religion Explorer*

As we can see in Figs. 2, 3, and 4, a different sorting of the provinces and data rows in these LM plots can reveal different aspects about the data that otherwise would not be visible. However, to make such changes, the user needs to manually modify the R code, e.g., update arguments for the *mmplot* function, replace the name of the sorting variable, etc. This naturally leads to the concept of interactive LM plots, further discussed in this section.

As summarized in Symanzik (2004), when we speak of interactive statistical graphics, this means that the user manipulates the currently visible graphic with various input devices such as the mouse, keyboard, etc., but without modifying any underlying computer code. In particular, for interactive LM plots, Symanzik (2004, p. 321) indicates: *"Micromap implementations that allow the user to create new LM plots 'on the fly' often provide features to switch from one geographic region or subregion to another, choose among several variables, resort the data increasingly or decreasingly according to different statistics (such as mean, median, minimum, or maximum of the data values in the underlying geographic region), and display different graphical summaries of the data (e.g., dotplots, boxplots, confidence intervals, or even time series)."*

The idea to access interactive LM plots on the Web is almost as old as LM plots themselves. In 1998, the U.S. Environmental Protection Agency (EPA) planned to give the general public access to its hazardous air pollutant (HAP) data set at different geographic locations and at different levels of geographic resolution (e.g., state, county, census tract level in the United States) via interactive tables and micromaps (Symanzik et al., 1999a,b, 2000). Due to outside concerns that the underlying data were outdated at the time of the planned release of this web site in 1999, the interactive LM plots were never made available to the general public and only a prototype was accessible for researchers at the EPA.

The U.S. Department of Agriculture—National Agricultural Statistics Service (USDA–NASS), Research and Development Division, released a Web site (http://www.nass.usda.gov/research/sumpant.htm) in September 1999 that uses interactive LM plots to display data from the 1997 Census of Agriculture. This USDA–NASS Web site, still accessible today, displays acreage, production, and yield of harvested cropland for corn, soybeans, wheat, hay, and cotton.

The National Cancer Institute (NCI) released the State Cancer Profiles Web site in April 2003 that provided interactive access to the NCI cancer data via LM plots. This Web site was Java-based and created micromaps "on the fly" (Carr et al., 2003, 2002; Wang et al., 2002).

4.1 Previous Software Developments at the CDC

Since 2009, researchers at the CDC have developed a series of closely related online software products for the analysis of data in different geographic regions. These software products include *China Geo-Explorer I & II*, *Urban and Regional Explorer*, *Religion Explorer*, and *US Geo-Explorer* (Bao et al., 2014; She et al., 2010, 2011; Zhang et al., 2010, 2009). While some of them are freely accessible, others are only accessible for researchers affiliated with the CDC. A common gateway to all of these software products is http://chinadataonline.org/.

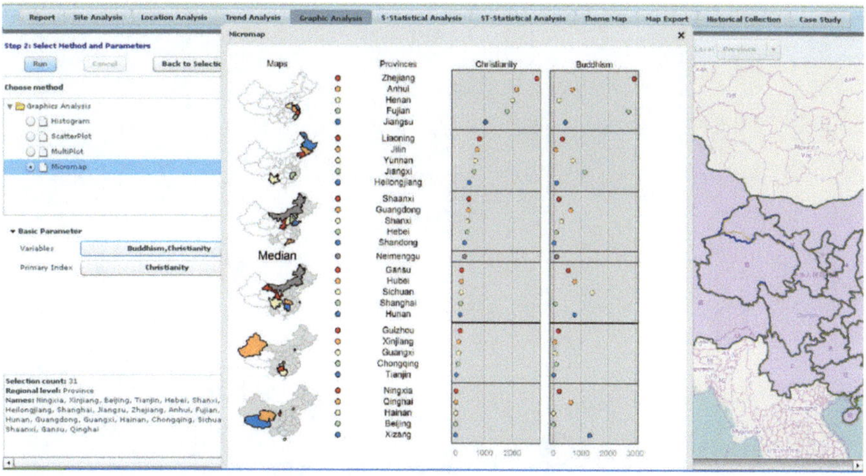

Fig. 5 LM Plot of Chinese religions in the *Religion Explorer* software. The background map is rendered with *OpenStreetMap*

4.2 LM Plots in the Religion Explorer Software

In a prototypic implementation, interactive LM plots were first added to the *Religion Explorer* software at the CDC. The overall workflow for the creation and display of LM plots in this environment can be summarized as follows: A user on the client site selects regions, variables of interest, and display attributes via a Web browser. This information is further processed, packaged, and sent to the server. On the server site, queries are made to the underlying data bases to extract relevant geographic and statistical data. These data are packed into XML (eXtended Markup Language) format and are sent to Rserve, a TCP/IP server which allows other programs to use facilities of R (http://rforge.net/Rserve/). After unpacking the data, a LM plot is produced in R, returned to the server, and finally displayed in the Web browser on the client site. This prototype is accessible at http://www.chinadataonline.org/religionexplorer2/. LM plots can be produced via the *Graphic Analysis* menu after selecting the regions of interest (see Fig. 5). In this example, Christianity and Buddhism have been selected and Christianity has been used as sorting variable for the provinces and data rows. In the background, the main window of the *Religion Explorer* software can be seen.

5 Google Maps of Chinese Religions

The R package *RgoogleMaps* (Loecher, 2015), further described in Loecher (2012) and Loecher and Ropkins (2015), provides an R interface to query the Google map server for static maps and to use these maps as background images for other plots in

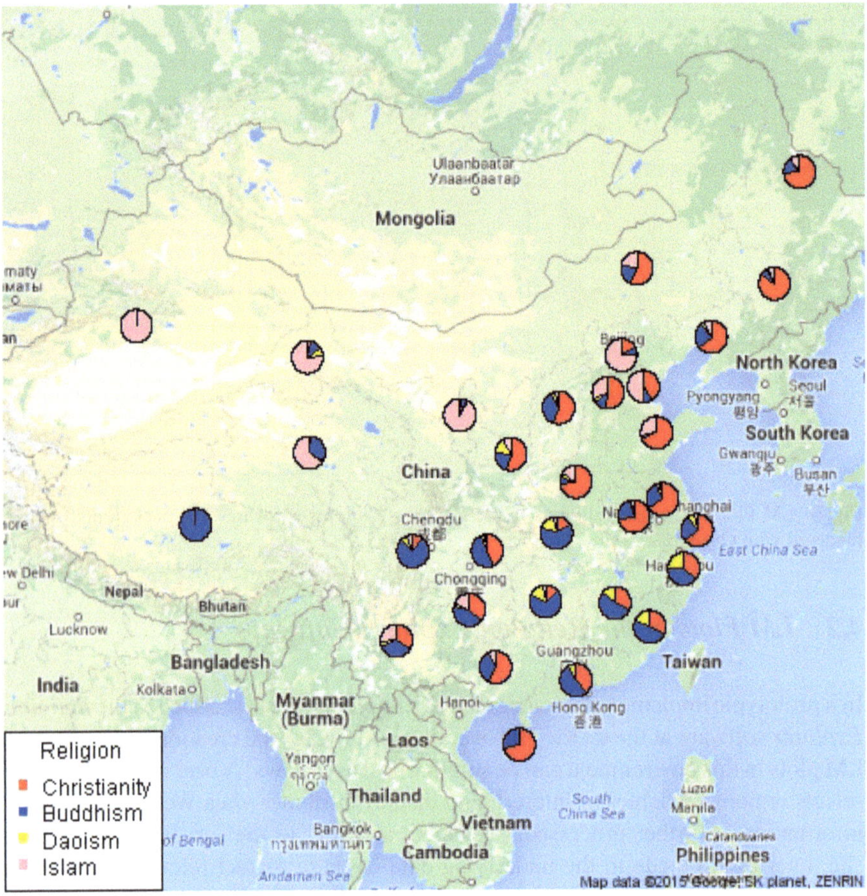

Fig. 6 Chinese religions overlayed on a Google map

R. It is possible to display spatial point patterns on these maps and to overlay more advanced plot types such as bar charts, histograms, pie charts, and fourfold plots for different subregions on these maps (Ahn and Park, 2013; Mun et al., 2013). Several other uses of Google maps as a background for statistical data exist (Ibraliu et al., 2011a,b; Lee and Marcovitz, 2011; Li et al., 2011; Yazdanparast et al., 2011).

Based on the R code developed by Mun et al. (2013), a Google map overlay for Chinese religions is shown in Fig. 6. For each of the 31 provinces from mainland China, a pie chart is shown in the geographic centers of the provinces. This figure shows that Christianity is dominant in the coastal and some interior provinces in the east, Buddhism is dominant in most of the southern and the remaining interior provinces, and Islam is dominant in the western and northern provinces of China. Daoism isn't dominant in any of these 31 provinces and doesn't contribute to more than 25 % of the number of religious sites and organizations in any province.

6 Discussion and Outlook

In this article, we have described the steps that are necessary to modify shapefiles to be able to produce meaningful LM plots for China. With these adjusted shapefiles, Chinese LM plots can now be created via the *micromap* R package and via the online *Religion Explorer* software at the CDC. This makes China the second country in Asia for which meaningful LM plots can be produced, in addition to previously introduced LM plots for Korea (Ahn, 2013; Han et al., 2014).

As indicated in Sect. 4.2, so far only a prototypic implementation of interactive LM plots in *Religion Explorer* exists. It is necessary to further enhance, test, and debug the current implementation. Eventually, the LM plot functionality will be added to some of the other software products developed at the CDC.

Acknowledgements We would like to acknowledge the contributions of Marc H. Weber, Michael G. McManus, Quinn Payton, Jeong Yong Ahn, and Se Jin Park to the recent advancements of linked micromap plots and Google map overlays that form the basis of this article.

References

Ahn, J. Y. (2013). Visualizing statistical information using Korean linked micromap plots. In: S. H. Cho (Ed.), *Proceedings of IASC–Satellite Conference for the 59th ISI WSC & The 8th Conference of IASC–ARS, Asian Regional Section of the IASC* (pp. 219–221). http://hbutton.com/IASC/iascproceedings/proceeding_pdf/Proceedings.pdf.

Ahn, J. Y., & Park, S. J. (2013). Map overlays based on Google maps and R. In: S. H. Cho (Ed.), *Proceedings of IASC–Satellite Conference for the 59th ISI WSC & The 8th Conference of IASC–ARS, Asian Regional Section of the IASC* (pp. 222–224). http://hbutton.com/IASC/iascproceedings/proceeding_pdf/Proceedings.pdf.

Andrienko, G. L., & Andrienko, N. V. (1999). Interactive maps for visual data exploration. *International Journal of Geographical Information Science, 13*(4), 355–374.

Andrienko, N., Andrienko, G., Savinov, A., Voss, H., & Wettschereck, D. (2001). Exploratory analysis of spatial data using interactive maps and data mining. *Cartography and Geographic Information Science, 28*(3), 151–165.

Anselin, L. (1994). Exploratory spatial data analysis and geographic information systems. In: M. Painho (Ed.), *New tools for spatial analysis*, Eurostat, Luxembourg (pp. 45–54).

Bao, S., Wang, C., & Shui, M. (2014). Spatial study of religion with spatial Religion Explorer. In: *22nd International Conference on Geoinformatics* (pp. 1–8). New York: IEEE.

Bivand, R. S. (2010). Exploratory spatial data analysis. In: M. M. Fischer & A. Getis (Eds.), *Handbook of applied spatial analysis: Software tools, methods and applications* (pp. 219–254). Berlin, Heidelberg: Springer.

Bivand, R. S., & Lewin-Koh, N. (2014). maptools: Tools for reading and handling spatial objects. R package version 0.8–29. http://CRAN.R-project.org/package=maptools.

Carr, D. B., Bell, B. S., Pickle, L. W., Zhang, Y., & Li, Y. (2003). The state cancer profiles web site and extensions of linked micromap plots and conditioned choropleth map plots. In: *Proceedings of the Third National Conference on Digital Government Research, Digital Government Research Center (DGRC)* (pp. 269–273). http://dl.acm.org/citation.cfm?id=1123196.

Carr, D. B., Chen, J., Bell, B. S., Pickle, L. W., & Zhang, Y. (2002). Interactive linked micromap plots and dynamically conditioned choropleth maps. In: *Proceedings of the Second National Conference on Digital Government Research, Digital Government Research Center (DGRC)* (pp. 61–67). http://dl.acm.org/citation.cfm?id=1123098.

Carr, D. B., & Pearson, J. B., Jr. (2015). micromapST: Linked micromap plots for U.S. States. R package version 1.0.5. http://CRAN.R-project.org/package=micromapST.

Carr, D. B., & Pickle, L. W. (2010). *Visualizing data patterns with micromaps*. Boca Raton, FL: Chapman & Hall/CRC.

Carr, D. B., & Pierson, S. M. (1996). Emphasizing statistical summaries and showing spatial context with micromaps. *Statistical Computing and Statistical Graphics Newsletter, 7*(3), 16–23.

Douglas, D. H., & Peucker, T. K. (1973). Algorithms for the reduction of the number of points required to represent a digitized line or its caricature. *The Canadian Cartographer, 10*(2), 112–122.

Gebreab, S. Y., Gillies, R. R., Munger, R. G., & Symanzik, J. (2008). Visualization and interpretation of birth defects data using linked micromap plots. *Birth Defects Research (Part A): Clinical and Molecular Teratology, 82*, 110–119.

Hackett, C., Grim, B. J., Skirbekk, V., Stonawski, M., & Goujon, A. (2011). Global Christianity: A report on the size and distribution of the world's Christian population. Report. Pew Research Center's Forum on Religion & Public Life, Washington, D.C.

Han, K. S., Park, S. J., Mun, G. S., Choi, S. H., Symanzik, J., & Gebreab, S., et al. (2014). Linked micromaps for the visualization of geographically referenced data. *ICIC Express Letters, 8*(2), 443–448.

Ibraliu, A., Mi, X., & Elezi, F. (2011a). Variation in essential oils to study the biodiversity in *satureja montana l. Journal of Medicinal Plants Research, 5*(14), 2978–2989.

Ibraliu, A., Mi, X., Ristić, M., Stefanovic, Z. D., & Shehu, J. (2011b). Analysis of essential oils of three wild medicinal plants in Albania. *Journal of Medicinal Plants Research, 5*(1), 58–62.

Lai, H. H. (2003). The religious revival in China. *Copenhagen Journal of Asian Studies, 18*, 40–64.

Lee, B. H., & Marcovitz, M. S. (2011). When oil and water mix: Temperature and salinity changes in the Gulf after the BP catastrophe. In: *2011 JSM Proceedings, American Statistical Association, Alexandria, VA, (CD).*

Li, T., Gao, C., & Xu, M. (2011). Analysis on Deepwater Horizon oil spoil by boosting tree and varying coefficient logistic regression. In: *2011 JSM Proceedings, American Statistical Association, Alexandria, VA, (CD).*

Loecher, M. (2012). Identifying and visualizing spatiotemporal clusters on map tiles. In: *2012 JSM Proceedings, American Statistical Association, Alexandria, VA, (CD).*

Loecher, M. (2015). RgoogleMaps: Overlays on Google map tiles in R. R package version 1.2.0.7. http://CRAN.R-project.org/package=RgoogleMaps.

Loecher, M., & Ropkins, K. (2015). RgoogleMaps and loa: Unleashing R graphics power on map tiles. *Journal of Statistical Software, 63*(4). http://www.jstatsoft.org/v63/i04/.

MacEachren, A. M., Gahegan, M., Pike, W., Brewer, I., Cai, G., & Lengerich, E., et al. (2004). Geovisualization for knowledge construction and decision support. *IEEE Computer Graphics and Applications, 24*(1), 13–17.

MacEachren, A. M., Wachowicz, M., Edsall, R., Haug, D., & Masters, R. (1999). Constructing knowledge from multivariate spatiotemporal data: Integrating geographical visualization with knowledge discovery in database methods. *International Journal of Geographical Information Science, 13*(4), 311–334.

Mun, G. S., Park, S. J., Symanzik, J., & Ahn, J.Y. (2013). Visualizing statistical information using Google static maps and R. *ICIC Express Letters, 7*(3A), 729–734.

Olsen, A. R., Carr, D. B., Courbois, J. P., & Pierson, S.M. (1996). Presentation of data in linked attribute and geographic space. In: *1996 Abstracts, Joint Statistical Meetings, Chicago, IL* (p. 271). Alexandria, VA: American Statistical Association.

Payton, Q. C., McManus, M. G., Weber, M. H., Olsen, A. R., & Kincaid, T.M. (2015). micromap: A package for linked micromaps. *Journal of Statistical Software, 63*(2). http://www.jstatsoft.org/v63/i02/.

Payton, Q. C., & Olsen, A. R. (2015). micromap: linked micromap plots. R package version 1.9.1. http://CRAN.R-project.org/package=micromap.

Payton, Q. C., Weber, M. H., McManus, M. G., & Olsen, A. R. (2012). Linked micromaps: Statistical summaries in a spatial context. In: *Water: One resource — shared effort — common future. 8th National Monitoring Conference, April 30–May 4, 2012, Portland, OR*. National Water Quality Monitoring Council. http://acwi.gov/monitoring/conference/2012/posters/posters_2012_conference.pdf.

Pickle, L. W., Pearson, J. B., Jr., & Carr, D. B. (2015). micromapST: Exploring and communicating geospatial patterns in U.S. State data. *Journal of Statistical Software, 63*(3). http://www.jstatsoft.org/v63/i03/.

R Core Team (2014). R: A language and environment for statistical computing. R Foundation for Statistical Computing, Vienna. http://www.R-project.org/.

Roth, R. E. (2013). Interactive maps: What we know and what we need to know. *Journal of Spatial Information Science, 6*, 59–115.

She, B., Zhu, X., & Bao, S. (2010). Spatial data integration and analysis with spatial intelligence. In: *18th International Conference on Geoinformatics, 2010* (pp 1–6). New York: IEEE.

She, B., Zhu, X., & Bao, S. (2011). Urban and Regional Explorer with spatial intelligence. In: *19th International Conference on Geoinformatics, 2011* (pp. 1–5). New York: IEEE.

Symanzik, J. (2004). Interactive and dynamic graphics. In: J. E. Gentle, W. Härdle, & Y. Mori (Eds.), *Handbook of computational statistics — concepts and methods*. Berlin, Heidelberg: Springer.

Symanzik, J. (2014). Exploratory spatial data analysis. In: M. M. Fischer & P. Nijkamp (Eds.), *Handbook of regional science* (pp. 1295–1310). Berlin, Heidelberg: Springer.

Symanzik, J., Axelrad, D. A., Carr, D. B., Wang, J., Wong, D., & Woodruff, T. J. (1999a). HAPs, micromaps and GPL — visualization of geographically referenced statistical summaries on the world wide web. In: *Annual Proceedings (ACSM–WFPS–PLSO–LSAW 1999 Conference CD), American Congress on Surveying and Mapping*.

Symanzik, J., & Carr, D. B. (2008). Interactive linked micromap plots for the display of geographically referenced statistical data. In: C. Chen, W. Härdle, & A. Unwin (Eds.), *Handbook of data visualization* (pp. 267–294 & 2 Color Plates). Berlin, Heidelberg: Springer.

Symanzik, J., & Carr, D. B. (2013). Linked micromap plots in R. In: Cho, S. H. (Ed.), *Proceedings of IASC–Satellite Conference for the 59th ISI WSC & The 8th Conference of IASC–ARS, Asian Regional Section of the IASC* (pp. 213–218). http://hbutton.com/IASC/iascproceedings/proceeding_pdf/Proceedings.pdf.

Symanzik, J., Carr, D. B., Axelrad, D. A., Wang, J., Wong, D., & Woodruff, T. J. (1999b). Interactive tables and maps — a glance at EPA's cumulative exposure project web page (pp. 94–99). In: *1999 Proceedings of the Section on Statistical Graphics*. Alexandria, VA: American Statistical Association.

Symanzik, J., Dai, X., Weber, M. H., Payton, Q., & McManus, M. G. (2014). Linked micromap plots for South America — general design considerations and specific adjustments. *Revista Colombiana de Estadística, 37*(2), 451–469.

Symanzik, J., Wong, D., Wang, J., Carr, D. B., Woodruff, T. J., & Axelrad, D. A. (2000). Web–based access and visualization of hazardous air pollutants. In: *Geographic Information Systems in Public Health: Proceedings of the Third National Conference August 18–20, 1998, San Diego, CA*. Agency for Toxic Substances and Disease Registry. http://webharvest.gov/peth04/20041020204613/http://www.atsdr.cdc.gov/gis/conference98/index.html.

Wang, X., Chen, J. X., Carr, D. B., Bell, B. S., & Pickle, L.W. (2002). Geographic statistics visualization: Web–based linked micromap plots. *Computing in Science & Engineering, 4*(3), 90–94.

Yazdanparast, A., Tran, T., & Suess, E. A. (2011). Effect of oil spill on birds: A graphical assay of the Deepwater Horizon oil spill's impact on birds. In: *2011 JSM Proceedings*. Alexandria, VA: American Statistical Association (CD).

Zhang, X., Bao, S., Zhu, X., & Su, K. (2010). Spatial intelligence with spatial statistics. In: *18th International Conference on Geoinformatics, 2010* (pp. 1–6). New York: IEEE.

Zhang, X., Zhu, X., She, B., & Bao, S. (2009). The spatial data integration and analysis with China Geo–Explorer. In: *17th International Conference on Geoinformatics, 2009* (pp. 1–8). New York: IEEE.

Zhu, X., Wang, C., Bao, S., & She, B. (2014). Spatial studies of Chinese religions and society. Report. China Data Center, University of Michigan, Ann Arbor, MI.

The Efficiency of Next-Generation Gibbs-Type Samplers: An Illustration Using a Hierarchical Model in Cosmology

Xiyun Jiao, David A. van Dyk, Roberto Trotta, and Hikmatali Shariff

Abstract Supernovae occur when a star's life ends in a violent thermonuclear explosion, briefly outshining an entire galaxy before fading from view over a period of weeks or months. Because so-called Type Ia supernovae occur only in a particular physical scenario, their explosions have similar intrinsic brightnesses which allows us to accurately estimate their distances. This in turn allows us to constrain the parameters of cosmological models that characterize the expansion history of the universe. In this paper, we show how a cosmological model can be embedded into a Gaussian hierarchical model and fit using observations of Type Ia supernovae. The overall model is an ideal testing ground of new computational methods. Ancillarity-Sufficiency Interweaving Strategy (ASIS) and Partially Collapsed Gibbs (PCG) are effective tools to improve the convergence of Gibbs samplers. Besides using either of them alone, we can combine PCG and/or ASIS along with Metropolis-Hastings algorithm to simplify implementation and further improve convergence. We use four samplers to draw from the posterior distribution of the cosmological hierarchical model, and confirm the efficiency of both PCG and ASIS. Furthermore, we find that we can gain more efficiency by combining two or more strategies into one sampler.

1 Introduction

The Physics Nobel Prize (2011) was awarded for the discovery that the expansion of the universe is accelerating, a phenomenon attributed to the existence of "dark energy". Type Ia supernova (SN) observations have been instrumental in this discovery and remain an important tool to quantify the characteristics of dark energy (March et al. 2011). Although details remain unclear, it is thought that a Type Ia SN occurs when a compact, carbon-oxygen white dwarf star accumulates extra

X. Jiao (✉) • D.A. van Dyk
Statistics Section, Imperial College, London, UK
e-mail: x.jiao12@imperial.ac.uk; d.van-dyk@imperial.ac.uk

R. Trotta • H. Shariff
Astrophysics Group, Imperial College, London, UK

Z. Jin et al. (eds.), *New Developments in Statistical Modeling, Inference and Application*, ICSA Book Series in Statistics, DOI 10.1007/978-3-319-42571-9_9

material until its mass approaches a critical threshold ("Chandrasekhar threshold": 1.44 $M_\odot$, where $M_\odot$ is the mass of the sun). Because of their common formation mechanism, all Type Ia SNe have similar absolute luminosity (which is measured in absolute magnitudes, i.e., the negative logarithm of flux). This means that their distance can be estimated from their apparent magnitude (i.e., their brightness as viewed from earth). We can also directly measure their redshift due to the expansion of the universe, a stretching of the wavelength of light emanating from objects moving away from us. The underlying cosmological models of interest predict the relationship between redshift and the difference between apparent and absolute magnitudes, called "distance modulus". We embed the cosmological model into a Gaussian hierarchical model that naturally represents the structure of the problem and dependence among its parameters. (See March et al. (2011) for more details on the formation of Type Ia SNe and their utility in fitting cosmological models.)

Markov Chain Monte Carlo (MCMC) methods have greatly facilitated the development of Bayesian inference, since they make it possible to sample from the distributions of highly-structured models. Gibbs sampling (Geman and Geman 1984) and the Data Augmentation (DA) algorithm (Tanner and Wong 1987; van Dyk and Meng 2001), which is a special case of the Gibbs sampler, are both widely used MCMC methods. However, their sometimes slow convergence rate can be problematic. To improve their efficiency, a variety of extensions have been proposed. Among them, the Ancillarity-Sufficiency Interweaving Strategy (ASIS) (Yu and Meng 2011) is an effective tool to improve the convergence properties of the DA algorithm, and the Partially Collapsed Gibbs (PCG) sampler (van Dyk and Park 2008) can improve the convergence of Gibbs samplers. Note that in a Gibbs-type sampler, we often need the help of the Metropolis-Hastings (MH) algorithm (Hastings 1970; Metropolis et al. 1953), when sampling from a conditional distribution that is not standard. In this paper, we explore the relative efficiencies of these strategies when fitting our Bayesian hierarchical model. In particular, we consider four samplers, MH within Gibbs, MH within PCG, ASIS and PCG within ASIS. By comparing their convergence, we demonstrate the higher efficiency of PCG and ASIS. Moreover, we obtain further efficiency by combining these strategies into a single sampler. Our general strategy for combining PCG and ASIS will appear in a separate paper that is currently in preparation (Jiao and van Dyk 2016).

This paper is organized as follows. In Sect. 2, we present the Bayesian cosmological hierarchical model. In Sect. 3, we review the DA algorithm, the Gibbs sampler, and their extensions—ASIS and PCG sampling, and then introduce the four samplers designed to sample from the posterior of the cosmological hierarchical model. In Sect. 4, we use a real-data analysis to illustrate the varying efficiency of the four samplers. Concluding remarks appear in Sect. 5.

2 Bayesian Hierarchical Model for Supernova Cosmology

We assume the absolute magnitudes of Type Ia SNe follow a Gaussian population distribution, that is,

$$M_i^o \overset{\text{iid}}{\sim} \mathrm{N}(M_0, \sigma_0^2), \text{ for } i = 1, \ldots, n. \tag{1}$$

Since the absolute magnitudes are similar, σ_0 is relatively small, but still too large to use Type Ia SNe as distance indicators without further adjustment. This intrinsic variability in the absolute magnitudes is due to variations in the properties of the progenitor star (e.g., mass and composition) and/or its environment. Fortunately, we can adjust for two covariates, the stretch parameter, x_i, and the color correction parameter, c_i, to reduce this scatter; these empirical adjustments are known as "Phillips corrections", see (Phillips 1993; Phillips et al. 1999) for details. Specifically,

$$M_i^o = M_i - \alpha x_i + \beta c_i, \text{ for } i = 1, \ldots, n, \text{ with } M_i \overset{\text{iid}}{\sim} \mathrm{N}(M_0, \sigma_{\text{res}}^2), \tag{2}$$

where M_i is the adjusted absolute magnitude and $\sigma_{\text{res}}^2 \ll \sigma_0^2$. (Because of their similar adjusted absolute magnitudes, Type Ia SNe are called "standardizable candles".)

For Type Ia SN i ($i = 1, \ldots, n$), four quantities are observed with error, the apparent magnitude $\hat{m}_{Bi}$, the *observed* stretch and color correction parameters, $\hat{x}_i$ and $\hat{c}_i$, and the redshift z_i.[1] That is,

$$\begin{pmatrix} \hat{c}_i \\ \hat{x}_i \\ \hat{m}_{Bi} \end{pmatrix} \sim \mathrm{N}\left[\begin{pmatrix} c_i \\ x_i \\ m_{Bi} \end{pmatrix}, \hat{C}_i\right], \text{ for } i = 1, \ldots, n. \tag{3}$$

Because its measurement error is very small, in this article, we assume z_i is known. For illustration, we ignore the small correlations among the observed quantities and take the matrix $\hat{C}_i$ to be diagonal, i.e., $\hat{C}_i = \mathrm{Diag}\left(\hat{\sigma}_{c_i}^2, \hat{\sigma}_{x_i}^2, \hat{\sigma}_{m_{Bi}}^2\right)$. The distance modulus is defined to be $\mu_i = m_{Bi} - M_i^o$, so that (2) can be written as

$$m_{Bi} = \mu_i + M_i - \alpha x_i + \beta c_i, \text{ for } i = 1, \ldots, n. \tag{4}$$

[1]The raw data are time-series observations of the evolving SN explosion in each of several color bands. These observations are summarized into the apparent magnitude, stretch parameter and color parameter using the SALT-II method (Guy et al. 2007). The apparent magnitude is the peak magnitude in the B-band.

This forms the first level of our hierarchical model and because of (3), it can be viewed as an *errors-in-variables* regression model (Carroll et al. 2006). The second level of the hierarchical model describes the population distribution of the SNe,

$$M_i \sim \mathrm{N}(M_0, \sigma^2_{\text{res}}),\ x_i \sim \mathrm{N}(x_0, R_x^2),\ c_i \sim \mathrm{N}(c_0, R_c^2),\ \text{for } i = 1, \ldots, n. \tag{5}$$

We use the ΛCDM cosmological model which predicts that the distance modulus, μ_i, as a deterministic function of the dark energy density Ω_Λ, matter density Ω_m, Hubble constant H_0, and redshift z_i. Specifically,

$$\mu_i = 25 + 5\log_{10}\left[\frac{c}{H_0} d_L(z_i, \Omega_\Lambda, \Omega_m, H_0)\right], \tag{6}$$

where the speed of light $c = 3 \times 10^5$ km/s, and

$$d_L(z_i, \Omega_\Lambda, \Omega_m, H_0) = \frac{(1+z_i)}{\sqrt{|\Omega_\kappa|}} \text{sinn}\left\{\sqrt{|\Omega_\kappa|}\int_0^{z_i}\left[(1+z')^3\Omega_m + \Omega_\Lambda + (1+z')^2\Omega_\kappa\right]^{-1/2} \mathrm{d}z'\right\}, \tag{7}$$

with Ω_κ the curvature parameter that is completely determined by Ω_Λ and Ω_m via $\Omega_\kappa = 1 - \Omega_\Lambda - \Omega_m$; $\text{sinn}(x) = x$, $\text{sinn}(x) = \sin(x)$, or $\text{sinn}(x) = \sinh(x)$ for $\Omega_\kappa = 0$, $\Omega_\kappa < 0$, and $\Omega_\kappa > 0$, respectively. Because the Hubble constant, H_0, is completely degenerate with M_0, we fix its value at 72 km/s/mpc (as determined by other measurements) and we write $\mu_i = \mu(z_i, \Omega_\Lambda, \Omega_m)$.

Finally, we specify weakly informative prior distributions for model parameters,

$$M_0 \sim \mathrm{N}(M_m, \sigma^2_{M_0}),\ x_0 \sim \mathrm{N}(0, \sigma^2_{x0}),\ c_0 \sim \mathrm{N}(0, \sigma^2_{c0}), \tag{8}$$

where $M_m = -19.3$, $\sigma_{M_0} = 2$, $\sigma_{x_0} = 10$ and $\sigma_{c_0} = 1$. According to March et al. (2011), these variances are large enough to make the priors for M_0, x_0 and c_0 sufficiently diffuse. They also find that the choice of mean and variance in the prior distribution of M_0 has little influence on numerical results. Furthermore, we specify $\log(\sigma_{\text{res}}) \sim \text{Unif}(-5, 2)$, $\log(R_x) \sim \text{Unif}(-5, 2)$, $\log(R_c) \sim \text{Unif}(-5, 2)$, $\alpha \sim \text{Unif}(0, 1)$, $\beta \sim \text{Unif}(0, 4)$, $\Omega_\Lambda \sim \text{Unif}(0, 2)$, and $\Omega_m \sim \text{Unif}(0, 1)$. We choose ranges of these uniform priors following March et al. (2011), which states that they generously cover all scientifically plausible values of the parameters.

3 Statistical Computation

3.1 Algorithm Review

Suppose we wish to obtain a Monte Carlo sample from the posterior distribution $p(\psi|Y_{\text{obs}})$, where ψ is an unknown model parameter and Y_{obs} is the observed data. The Gibbs sampler partitions ψ into $\psi = (\psi_1, \ldots, \psi_N)$, where $N \geq 2$, and samples each component of ψ from its *complete conditional distribution* in turn. That is, at each iteration, each ψ_i is sampled from its conditional posterior distribution given the current value of the other components of ψ. (We consider systematic-scan samplers, where the components are updated in a fixed order, see Liu et al. (1995).) After suitable burn-in, $\{\psi^{(t)}, t = T_b + 1, T_b + 2, \ldots, T\}$ can be regarded as a Monte Carlo sample from $p(\psi|Y_{\text{obs}})$, see e.g., Robert and Casella (2004), for details, conditions, and practical advice.

When $N = 2$, the Gibbs sampler is sometimes called the Data Augmentation Algorithm. To be consistent with the notation of the DA algorithm, we write $\psi = (\theta, Y_{\text{mis}})$ in this case. When the DA algorithm is used, the target posterior distribution is typically $p(\theta|Y_{\text{obs}})$ and Y_{mis} is introduced to enable Gibbs-type sampling. As mentioned in Sect. 1, ASIS and PCG can dramatically improve the convergence of the DA algorithm and Gibbs sampler.

3.1.1 Ancillarity-Sufficiency Interweaving Strategy

ASIS combines a pair of special DA schemes, each with a different choice of Y_{mis}. One uses a sufficient augmentation, $Y_{\text{mis},S}$, which means $p(Y_{\text{obs}}|Y_{\text{mis},S}, \theta)$ is free of θ. The other uses an ancillary augmentation, $Y_{\text{mis},A}$, for which $p(Y_{\text{mis},A}|\theta)$ does not depend on θ. Normally, given θ, $Y_{\text{mis},S}$ is related to $Y_{\text{mis},A}$ via a one-to-one mapping, $\mathscr{F}_\theta$, that is, $Y_{\text{mis},A} = \mathscr{F}_\theta(Y_{\text{mis},S})$ (but see Yu and Meng (2011) for an exception). We assume $\mathscr{F}_\theta$ is differentiable when $Y_{\text{mis},S}$ is continuous. In practice, it is often the case that if the sampler constructed via one of these two augmentations is fast, the other is slow. ASIS takes advantage of this "beauty-and-beast" feature of the two DA algorithms by interweaving them to produce a more powerful sampler (Yu and Meng 2011). The algorithm proceeds as

Step 1: $Y_{\text{mis},S}^{(t+1)} \sim p(Y_{\text{mis},S}|\theta^{(t)}, Y_{\text{obs}})$, (Sampler 3.1)
Step 2: $\theta^{(t+1/2)} \sim p(\theta|Y_{\text{mis},S}^{(t+1)}, Y_{\text{obs}})$; $Y_{\text{mis},A}^{(t+1)} = \mathscr{F}_{\theta^{(t+1/2)}}(Y_{\text{mis},S}^{(t+1)})$,
Step 3: $\theta^{(t+1)} \sim p(\theta|Y_{\text{mis},A}^{(t+1)}, Y_{\text{obs}})$,

where $\theta^{(t+1/2)}$ represents the intermediate draw that facilitates the transition from $\theta^{(t)}$ to $\theta^{(t+1)}$; it is not part of the marginal chain for θ. Because $Y_{\text{mis},S}$ and $Y_{\text{mis},A}$ are both legitimate augmentation schemes, $p(Y_{\text{mis},S}, \theta|Y_{\text{obs}})$ and $p(Y_{\text{mis},A}, \theta|Y_{\text{obs}})$ share the same marginal distribution of θ, i.e., $p(\theta|Y_{\text{obs}})$. Since Step 2 of Sampler 3.1 is equivalent to sampling $Y_{\text{mis},A}^{(t+1)}$ from $p(Y_{\text{mis},A}|Y_{\text{mis},S}^{(t+1)}, Y_{\text{obs}})$, the marginal Markov transition kernel of θ is

$$\mathscr{K}(\theta^{(t+1)}|\theta^{(t)}) = \tag{9}$$

$$\int\int p(\theta^{(t+1)}|Y_{\text{mis},A}^{(t+1)}, Y_{\text{obs}}) p(Y_{\text{mis},A}^{(t+1)}|Y_{\text{mis},S}^{(t+1)}, Y_{\text{obs}}) p(Y_{\text{mis},S}^{(t+1)}|\theta^{(t)}, Y_{\text{obs}}) \mathrm{d}Y_{\text{mis},S}^{(t+1)} \mathrm{d}Y_{\text{mis},A}^{(t+1)}.$$

(a) Gibbs Sampler	(b) Marginalization	(c) Permute	(d) Trim
1. $p(\psi_1 \mid \psi_2', \psi_3', \psi_4')$	1. $p(\psi_1, \psi_3^\star \mid \psi_2', \psi_4')$	1. $p(\psi_2 \mid \psi_1', \psi_3', \psi_4')$	1. $p(\psi_2 \mid \psi_1', \psi_3', \psi_4')$
2. $p(\psi_2 \mid \psi_1, \psi_3', \psi_4')$	2. $p(\psi_2 \mid \psi_1, \psi_3^\star, \psi_4')$	2. $p(\psi_1, \psi_3^\star \mid \psi_2, \psi_4')$	2. $p(\psi_1 \mid \psi_2, \psi_4')$
3. $p(\psi_3, \psi_4 \mid \psi_1, \psi_2)$	3. $p(\psi_3, \psi_4 \mid \psi_1, \psi_2)$	3. $p(\psi_3, \psi_4 \mid \psi_1, \psi_2)$	3. $p(\psi_3, \psi_4 \mid \psi_1, \psi_2)$

Fig. 1 An example of using three stages to transform a Gibbs sampler into a proper PCG sampler. The conditional distributions sampled in each step of the samplers are given; a prime in the superscript denotes the current state of a parameter. The parent Gibbs sampler appears in (**a**). The sampler in (**b**) updates ψ_3 rather than conditioning on it in Step 1. The steps of this sampler are permuted in (**c**) to make the draw of $\psi_3^\star$—in Step 2 of (**c**)—redundant. Trimming $\psi_3^\star$, we obtain the proper PCG sampler in (**d**)

It is easy to verify that the stationary distribution of $\mathscr{K}(\theta^{(t+1)} \mid \theta^{(t)})$ is $p(\theta \mid Y_{\text{obs}})$, see Yu and Meng (2011) for details.

Yu and Meng (2011) find that Steps 1–3 of Sampler 3.1 can be regarded as sampling $(\theta, Y_{\text{mis},S})$ along different directions. ASIS selects a particular combination of sampling directions (defined by the ancillary and sufficient augmentations) that yields substantial improvement over both parent DA samplers, while the additional computational expense is fairly small, see Yu and Meng (2011).

3.1.2 Partially Collapsed Gibbs Sampler

The PCG sampler improves convergence by reducing conditioning, that is, replacing some complete conditional distributions of an ordinary Gibbs sampler with the complete conditionals of marginal distributions of the target joint posterior distribution (van Dyk and Park 2008). This generally leads to larger variance of the conditional distribution, and hence bigger jumps.

Care must be taken to make sure that the stationary distribution of a PCG sampler is the desired target. We review the three stages used to transform a Gibbs sampler into a PCG sampler, while maintaining the target distribution. They are provided by van Dyk and Park (2008) and named as *marginalization*, *permutation* and *trimming* respectively. Here we refer to a sampler as *proper* if its stationary distribution is the target and *improper* otherwise. For illustration, suppose we sample from $p(\psi \mid Y_{\text{obs}})$ with the (proper) Gibbs sampler in Fig. 1(a), with $\psi = (\psi_1, \ldots, \psi_4)$. In the marginalization stage we replace one or more steps of the Gibbs sampler, with steps that sample some components of ψ that were conditioned upon in the original Gibbs, see Step 1 in Fig. 1(b). This results in the same component sampled in two or more steps. Note that we use the superscript "$\star$" to indicate the *intermediate quantities* which are updated in a sampler but not part of the final output, e.g., ψ_3 in Step 1 of Fig. 1(b). Then we *permute* the steps of the marginalized sampler to make as many intermediate updates as possible to be *redundant quantities*, which are intermediate quantities not conditioned on in any subsequent draws. The value of redundant quantities does not affect the transition kernel of the sampler; $\psi_3^\star$ in Step 2 of Fig. 1(c) is an example of a redundant quantity. Finally, we trim the redundant quantities resulting in a step that samples from the conditional distribution of a marginal of $p(\psi|Y_{\text{obs}})$, i.e., Step 2 in Fig. 1(d). We refer to such steps as *reduced steps*. Since all three stages preserve the stationary distribution of the parent Gibbs sampler, the resulting PCG sampler is proper. More details and examples of implementing the three stages can be found in van Dyk and Park (2008), Park and van Dyk (2009) and van Dyk and Jiao (2015).

In some cases the PCG sampler is simply a blocked or collapsed version of the parent Gibbs sampler (Liu et al. 1994). In other cases, however, it is composed of samples from a set of *incompatible conditional distributions*. That is, there is no joint distribution corresponding to this set of conditional distributions, e.g., the PCG sampler in Fig. 1(d). The incompatibility is introduced by trimming. Unlike the Gibbs sampler, changing the order of the steps of a PCG sampler may alter its stationary distribution.

Marginalization can significantly improve the rate of convergence, while permutation typically has a minor effect and trimming has no effect on the rate of convergence (van Dyk and Park 2008). Thus, we generally expect the PCG sampler to exhibit better and often much better convergence properties than its parent Gibbs sampler.

3.2 *Bayesian Fitting of the Cosmological Hierarchical Model*

We now show how ASIS and PCG can be implemented to fit the model in Sect. 2, and illustrate how they can be combined to further improve convergence. To simplify notation, we let Y denote the $(3n \times 1)$ vector of observed quantities, i.e., $Y = (\hat{c}_1, \hat{x}_1, \hat{m}_{B1}, \ldots, \hat{c}_n, \hat{x}_n, \hat{m}_{Bn})$, ξ denote the (3×1) mean vector of the distribution in the second level of the hierarchical model, i.e., $\xi = (c_0, x_0, M_0)$, and X denote the $(3n \times 1)$ vector of latent variables, i.e., $X = (c_1, x_1, M_1, \ldots, c_n, x_n, M_n)$.

Sampler 1 is a standard Gibbs sampler, where each (sometimes multivariate) component is updated from its complete conditional distribution. We list the steps of Sampler 1 in the top-left panel of Fig. 2. We sample $(\Omega_m, \Omega_\Lambda)$ with the help of MH because its conditional distribution is not in closed form. (It is evaluated numerically.) Details of this and the other samplers, including the MH updates, appear in the Appendix.

In order to improve the convergence of the parameters $(\Omega_m, \Omega_\Lambda)$ and (α, β), we consider three other samplers. Sampler 2 is an MH within PCG sampler. It uses MH to update $(\Omega_m, \Omega_\Lambda)$ and (α, β) without conditioning on ξ or X, see the top-right panel of Fig. 2. While using MH within Gibbs samplers is a standard strategy, embedding MH into PCG samplers leads to subtleties in both theory and application, see van Dyk and Jiao (2015). We derive Sampler 2 from Sampler 1 using the three stages exactly as described in van Dyk and Jiao (2015), see Fig. 3. This guarantees that Sampler 2 has the target stationary distribution. Note that in Step 2 of Fig. 3(b), we sample $(\Omega_m, \Omega_\Lambda)$ together with (ξ, X). This full step is in fact composed of two

MH within Gibbs (Sampler 1)

1. $p(\xi, X|Y, \Omega'_m, \Omega'_\Lambda, \alpha', \beta', R'_c, R'_x, \sigma'_{\text{res}})$
2. $\mathscr{M}(\Omega_m, \Omega_\Lambda|Y, \xi, X, \alpha', \beta', R'_c, R'_x, \sigma'_{\text{res}})$
3. $p(\alpha, \beta|Y, \xi, X, \Omega_m, \Omega_\Lambda, R'_c, R'_x, \sigma'_{\text{res}})$
4. $p(R_c|Y, \xi, X, \Omega_m, \Omega_\Lambda, \alpha, \beta, R'_x, \sigma'_{\text{res}})$
5. $p(R_x|Y, \xi, X, \Omega_m, \Omega_\Lambda, \alpha, \beta, R_c, \sigma'_{\text{res}})$
6. $p(\sigma_{\text{res}}|Y, \xi, X, \Omega_m, \Omega_\Lambda, \alpha, \beta, R_c, R_x)$

MH within PCG (Sampler 2)

1. $\mathscr{M}(\Omega_m, \Omega_\Lambda|Y, \alpha', \beta', R'_c, R'_x, \sigma'_{\text{res}})$
2. $\mathscr{M}(\alpha, \beta|Y, \Omega_m, \Omega_\Lambda, R'_c, R'_x, \sigma'_{\text{res}})$
3. $p(\xi, X|Y, \Omega_m, \Omega_\Lambda, \alpha, \beta, R'_c, R'_x, \sigma'_{\text{res}})$
4. $p(R_c|Y, \xi, X, \Omega_m, \Omega_\Lambda, \alpha, \beta, R'_x, \sigma'_{\text{res}})$
5. $p(R_x|Y, \xi, X, \Omega_m, \Omega_\Lambda, \alpha, \beta, R_c, \sigma'_{\text{res}})$
6. $p(\sigma_{\text{res}}|Y, \xi, X, \Omega_m, \Omega_\Lambda, \alpha, \beta, R_c, R_x)$

ASIS (Sampler 3)

1. $p(\xi, X^\star|Y, \Omega'_m, \Omega'_\Lambda, \alpha', \beta', R'_c, R'_x, \sigma'_{\text{res}})$
2. $\mathscr{M}(\Omega^\star_m, \Omega^\star_\Lambda|Y, \xi, X^\star, \alpha', \beta', R'_c, R'_x, \sigma'_{\text{res}})$;
   Use $(\Omega^\star_m, \Omega^\star_\Lambda)$ to construct $L^\star$
3. $p(\alpha^\star, \beta^\star|Y, \xi, X^\star, \Omega^\star_m, \Omega^\star_\Lambda, R'_c, R'_x, \sigma'_{\text{res}})$;
   Use $(\alpha^\star, \beta^\star)$ to construct $A^\star$.
   Then set $\tilde{X} = A^\star X^\star + L^\star$
4. $\mathscr{M}(\Omega_m, \Omega_\Lambda|Y, \xi, \tilde{X}, \alpha^\star, \beta^\star, R'_c, R'_x, \sigma'_{\text{res}})$;
   Use $(\Omega_m, \Omega_\Lambda)$ to construct L
5. $p(\alpha, \beta|Y, \xi, \tilde{X}, \Omega_m, \Omega_\Lambda, R'_c, R'_x, \sigma'_{\text{res}})$;
   Use (α, β) to construct A.
   Then set $X = A^{-1}(\tilde{X} - L)$
6. $p(R_c|Y, \xi, X, \Omega_m, \Omega_\Lambda, \alpha, \beta, R'_x, \sigma'_{\text{res}})$
7. $p(R_x|Y, \xi, X, \Omega_m, \Omega_\Lambda, \alpha, \beta, R_c, \sigma'_{\text{res}})$
8. $p(\sigma_{\text{res}}|Y, \xi, X, \Omega_m, \Omega_\Lambda, \alpha, \beta, R_c, R_x)$

PCG within ASIS (Sampler 4)

1. $\mathscr{M}(\Omega_m, \Omega_\Lambda|Y, \alpha', \beta', R'_c, R'_x, \sigma'_{\text{res}})$;
   Use $(\Omega_m, \Omega_\Lambda)$ to construct L
2. $p(\xi, X^\star|Y, \Omega_m, \Omega_\Lambda, \alpha', \beta', R'_c, R'_x, \sigma'_{\text{res}})$
3. $p(\alpha^\star, \beta^\star|Y, \xi, X^\star, \Omega_m, \Omega_\Lambda, R'_c, R'_x, \sigma'_{\text{res}})$;
   Use $(\alpha^\star, \beta^\star)$ to construct $A^\star$.
   Then set $\tilde{X} = A^\star X^\star + L$
4. $p(\alpha, \beta|Y, \xi, \tilde{X}, \Omega_m, \Omega_\Lambda, R'_c, R'_x, \sigma'_{\text{res}})$;
   Use (α, β) to construct A.
   Then set $X = A^{-1}(\tilde{X} - L)$
5. $p(R_c|Y, \xi, X, \Omega_m, \Omega_\Lambda, \alpha, \beta, R'_x, \sigma'_{\text{res}})$
6. $p(R_x|Y, \xi, X, \Omega_m, \Omega_\Lambda, \alpha, \beta, R_c, \sigma'_{\text{res}})$
7. $p(\sigma_{\text{res}}|Y, \xi, X, \Omega_m, \Omega_\Lambda, \alpha, \beta, R_c, R_x)$

Fig. 2 Samplers 1–4. The *top-left, top-right, bottom-left and bottom-right panels* show the steps of the MH within Gibbs sampler (Sampler 1), the proper MH within PCG sampler (Sampler 2), the ASIS sampler (Sampler 3) and the PCG within ASIS sampler (Sampler 4), respectively

sub-steps: (1) MH is used to update $(\Omega_m, \Omega_\Lambda)$ from the reduced step with ξ and X integrated out; and (2) (ξ, X) is sampled from its complete conditional distribution. The joint update is denoted by $\mathscr{M}^\star$; Step 3 of Fig. 3(b) has the same structure.

Next, we construct an ASIS sampler. We derive the sufficient and ancillary augmentations for $(\Omega_m, \Omega_\Lambda)$ and (α, β) conditioning on the other parameters ξ, R_c, R_x and σ_{res}. The distribution of X conditioning on $(\Omega_m, \Omega_\Lambda)$ and (α, β) is

$$X|\Omega_m, \Omega_\Lambda, \alpha, \beta \sim \mathrm{N}(J\xi, \Sigma_P), \tag{10}$$

where $J_{(3n\times 3)} = (I, \ldots, I)^T$ with $I = \mathrm{Diag}(1, 1, 1)$, and $\Sigma_{P(3n\times 3n)} = \mathrm{Diag}(S, \ldots, S)$ with $S = \mathrm{Diag}(R_c^2, R_x^2, \sigma_{\text{res}}^2)$. Because this distribution is free of $(\Omega_m, \Omega_\Lambda)$ and (α, β), X is an ancillary augmentation for both of them. To derive a sufficient augmentation, we set $\tilde{X} = AX + L$, where $A_{(3n\times 3n)} = \mathrm{Diag}(T, \ldots, T)$ with

(a) MH within Gibbs (Sampler 1)	(b) Marginalization
1. $p(\xi, X \mid Y, \Omega_m', \Omega_\Lambda', \alpha', \beta', R_c', R_x', \sigma_{\text{res}}')$	1. $p(\xi^\star, X^\star \mid Y, \Omega_m', \Omega_\Lambda', \alpha', \beta', R_c', R_x', \sigma_{\text{res}}')$
2. $\mathscr{M}(\Omega_m, \Omega_\Lambda \mid Y, \xi, X, \alpha', \beta', R_c', R_x', \sigma_{\text{res}}')$	2. $\mathscr{M}^\star(\Omega_m, \Omega_\Lambda, \xi^\star, X^\star \mid Y, \alpha', \beta', R_c', R_x', \sigma_{\text{res}}')$
3. $p(\alpha, \beta \mid Y, \xi, X, \Omega_m, \Omega_\Lambda, R_c', R_x', \sigma_{\text{res}}')$	3. $\mathscr{M}^\star(\alpha, \beta, \xi, X \mid Y, \Omega_m, \Omega_\Lambda, R_c', R_x', \sigma_{\text{res}}')$
4. $p(R_c \mid Y, \xi, X, \Omega_m, \Omega_\Lambda, \alpha, \beta, R_x', \sigma_{\text{res}}')$	4. $p(R_c \mid Y, \xi, X, \Omega_m, \Omega_\Lambda, \alpha, \beta, R_x', \sigma_{\text{res}}')$
5. $p(R_x \mid Y, \xi, X, \Omega_m, \Omega_\Lambda, \alpha, \beta, R_c, \sigma_{\text{res}}')$	5. $p(R_x \mid Y, \xi, X, \Omega_m, \Omega_\Lambda, \alpha, \beta, R_c, \sigma_{\text{res}}')$
6. $p(\sigma_{\text{res}} \mid Y, \xi, X, \Omega_m, \Omega_\Lambda, \alpha, \beta, R_c, R_x)$	6. $p(\sigma_{\text{res}} \mid Y, \xi, X, \Omega_m, \Omega_\Lambda, \alpha, \beta, R_c, R_x)$

(c) Permute	(d) Trim (Sampler 2)
1. $\mathscr{M}^\star(\Omega_m, \Omega_\Lambda, \xi^\star, X^\star \mid Y, \alpha', \beta', R_c', R_x', \sigma_{\text{res}}')$	1. $\mathscr{M}(\Omega_m, \Omega_\Lambda \mid Y, \alpha', \beta', R_c', R_x', \sigma_{\text{res}}')$
2. $\mathscr{M}^\star(\alpha, \beta, \xi^\star, X^\star \mid Y, \Omega_m, \Omega_\Lambda, R_c', R_x', \sigma_{\text{res}}')$	2. $\mathscr{M}(\alpha, \beta \mid Y, \Omega_m, \Omega_\Lambda, R_c', R_x', \sigma_{\text{res}}')$
3. $p(\xi, X \mid Y, \Omega_m, \Omega_\Lambda, \alpha, \beta, R_c', R_x', \sigma_{\text{res}}')$	3. $p(\xi, X \mid Y, \Omega_m, \Omega_\Lambda, \alpha, \beta, R_c', R_x', \sigma_{\text{res}}')$
4. $p(R_c \mid Y, \xi, X, \Omega_m, \Omega_\Lambda, \alpha, \beta, R_x', \sigma_{\text{res}}')$	4. $p(R_c \mid Y, \xi, X, \Omega_m, \Omega_\Lambda, \alpha, \beta, R_x', \sigma_{\text{res}}')$
5. $p(R_x \mid Y, \xi, X, \Omega_m, \Omega_\Lambda, \alpha, \beta, R_c, \sigma_{\text{res}}')$	5. $p(R_x \mid Y, \xi, X, \Omega_m, \Omega_\Lambda, \alpha, \beta, R_c, \sigma_{\text{res}}')$
6. $p(\sigma_{\text{res}} \mid Y, \xi, X, \Omega_m, \Omega_\Lambda, \alpha, \beta, R_c, R_x)$	6. $p(\sigma_{\text{res}} \mid Y, \xi, X, \Omega_m, \Omega_\Lambda, \alpha, \beta, R_c, R_x)$

Fig. 3 Three-stage framework used to derive Sampler 2 from its parent MH within Gibbs sampler, i.e., Sampler 1. The parent sampler appears in (**a**) with Step 2 requiring MH. Steps 2 and 3 are marginalized in (**b**). The steps are permuted in (**c**) to allow redundant draws of (ξ, X) to be trimmed in Steps 1–2. The resulting proper MH within PCG sampler, that is, Sampler 2, appears in (**d**)

$T_{(3\times 3)} = \begin{bmatrix} 1 & 0 & 0 \\ 0 & 1 & 0 \\ \beta & -\alpha & 1 \end{bmatrix}$, and let L denote the $(3n\times 1)$ vector $(0, 0, \mu_1, \ldots, 0, 0, \mu_n)$, which is a deterministic function of $(\Omega_m, \Omega_\Lambda)$. The distribution of observed quantities Y conditioning on $\tilde{X}$, $(\Omega_m, \Omega_\Lambda)$ and (α, β) is

$$Y \mid \tilde{X}, \Omega_m, \Omega_\Lambda, \alpha, \beta \sim \mathrm{N}(\tilde{X}, \Sigma_C), \tag{11}$$

where $\Sigma_{C(3n\times 3n)} = \mathrm{Diag}(\hat{C}_1, \ldots, \hat{C}_n)$. Because this distribution is free of $(\Omega_m, \Omega_\Lambda)$ and (α, β), $\tilde{X}$ is a sufficient augmentation for both parameters. Sampler 3 is the ASIS sampler corresponding to this pair of sufficient and ancillary augmentations. Specifically, we implement ASIS conditioning on ξ, R_c, R_x and σ_{res}: (1) (ξ, X) is sampled from its complete conditional distribution; (2) $(\Omega_m, \Omega_\Lambda)$ and (α, β) are updated conditioning on X, and X is transformed to $\tilde{X}$ conditioning on $(\Omega_m, \Omega_\Lambda)$ and (α, β); and (3) $(\Omega_m, \Omega_\Lambda)$ and (α, β) are updated again but conditioning on $\tilde{X}$. Both of the updates of $(\Omega_m, \Omega_\Lambda)$ require MH. See the bottom-left panel of Fig. 2 for the steps of Sampler 3.

Sampler 4 combines MH within PCG and ASIS. Conditioning on (α, β), we update $(\Omega_m, \Omega_\Lambda)$ with MH within PCG, and then conditioning on $(\Omega_m, \Omega_\Lambda)$, we update (α, β) with ASIS. See the bottom-right panel of Fig. 2 for its steps. It is easy to verify that Sampler 4 is proper. Assume $(\xi', X', \Omega_m', \Omega_\Lambda', \alpha', \beta', R_c', R_x', \sigma_{\text{res}}')$ is a draw from the target distribution. Although in Step 1 of Sampler 4, we sample $(\Omega_m, \Omega_\Lambda)$ without conditioning on (ξ, X), the marginal distribution of $(\Omega_m, \Omega_\Lambda, \alpha', \beta', R_c', R_x', \sigma_{\text{res}}')$ is still that of the target. After updating (ξ, X) from its complete conditional distribution in Step 2, $(\xi, X, \Omega_m, \Omega_\Lambda, \alpha', \beta', R_c', R_x', \sigma_{\text{res}}')$ follows the target distribution. Since the distribution of (X, α, β) is equivalent to that of $(\tilde{X}, \alpha, \beta)$ conditioning on the other parameters, when we transform back to (X, α, β) at the end of Step 4, $(\xi, X, \Omega_m, \Omega_\Lambda, \alpha, \beta, R_c', R_x', \sigma_{\text{res}}')$ follows the target distribution. In addition, the steps that sample R_c, R_x and σ_{res} are standard Gibbs steps which preserve the target stationary distribution. Thus, Sampler 4 is proper.

4 Analysis of Observed Type Ia SNe

To illustrate the relative efficiencies of Samplers 1–4, we use a data set consisting of 288 Type Ia SN observations compiled by Kessler (2009). To sample from the posterior distribution of the hierarchical Gaussian model, we run each of Samplers 1–4, starting with the same sets of initial values.[2] While we run Samplers 2–4 for 11,000 iterations with a burn-in of 1000, we run Sampler 1 for 12,000 iterations with a burn-in of 2000. We double the length of burn-in for Sampler 1 to obtain satisfactory convergence.[3]

Figures 4 and 5 show the convergence properties of Samplers 1–4. For each sampler, we display the time-series plots (left column) and autocorrelation plots (right column) for Ω_m, Ω_Λ, α and β. For all four parameters, Samplers 2–4 produce chains with much faster mixing and lower autocorrelation than Sampler 1. To further compare the convergence, we estimate the effective sample size (ESS),

$$\text{ESS}(\psi) = \frac{T}{1 + 2\sum_{t=1}^{\infty} \rho_t(\psi)}, \tag{12}$$

where T is the total posterior sample size and $\rho_t(\psi)$ is the lag-t autocorrelation of the parameter ψ. The ESS approximates the size of an independent sample with equivalent information in terms of the Monte Carlo variance of the sample mean, and is indicative of how well the chain mixes, see Kass et al. (1998) and Liu (2001). We use the function "effectiveSize" in the R package `coda` to estimate the ESS. We display the ESS (in parentheses) and ESS per second of Ω_m, Ω_Λ, α and β in Table 1. (The total CPU time required by each sampler is also reported in Table 1.) The larger the ESS per second, the more efficient is the sampler. By this measurement, Samplers 2–4 all substantially improve the convergence properties of Sampler 1.

[2] We use Python to implement all the samplers, and all the chains are run on a Macbook Pro with a system of OS X 10.8.5 and a processor of 2.5 GHz Intel Core i5.

[3] To check convergence, we ran each sampler with three different overdispersed initial values. The Gelman-Rubin statistic (Gelman et al. 2013; Gelman and Rubin 1992) suggested adequate convergence after only a few iterations for Samplers 2–4. (A burn-in of 1000 iterations was quite conservative for Samplers 2–4.) For Sampler 1, however, a burn-in of 2000 iterations was required.

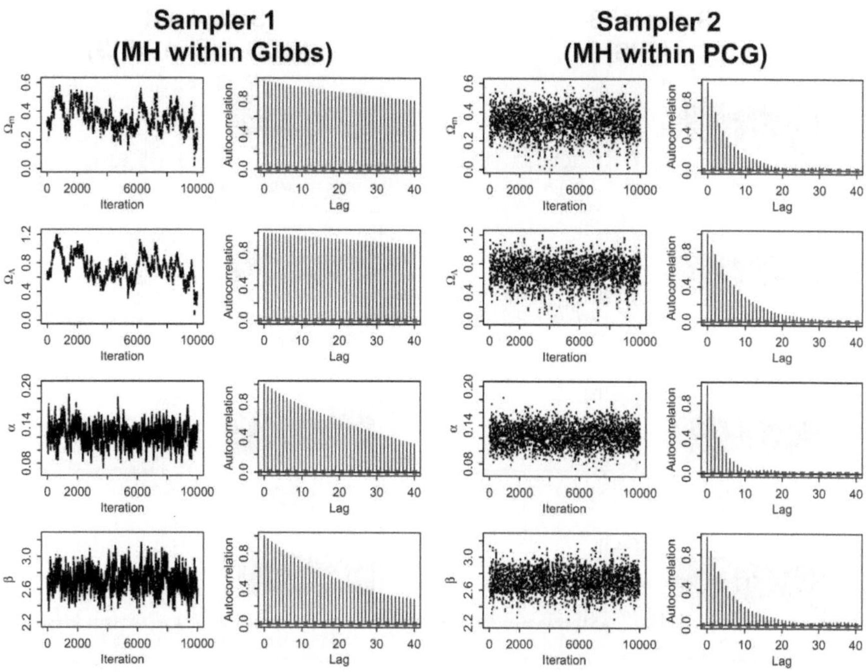

Fig. 4 The sampling results of Samplers 1 and 2. The *left two columns* are the time-series and autocorrelation plots for the posterior draws of Ω_m, Ω_Λ, α and β respectively from Sampler 1, while the *right two columns* are those from Sampler 2

Thus we confirm that both PCG and ASIS are efficient in improving convergence. More interestingly, ASIS is less efficient in improving the convergence of $(\Omega_m, \Omega_\Lambda)$ than MH within PCG, while better in improving the convergence of (α, β). When we combine these two strategies into Sampler 4, the result outperforms both Samplers 2 and 3 in terms of ESS per second. (Although Sampler 3 is slightly better than Sampler 4 for α, it takes around 15% longer to obtain the same ESS for β, and more than four times longer for both Ω_m and Ω_Λ.) Even though CPU time can vary somewhat from run to run, the ESS also clearly shows the advantage of Sampler 4. See Jiao and van Dyk (2016) for more on a general strategy for combining several state-of-the-art strategies into a single sampler.

Finally, in Table 2, we report the posterior means and standard deviations of Ω_m, Ω_Λ, α, β, σ_{res}, R_c and R_x for Samplers 1–4. We also plot the 68% and 95% contours of the joint posterior distribution of Ω_m and Ω_Λ, and the marginal posterior densities of Ω_m, Ω_Λ, α and β computed with Samplers 1–4, see Fig. 6. Although the samplers all give similar estimates of the posterior moments, Samplers 2–4 better represent the shape of the joint posterior distribution of Ω_m and Ω_Λ; see left panel of Fig. 6.

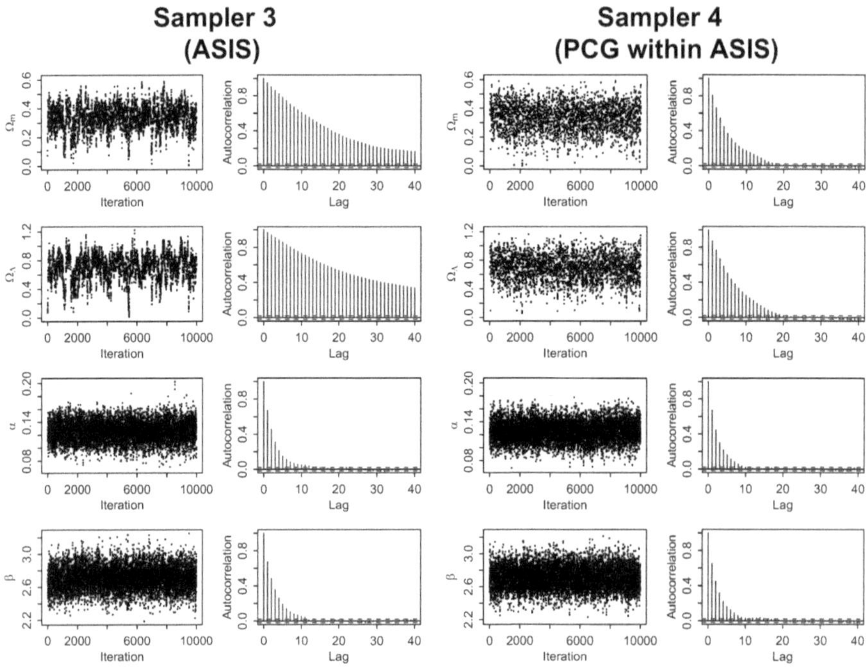

Fig. 5 The sampling results of Samplers 3 and 4. The *left two columns* are the time-series and autocorrelation plots for the posterior draws of Ω_m, Ω_Λ, α and β respectively from Sampler 3, while the *right two columns* are those from Sampler 4

Table 1 The ESS per second and ESS (in parentheses) of Ω_m, Ω_Λ, α and β for Samplers 1–4

	Sampler 1	Sampler 2	Sampler 3	Sampler 4
Ω_m	0.0017 (32.0544)	0.0366 (1030.40)	0.0097 (251.552)	0.0411 (1021.14)
Ω_Λ	0.0010 (18.2937)	0.0229 (643.963)	0.0060 (155.240)	0.0269 (667.807)
α	0.0075 (139.844)	0.0507 (1428.54)	0.0759 (1976.15)	0.0731 (1816.16)
β	0.0096 (178.910)	0.0285 (801.793)	0.0643 (1673.59)	0.0737 (1829.53)
CPU time (s)	18630.82	28178.60	26021.07	24832.64

The CPU time consumed by each of the four samplers is reported in the last row

Table 2 Posterior means (and standard deviations) of Ω_m, Ω_Λ, α, β, σ_{res}, R_c and R_x computed with Samplers 1–4

	Sampler 1	Sampler 2	Sampler 3	Sampler 4
Ω_m	0.353 (0.085)	0.337 (0.085)	0.335 (0.086)	0.341 (0.090)
Ω_Λ	0.730 (0.172)	0.706 (0.167)	0.701 (0.177)	0.710 (0.174)
α	0.124 (0.016)	0.125 (0.015)	0.125 (0.015)	0.125 (0.015)
β	2.710 (0.136)	2.710 (0.132)	2.709 (0.138)	2.713 (0.135)
σ_{res}	0.127 (0.011)	0.127 (0.011)	0.127 (0.011)	0.127 (0.011)
R_c	0.101 (0.005)	0.102 (0.006)	0.101 (0.005)	0.101 (0.006)
R_x	0.904 (0.052)	0.905 (0.050)	0.904 (0.050)	0.903 (0.050)

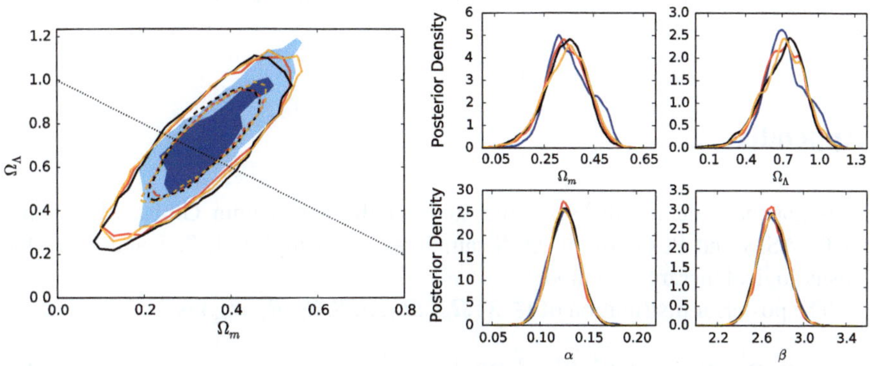

Fig. 6 Graphical representation of the posterior distribution computed with each of Samplers 1–4. The *left panel* gives the 68% and 95% contours of the joint posterior distribution of Ω_m and Ω_Λ. (These correspond to highest posterior density regions.) The *right panel* gives the marginal posterior distributions of Ω_m, Ω_Λ, α and β. *Blue, red, black and orange* represent Samplers 1, 2, 3 and 4 respectively. For Sampler 1, we use *dark and light blue* to represent the 68% and 95% contours; for the other samplers we use *dashed* and *solid lines* to distinguish

5 Conclusion

To explore the acceleration of the expansion of the universe, we analyze Type Ia SN data by embedding a cosmological model into a Bayesian hierarchical Gaussian model. This hierarchical model naturally reflects the structure of the problem and treats the uncertainties in a more consistent way.

Because of its complexity, the hierarchical model is an ideal testing ground for our new algorithms. By comparing the performance of four samplers, we confirm the efficiency of both PCG and ASIS in improving convergence properties of Gibbs-type samplers. Furthermore, we find that we can gain more efficiency by combining two or more strategies into a single sampler. Sometimes, it is necessary to do this. For example, when using an MH algorithm within a Gibbs-type sampler because direct sampling from some conditionals is difficult (Gilks et al. 1995; van Dyk and Jiao 2015). But more intriguingly, when there is more than one parameter whose convergence requires improvement, it is sometimes the case that one strategy can significantly improve the convergence of one parameter but has little effect on other parameters, while another strategy has the opposite effect. Under this circumstance, we can gain more efficiency by combining two or more strategies than by using either alone. Even if one strategy alone is fairly good for all the parameters, we prefer to use a combination, as long as the gained efficiency can compensate the extra computational burden.

Acknowledgements David van Dyk acknowledges partial support for this work from a Wolfson Research Merit Award (WM110023) provided by the British Royal Society and from a Marie-Curie Career Integration Grant (FP7-PEOPLE-2012-CIG-321865) provided by the European Commission; Roberto Trotta acknowledges partial support from an EPSRC "Pathways to Impact" grant.

Appendix

This appendix details the sampling steps of the MH within Gibbs, MH within PCG, ASIS and PCG within ASIS samplers, i.e., Samplers 1, 2, 3 and 4, for the cosmological hierarchical model.

The posterior distribution of $(\xi, X, \Omega_m, \Omega_\Lambda, \alpha, \beta, R_c^2, R_x^2, \sigma_{\rm res}^2)$ is

$$\begin{aligned} & p(\xi, X, \Omega_m, \Omega_\Lambda, \alpha, \beta, R_c^2, R_x^2, \sigma_{\rm res}^2 | Y) \\ & \propto |\Sigma_C|^{-1/2} |\Sigma_P|^{-1/2} |\Sigma_0|^{-1/2} \exp\Bigg\{ -\frac{1}{2} \big[(Y - AX - L)^T \Sigma_C^{-1} (Y - AX - L) \\ & + (X - J\xi)^T \Sigma_P^{-1} (X - J\xi) + (\xi - \xi_m)^T \Sigma_0^{-1} (\xi - \xi_m) \big] \Bigg\} \frac{1}{R_c^2} \frac{1}{R_x^2} \frac{1}{\sigma_{\rm res}^2}, \end{aligned} \tag{13}$$

where $\xi_m = (0, 0, M_m)$ and $\Sigma_0 = \text{Diag}(\sigma_{c0}^2, \sigma_{x0}^2, \sigma_{M_0}^2)$; Σ_C, Σ_P, J, A and L are defined in Sect. 3.2. Setting $\tilde{X} = AX + L$, the joint posterior distribution of $(\xi, \tilde{X}, \Omega_m, \Omega_\Lambda, \alpha, \beta, R_c^2, R_x^2, \sigma_{\rm res}^2)$ is

$$\begin{aligned} & p(\xi, \tilde{X}, \Omega_m, \Omega_\Lambda, \alpha, \beta, R_c^2, R_x^2, \sigma_{\rm res}^2 | Y) \\ & \propto |\Sigma_C|^{-1/2} |\Sigma_P|^{-1/2} |\Sigma_0|^{-1/2} \exp\Bigg\{ -\frac{1}{2} \Big[(Y - \tilde{X})^T \Sigma_C^{-1} (Y - \tilde{X}) \\ & + (A^{-1}\tilde{X} - A^{-1}L - J\xi)^T \Sigma_P^{-1} (A^{-1}\tilde{X} - A^{-1}L - J\xi) \\ & + (\xi - \xi_m)^T \Sigma_0^{-1} (\xi - \xi_m) \Big] \Bigg\} \frac{1}{R_c^2} \frac{1}{R_x^2} \frac{1}{\sigma_{\rm res}^2}. \end{aligned} \tag{14}$$

Furthermore, integrating out (ξ, X), the marginal distribution of $(\Omega_m, \Omega_\Lambda, \alpha, \beta, R_c^2, R_x^2, \sigma_{\rm res}^2)$ is

$$
\begin{aligned}
&p(\Omega_m, \Omega_\Lambda, \alpha, \beta, R_c^2, R_x^2, \sigma_{\text{res}}^2 | Y) \\
&\quad \propto |\Sigma_C|^{-1/2} |\Sigma_P|^{-1/2} |\Sigma_A|^{1/2} |K|^{1/2} |\Sigma_0|^{-1/2} \frac{1}{R_c^2} \frac{1}{R_x^2} \frac{1}{\sigma_{\text{res}}^2} \\
&\quad \times \exp\left\{ -\frac{1}{2} \left[(Y-L)^T \Sigma_C^{-1} (Y-L) - \Delta^T \Sigma_A \Delta - k_0^T K^{-1} k_0 + \xi_m^T \Sigma_0^{-1} \xi_m \right] \right\},
\end{aligned} \tag{15}
$$

where $\Sigma_A^{-1} = A^T \Sigma_C^{-1} A + \Sigma_P^{-1}$, $K^{-1} = -J^T \Sigma_P^{-1} \Sigma_A \Sigma_P^{-1} J + J^T \Sigma_P^{-1} J + \Sigma_0^{-1}$, $\Delta = A^T \Sigma_C^{-1}(Y - L)$, and $k_0 = K(J^T \Sigma_P^{-1} \Sigma_A \Delta + \Sigma_0^{-1} \xi_m)$.

When MH updates are required in any of the samplers, we use truncated normal distributions as the proposal distributions. These distributions are centered at the current draws with variance-covariance matrices adjusted to obtain an acceptance rate of around 25%. The truncation enforces prior constraints and in all cases the MH updates are bivariate.

When generating parameters from a truncated distribution, we repeat drawing from the corresponding unconstrained distribution until the truncation condition is satisfied. In the cosmological example, rejection sampling is not computationally demanding, since the ranges of the prior distributions are fairly large.

The steps of Sampler 1 are

1. Sample (ξ, X), which consists of two sub-steps:
   - Sample ξ from $\text{N}(k_0, K)$;
   - Sample X from $\text{N}(\mu_A, \Sigma_A)$, where $\mu_A = \Sigma_A(\Delta + \Sigma_P^{-1} J\xi)$.
2. Use MH to sample $(\Omega_m, \Omega_\Lambda)$ from $p(\Omega_m, \Omega_\Lambda | Y, \xi, X, \alpha, \beta, R_c^2, R_x^2, \sigma_{\text{res}}^2)$, which is proportional to $p(\xi, X, \Omega_m, \Omega_\Lambda, \alpha, \beta, R_c^2, R_x^2, \sigma_{\text{res}}^2 | Y)$, under the constraint $(\Omega_m, \Omega_\Lambda) \in [0, 1] \times [0, 2]$.
3. Sample (α, β) from $\text{N}(\mu_B, \Sigma_B)$ with constraint $(\alpha, \beta) \in [0, 1] \times [0, 4]$, where

$$
\Sigma_B^{-1} = \begin{bmatrix} \sum_{i=1}^{n} \frac{x_i^2}{\hat{\sigma}_{mBi}^2} & \sum_{i=1}^{n} \frac{-x_i c_i}{\hat{\sigma}_{mBi}^2} \\ \sum_{i=1}^{n} \frac{-x_i c_i}{\hat{\sigma}_{mBi}^2} & \sum_{i=1}^{n} \frac{c_i^2}{\hat{\sigma}_{mBi}^2} \end{bmatrix} \text{ and } \mu_B = \Sigma_B \begin{bmatrix} \sum_{i=1}^{n} \frac{x_i(M_i - \hat{m}_{Bi} + \mu_i)}{\hat{\sigma}_{mBi}^2} \\ \sum_{i=1}^{n} \frac{-c_i(M_i - \hat{m}_{Bi} + \mu_i)}{\hat{\sigma}_{mBi}^2} \end{bmatrix}. \tag{16}
$$

4. Sample R_c^2 from Inv-Gamma $\left[\frac{n}{2}, \frac{\sum_{i=1}^{n}(c_i - c_0)^2}{2}\right]$ with $\log(R_c) \in [-5, 2]$.
5. Sample R_x^2 from Inv-Gamma $\left[\frac{n}{2}, \frac{\sum_{i=1}^{n}(x_i - x_0)^2}{2}\right]$ with $\log(R_x) \in [-5, 2]$.
6. Sample σ_{res}^2 from Inv-Gamma $\left[\frac{n}{2}, \frac{\sum_{i=1}^{n}(M_i - M_0)^2}{2}\right]$ with $\log(\sigma_{\text{res}}) \in [-5, 2]$.

The steps of Sampler 2 are

1. Use MH to sample $(\Omega_m, \Omega_\Lambda)$ from $p(\Omega_m, \Omega_\Lambda|Y, \alpha, \beta, R_c^2, R_x^2, \sigma_{\text{res}}^2)$, which is proportional to $p(\Omega_m, \Omega_\Lambda, \alpha, \beta, R_c^2, R_x^2, \sigma_{\text{res}}^2|Y)$, with $(\Omega_m, \Omega_\Lambda) \in [0, 1] \times [0, 2]$.
2. Use MH to sample (α, β) from $p(\alpha, \beta|Y, \Omega_m, \Omega_\Lambda, R_c^2, R_x^2, \sigma_{\text{res}}^2)$, which is proportional to $p(\Omega_m, \Omega_\Lambda, \alpha, \beta, R_c^2, R_x^2, \sigma_{\text{res}}^2|Y)$, with $(\alpha, \beta) \in [0, 1] \times [0, 4]$.
3. Sample (ξ, X), which consists of two sub-steps:
   - Sample ξ from $\mathrm{N}(k_0, K)$;
   - Sample X from $\mathrm{N}(\mu_A, \Sigma_A)$, where $\mu_A = \Sigma_A(\Delta + \Sigma_P^{-1}J\xi)$.
4. Sample R_c^2 from Inv-Gamma$\left[\frac{n}{2}, \frac{\sum_{i=1}^n (c_i - c_0)^2}{2}\right]$ with $\log(R_c) \in [-5, 2]$.
5. Sample R_x^2 from Inv-Gamma$\left[\frac{n}{2}, \frac{\sum_{i=1}^n (x_i - x_0)^2}{2}\right]$ with $\log(R_x) \in [-5, 2]$.
6. Sample σ_{res}^2 from Inv-Gamma$\left[\frac{n}{2}, \frac{\sum_{i=1}^n (M_i - M_0)^2}{2}\right]$ with $\log(\sigma_{\text{res}}) \in [-5, 2]$.

The steps of Sampler 3 are

1. Sample $(\xi, X^\star)$, which consists of two sub-steps:
   - Sample ξ from $\mathrm{N}(k_0, K)$;
   - Sample $X^\star$ from $\mathrm{N}(\mu_A, \Sigma_A)$, where $\mu_A = \Sigma_A(\Delta + \Sigma_P^{-1}J\xi)$.
2. Use MH to sample $(\Omega_m^\star, \Omega_\Lambda^\star)$ from $p(\Omega_m, \Omega_\Lambda|Y, \xi, X^\star, \alpha, \beta, R_c^2, R_x^2, \sigma_{\text{res}}^2)$, which is proportional to $p(\xi, X^\star, \Omega_m^\star, \Omega_\Lambda^\star, \alpha, \beta, R_c^2, R_x^2, \sigma_{\text{res}}^2|Y)$, under the constraint $(\Omega_m^\star, \Omega_\Lambda^\star) \in [0, 1] \times [0, 2]$; Use $(\Omega_m^\star, \Omega_\Lambda^\star)$ to construct $L^\star$.
3. Sample $(\alpha^\star, \beta^\star)$ from $\mathrm{N}(\mu_B, \Sigma_B)$ with constraint $(\alpha^\star, \beta^\star) \in [0, 1] \times [0, 4]$; Use $(\alpha^\star, \beta^\star)$ to construct $A^\star$. Then set $\tilde{X} = A^\star X^\star + L^\star$.
4. Use MH to sample $(\Omega_m, \Omega_\Lambda)$ from $p(\Omega_m, \Omega_\Lambda|Y, \xi, \tilde{X}, \alpha^\star, \beta^\star, R_c^2, R_x^2, \sigma_{\text{res}}^2)$, which is proportional to $p(\xi, \tilde{X}, \Omega_m, \Omega_\Lambda, \alpha^\star, \beta^\star, R_c^2, R_x^2, \sigma_{\text{res}}^2|Y)$, under the constraint $(\Omega_m, \Omega_\Lambda) \in [0, 1] \times [0, 2]$; Use $(\Omega_m, \Omega_\Lambda)$ to construct L.
5. Sample (α, β) from $\mathrm{N}(\mu_D, \Sigma_D)$ with constraint $(\alpha, \beta) \in [0, 1] \times [0, 4]$, where

$$\Sigma_D^{-1} = \begin{bmatrix} \sum\limits_{i=1}^n \frac{\tilde{x}_i^2}{\sigma_{\text{res}}^2} & \sum\limits_{i=1}^n \frac{-\tilde{x}_i\tilde{c}_i}{\sigma_{\text{res}}^2} \\ \sum\limits_{i=1}^n \frac{-\tilde{x}_i\tilde{c}_i}{\sigma_{\text{res}}^2} & \sum\limits_{i=1}^n \frac{\tilde{c}_i^2}{\sigma_{\text{res}}^2} \end{bmatrix} \text{ and } \mu_D = \Sigma_D \begin{bmatrix} \sum_{i=1}^n \frac{\tilde{x}_i(M_0 - \tilde{M}_i)}{\sigma_{\text{res}}^2} \\ \sum_{i=1}^n \frac{-\tilde{c}_i(M_0 - \tilde{M}_i)}{\sigma_{\text{res}}^2} \end{bmatrix}, \tag{17}$$

   where $\tilde{c}_i, \tilde{x}_i$ and $\tilde{M}_i$ are the $(3i-2)^{\text{th}}$, $(3i-1)^{\text{th}}$ and $(3i)^{\text{th}}$ components of $(\tilde{X} - L)$; Use (α, β) to construct A. Then set $X = A^{-1}(\tilde{X} - L)$.
6. Sample R_c^2 from Inv-Gamma$\left[\frac{n}{2}, \frac{\sum_{i=1}^n (c_i - c_0)^2}{2}\right]$ with $\log(R_c) \in [-5, 2]$.
7. Sample R_x^2 from Inv-Gamma$\left[\frac{n}{2}, \frac{\sum_{i=1}^n (x_i - x_0)^2}{2}\right]$ with $\log(R_x) \in [-5, 2]$.
8. Sample σ_{res}^2 from Inv-Gamma$\left[\frac{n}{2}, \frac{\sum_{i=1}^n (M_i - M_0)^2}{2}\right]$ with $\log(\sigma_{\text{res}}) \in [-5, 2]$.

The steps of Sampler 4 are

1. Use MH to sample $(\Omega_m, \Omega_\Lambda)$ from $p(\Omega_m, \Omega_\Lambda | Y, \alpha, \beta, R_c^2, R_x^2, \sigma_{\text{res}}^2)$, which is proportional to $p(\Omega_m, \Omega_\Lambda, \alpha, \beta, R_c^2, R_x^2, \sigma_{\text{res}}^2 | Y)$ with $(\Omega_m, \Omega_\Lambda) \in [0,1] \times [0,2]$; Use $(\Omega_m, \Omega_\Lambda)$ to construct L.
2. Sample $(\xi, X^\star)$, which consists of two sub-steps:
   - Sample ξ from $\mathrm{N}(k_0, K)$;
   - Sample $X^\star$ from $\mathrm{N}(\mu_A, \Sigma_A)$, where $\mu_A = \Sigma_A(\Delta + \Sigma_P^{-1} J \xi)$.
3. Sample $(\alpha^\star, \beta^\star)$ from $\mathrm{N}(\mu_B, \Sigma_B)$ with constraint $(\alpha^\star, \beta^\star) \in [0,1] \times [0,4]$; Use $(\alpha^\star, \beta^\star)$ to construct $A^\star$. Then set $\tilde{X} = A^\star X^\star + L$.
4. Sample (α, β) from $\mathrm{N}(\mu_D, \Sigma_D)$ with constraint $(\alpha, \beta) \in [0,1] \times [0,4]$; Use (α, β) to construct A. Then set $X = A^{-1}(\tilde{X} - L)$.
5. Sample R_c^2 from Inv-Gamma$\left[\frac{n}{2}, \frac{\sum_{i=1}^n (c_i - c_0)^2}{2}\right]$ with $\log(R_c) \in [-5, 2]$.
6. Sample R_x^2 from Inv-Gamma$\left[\frac{n}{2}, \frac{\sum_{i=1}^n (x_i - x_0)^2}{2}\right]$ with $\log(R_x) \in [-5, 2]$.
7. Sample σ_{res}^2 from Inv-Gamma$\left[\frac{n}{2}, \frac{\sum_{i=1}^n (M_i - M_0)^2}{2}\right]$ with $\log(\sigma_{\text{res}}) \in [-5, 2]$.

References

Carroll, R. J., Ruppert, D., Stefanski, L. A., & Crainiceanu, C. (2006). *Measurement error in nonlinear models: A modern perspective* (2nd ed.). Chapman & Hall/CRC monographs on statistics & applied probability. London: Chapman & Hall/CRC.

Gelman, A., Carlin, J. B., Stern, H. S., Dunson, D. B., Vehtari, A., & Rubin, D. B. (2013). *Bayesian data analysis* (3rd ed.). Chapman & Hall/CRC texts in statistical science. London: Chapman & Hall/CRC.

Gelman, A., & Rubin, D. B. (1992). Inference from iterative simulation using multiple sequences. *Statistical Science, 7*, 457–472.

Geman, S., & Geman, D. (1984). Stochastic relaxation, Gibbs distributions, and the Bayesian restoration of images. *IEEE Transactions on Pattern Analysis and Machine Intelligence, 6*, 721–741.

Gilks, W. R., Best, N. G., & Tan, K. K. C. (1995). Adaptive rejection Metropolis sampling within Gibbs sampling. *Journal of the Royal Statistical Society, 44*, 455–472.

Guy, J., Astier, P., Baumont, S., Hardin, D., Pain, R., Regnault, N., et al. (2007). SALT2: Using distant supernovae to improve the use of type Ia supernovae as distance indicators. *Astronomy and Astrophysics, 466*, 11–21.

Hastings, W. K. (1970). Monte Carlo sampling methods using Markov chains and their applications. *Biometrika, 57*, 97–109.

Jiao, X. Y., & van Dyk, D. A. (2016). Combining strategies for improving the performance of Gibbs-type samplers. In preparation.

Kass, R. E., Carlin, B. P., Gelman, A., & Neal, R. M. (1998). Markov Chain Monte Carlo in practice: A roundtable discussion. *The American Statistician, 52*, 93–100.

Kessler, R. (2009). First-year sloan digital sky survey-II supernova results: Hubble diagram and cosmological parameters. *The Astrophysical Journal Supplement, 185*, 32–84.

Liu, J. S. (2001). *Monte Carlo strategies in scientific computing*. New York: Springer.

Liu, J. S., Wong, W. H., & Kong, A. (1994). Covariance structure of the Gibbs sampler with applications to comparisons of estimators and augmentation schemes. *Biometrika, 81*, 27–40.

Liu, J. S., Wong, W. H., & Kong, A. (1995). Covariance structure and convergence rate of the Gibbs sampler with various scan. *Journal of the Royal Statistical Society, Series B. Statistical Methodology, 57*, 157–169.

March, M. C., Trotta, R., Berkes, P., Starkman, G. D., & Vaudrevange, P. M. (2011). Improved constraints on cosmological parameters from SNIa data. *Monthly Notices of the Royal Astronomical Society, 418*, 2308–2329.

Metropolis, N., Rosenbluth, A. W., Rosenbluth, M. N., Teller, A. H., & Teller, E. (1953). Equations of state calculations by fast computing machines. *The Journal of Chemical Physics, 21*, 1087–1092.

Park, T., & van Dyk, D. A. (2009). Partially collapsed Gibbs samplers: Illustrations and applications. *Journal of Computational and Graphical Statistics, 18*, 283–305.

Phillips, M. M. (1993). The absolute magnitudes of type Ia supernovae. *The Astrophysical Journal, 413*, L105–L108.

Phillips, M. M., Lira, P., Suntzeff, N. B., Schommer, R. A., Hamuy, M., & Maza, J. (1999). The reddening-free decline rate versus luminosity relationship for type Ia supernovae. *Astronomy Journal, 118*, 1766–1776.

Robert, C., & Casella, G. (2004). *Monte Carlo statistical methods* (2nd ed.). Springer texts in statistics. New York: Springer.

Tanner, M. A., & Wong, W. H. (1987). The calculation of posterior distributions by data augmentation (with discussion). *Journal of the American Statistical Association, 82*, 528–550.

van Dyk, D. A., & Jiao, X. Y. (2015). Metropolis-Hastings within partially collapsed Gibbs samplers. *Journal of Computational and Graphical Statistics, 24*, 301–327.

van Dyk, D. A., & Meng, X. L. (2001). The art of data augmentation (with discussion). *Journal of Computational and Graphical Statistics, 10*, 1–50.

van Dyk, D. A., & Park, T. (2008). Partially collapsed Gibbs samplers: Theory and methods. *Journal of the American Statistical Association, 103*, 790–796.

Yu, Y., & Meng, X. L. (2011). To center or not to center: That is not the question—an ancillarity-sufficiency interweaving strategy (ASIS) for boosting MCMC efficiency (with discussion). *Journal of Computational and Graphical Statistics, 20*, 531–570.

Dynamic Spatial Pattern Recognition in Count Data

Xia Wang, Ming-Hui Chen, Rita C. Kuo, and Dipak K. Dey

Abstract This study explores a Bayesian regression analysis for count data in the presence of spatial and temporal correlations. The contribution is to develop a regression model for count data that provides flexibility in modeling the complexity of zero-inflation, overdispersion, as well as spatial patterns in a dynamic manner. More importantly, it improves the computational efficiency via dimension reduction while handling the high-dimensional correlation structure in the data. The proposed model is applied to the survey data by the Northeast Fisheries Sciences Center (NEFSC) for estimation and prediction of the Atlantic cod in the Gulf of Maine—Georges Bank region. Both zero-inflated Poisson and negative binomial models are fitted. Model comparison shows the improvement in model fitting with consideration in the spatial-temporal correlation as well as the overdispersion in the count data.

1 Introduction

Count data are commonly available in the fields of ecology, epidemiology, marketing, political sciences, and many others. Quite often, the locations and the time stamps regarding the count data are also available. For instance, Wang et al. (2015) described a survey data by the Northeast Fisheries Sciences Center (NEFSC) in the Gulf of Maine—Georges Bank region during 1970–2008. Figure 1 shows a snapshot of data for the presence and the number of Atlantic cods caught in 1977, 1987, 1997, and 2007. There is a large proportion of zero counts in the number

X. Wang
Department of Mathematical Sciences, University of Cincinnati, Cincinnati, OH, USA
e-mail: xia.wang@uc.edu

M.-H. Chen (✉) • D.K. Dey
Department of Statistics, University of Connecticut, Storrs, CT, USA
e-mail: ming-hui.chen@uconn.edu; dipak.dey@uconn.edu

R.C. Kuo
Joint Genome Institute, Lawrence Berkeley National Laboratory, Walnut Creek, CA, USA
e-mail: rckuo@lbl.gov

Z. Jin et al. (eds.), *New Developments in Statistical Modeling, Inference and Application*, ICSA Book Series in Statistics, DOI 10.1007/978-3-319-42571-9_10

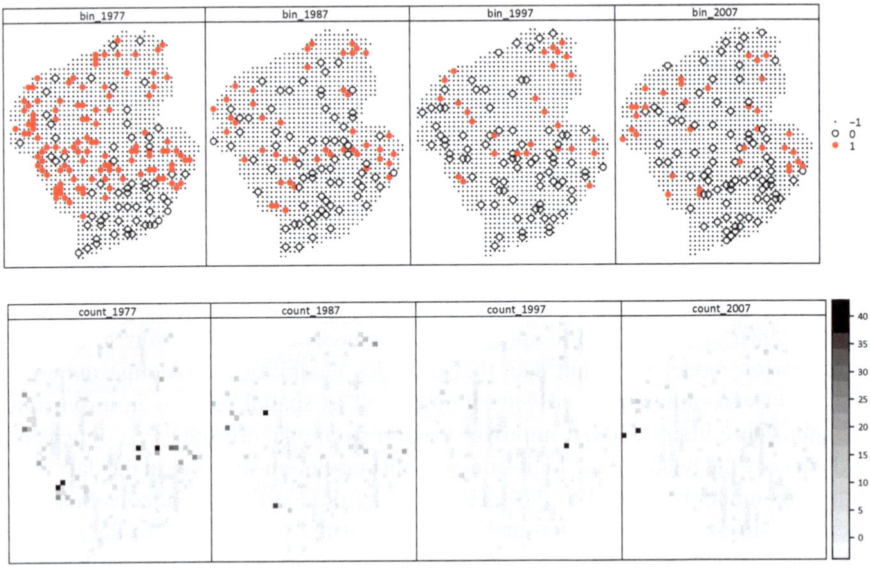

Fig. 1 A 40-year snapshot of survey locations, presence and abundance for the Atlantic cods in NEFSC survey data. *Upper panel*: surveyed grids with fish caught (*solid circle (1)*), surveyed grids without fish caught (*empty circle (0)*) and grids that were not surveyed (*dot (-1)*). *Lower panel*: counts of fish caught in the surveyed grids (capped at 40)

of cods caught in a tow, which can be clearly seen in Fig. 2 as a histogram for the counts. A few very large count values also suggest that there are potential extra overdispersion that cannot be accounted by the Poisson model. In an initial exploratory analysis, a simple zero-inflated Poisson model (ZIP) is fitted to these count data. The Pearson χ^2 statistic computed based on the ZIP model shows that $X^2 = 23545.74$ with 4852.61 degrees of freedom ($d.f.$), which is much larger than the one under the Poisson assumption (i.e., $X^2/d.f. \approx 1$). Thus, besides the potential spatial and temporal correlation features, these data, like many other count data, are also complicated by excess zeros and overdispersion.

This paper sets out to consider the task of modeling count data with the above complications, that is, spatially and temporally correlated count data in the presence of excess zeros and overdispersion. Particularly, our contributions lie in two aspects. First, it explores and compares the zero-inflated Poisson (ZIP) and the zero-inflated negative binomial (ZINB) models with dynamic and spatial correlated random effects. It is one of few studies that carry out this comparison directly. Second, it applies the newly developed Bayesian spatial-temporal model (Wang et al. 2015) to improve the computational efficiency with the overdispersion parameter introduced in the model.

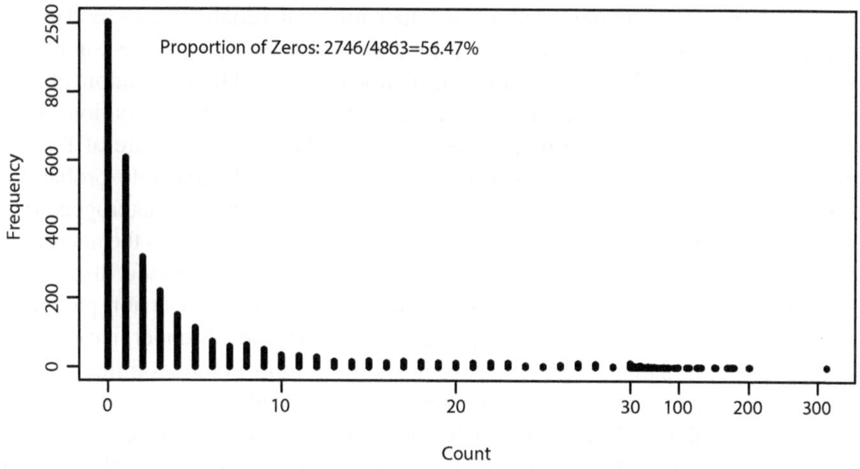

Fig. 2 The counts of Atlantic cod caught in a tow in the Gulf of Maine—Georges Bank region during 1970–2008

Zero counts in the data can have quite different scientific implications: a "true" zero when the surveyed subject truly does not exist or a "false" zero when the surveyed subject exists but was randomly sampled as zero due to imperfect detection or other mechanisms leading to insufficient information. Some data contain only "true" zeros, while other data contain a mixture of "true" and "false" zeros. How to model the excess zeros depends on the generating process of zeros in the data. A case with only "true" zeros is illustrated in Ver Hoef and Jansen (2007). In their study of haulout patterns of harbor seals on glacial ice, it is stated that it is highly likely for seals to be detected, if present, because of the good quality video showing a high contrast between the dark seals and the lighter-colored ice. In this case, it is reasonable to treat the zeros in data as true absence. When the zeros can only be true zeros, a two-stage model is applied first to model the zero versus nonzero observations and then to model the count process conditional on positive outcomes (Recta et al. 2012; Ver Hoef and Jansen 2007). In our motivating example, though, zeros may be either true absence or presence but not caught. The zero-inflated count model is a natural way to model the two types of zeros via a mixture of a Bernoulli distribution and a count distribution, such as ZIP or ZINB.

Compared to the ZIP model, the ZINB model provides flexibility in modeling overdispersion and explicitly accommodating heterogeneity. Overdispersion often presents in count data collected in a survey study, such as our motivating example, due to the presence of heterogeneity among the sampling units. For example, there may be a rich collection of environmental and individual characteristics that influence the count of a given species at a survey location. Ideally, a model should account for these characteristics. However, it is usually not possible in practice: information on these characteristics has not been or cannot be collected. This is then a source of the extra-Poisson variation in the data. That is, the observed variability is much larger than the observed mean. The additional variability can be partially accommodated by observation-specific random effects along with the conditional Poisson distribution. When a gamma distribution is assumed for the random effects, the marginal distribution of the count is a negative binomial (NB) distribution. When the NB distribution is constructed in the terms of the gamma mixture of Poisson distributions as above, it not only leads to an analytically tractable probability function but also provides a simple and intuitive accommodation of heterogeneity in the data. In addition, its overdispersion parameter explicitly measures the magnitude of overdispersion with respect to the Poisson variation. The Poisson distribution becomes a special case of the NB distribution with the overdispersion parameter approaching 0. In this study, we compare ZIP and ZINB models under five different spatial-temporal random effects structures, showing gains in model fitting through accommodating overdispersion by the NB distribution under various scenarios.

The zero-inflated Poisson model has been widely used to model the spatial (Agarwal et al. 2002; Fei and Rathbun 2006) or spatial-temporal correlated count data (Fernandes et al. 2009; Ver Hoef and Jansen 2007; Wang et al. 2015; Wikle and Anderson 2003). The literature on the zero-inflated negative binomial model, especially for spatial-temporal correlated count data, is still sparse. When overdispersion is in question, the prior studies have shown the better performance of the ZINB model compared to the ZIP model for spatially correlated data (Alexander et al. 2000; Lee and Bell 2009; Li 2008; Mohebbi et al. 2014). A recent study by Rumisha et al. (2014) developed a zero-inflated spatial-temporal negative binomial model for the study of malaria transmission heterogeneity. In their model, the spatial and temporal random effects are assumed to be additive. The current study is motivated by and extended from our previous study of the survey data by NEFSC (Wang et al. 2015), in which we propose a more flexible spatial-temporal correlation structure as well as a more efficient computation scheme. In our study, we focus on modeling the count data in the presence of both "true" and "false" zero counts. Our proposed algorithm, though, can be easily modified to fit the two-stage model with only "true" zeros.

For regression models on zero-inflated count data, researchers have developed both maximum likelihood methods (Kassahun et al. 2015; Min and Agresti 2005) and Bayesian approaches (Fu et al. 2015; Ghosh et al. 2006). Most of studies, though, used the Bayesian approach when comparing ZIP and ZINB models with spatial or spatial-temporal random effects (Alexander et al. 2000; Lee and Bell 2009; Li 2008; Mohebbi et al. 2014; Rumisha et al. 2014). This is because of several potentially attractive modeling and computational advantages provided by the Bayesian approach over the maximum likelihood-based approach, especially for modeling spatial and spatial-temporal data. First, the Bayesian hierarchial model is particularly useful in constructing a multiple-layer model that is easy to understand and compute for the complex data structure like the non-Gaussian, spatial-temporal data in our example (Banerjee et al. 2004). Secondly, with the high dimensionality of random effects, the optimization of the likelihood function usually involves high dimensional integrals, which are analytically intractable. The Bayesian approach overcomes this challenge via the Markov chain Monte Carlo (MCMC) simulation.

Finally, the Bayesian approach treats all parameters as random, which provides a straightforward mechanism to incorporate scientific knowledge into the statistical model through the prior distributions. In the current study, we choose to use the Bayesian approach given the complexity of our data and our proposed model. The main challenge in the MCMC simulation is the big "N" problem, which is common in modeling large-scale spatial-temporal data. One of our contributions is to improve computation efficiency by dimension reduction techniques.

The remainder of the paper is organized as follows. Within the generalized linear mixed model framework, the proposed zero-inflated spatial-temporal model is developed in Sect. 2. Also in Sect. 2, the priors and the values of hyperparameters are specified and the posterior computation and the model comparison are discussed. Section 3 presents the Atlantic cod data and provides the results on fitting a group of ZIP and ZINB models under the different structures of spatial and temporal random effects. Section 4 concludes the paper with discussion and future research problems.

2 The Model

Within the framework of the generalized linear mixed effects model, the proposed regression model for count data is composed of three modules: the random component, the systematic component, and the link function. The variations of the proposed regression model can be obtained by changing one or several modules. For example, in the classical setting of independent data, the generalized linear model (GLM) as introduced by Nelder and Wedderburn (1972) is obtained from an extension in the random component from Gaussian data to both Guassian and non-Gaussian data. The generalized linear mixed model (GLMM), as a further extension from GLM, changes the systematic component by introducing unobservable random effects into the linear systematic component (Breslow and Clayton 1993). Diggle et al. (1998) then specified the structure in the random components for modeling geostatistical data which leads to the spatial generalized linear model. It is presented as a natural extension of the mixed model by assuming the random effects as the underlying Gaussian signal process at each of the sample locations. The same GLMM framework is also used for areal or lattice data with a Gaussian Markov random field model (Banerjee et al. 2004). This module view of the regression model nicely unifies a rich family of regression models and further suggests potential new models, including the zero-inflated spatial-temporal model proposed here. It also greatly simplifies the algorithm development.

2.1 *Zero-Inflated Models: A Step-by-Step Journey*

We first introduce the notation used in the spatial-temporal model. Suppose data are collected from N areal units in the region of interest over T time points. Let $y_{t,i}$ denote the count data collected and $E_{t,i}$ be the binary indicator of whether the surveyed subject is truly presence/absence in the areal unit i in year t, $i = 1, \ldots, N$ and $t = 1, \ldots, T$. The presence status is unobservable if $y_{t,i} = 0$, and may be influenced by a rich collection of environmental and subject-specific characteristics. A hierarchical model can be built through three modules: data models, process models, and parameter models. The data model for zero-inflated data is usually specified as

$$E_{t,i} = \begin{cases} 1, & \text{with probability } p_{t,i}, \\ 0, & \text{with probability } 1 - p_{t,i}, \end{cases}$$

$$\text{Prob}(Y_{t,i} = y_{t,i} | E_{t,i}) = \begin{cases} 1, & \text{if } E_{t,i} = 0, \\ P_{\text{Count}}(y_{t,i} | \boldsymbol{\theta}_{t,i}), & \text{if } E_{t,i} = 1, \end{cases}$$

where $P_{\text{Count}}(y_{t,i} | \boldsymbol{\theta}_{t,i})$ is the probability mass function of a random variable $Y_{t,i}$ with distribution $P_{\text{Count}}(\cdot; \boldsymbol{\theta})$, whose mean and variance are decided by the parameter $\boldsymbol{\theta}$. It is assumed that, conditioned on $p_{t,i}$, the $E_{t,i}$'s are independent Bernoulli random variables with $\mathbb{E}(E_{t,i}) = p_{t,i}$. Given $E_{t,i} = 1$, the $Y_{t,i}$'s are conditionally independent.

Here we consider two count distributions: Poisson and negative binomial. The Poisson model is denoted by $\text{Poisson}(y_{t,i} | E_{t,i} = 1, \lambda_{t,i})$ under the assumption that the mean and the variance are equal, that is, $E(Y_{t,i}) = \text{Var}(Y_{t,i}) = \lambda_{t,i}$. The probability mass function is given as

$$P(Y_{t,i} = y_{t,i} | E_{t,i} = 1, \lambda_{t,i}) = \frac{\exp(-\lambda_{t,i}) \lambda_{t,i}^{y_{t,i}}}{\Gamma(y_{t,i} + 1)}. \tag{1}$$

The negative binomial model is denoted by $\text{NB}(y_{t,i} | E_{t,i} = 1, \lambda_{t,i}, a)$ with the probability mass function as

$$P(Y_{t,i} = y_{t,i} | E_{t,i} = 1, \lambda_{t,i}, a) = \frac{\Gamma(y_{t,i} + \frac{1}{a})}{\Gamma(y_{t,i} + 1)\Gamma(\frac{1}{a})} \left(\frac{\frac{1}{a}}{\frac{1}{a} + \lambda_{t,i}} \right)^{\frac{1}{a}} \left(\frac{\lambda_{t,i}}{\frac{1}{a} + \lambda_{t,i}} \right)^{y_{t,i}}. \tag{2}$$

The negative binomial distribution has its variance always greater than the mean and thus is used to model the extra-Poisson variability in the count data. The parameter a is an overdispersion parameter, with a larger value indicating higher heterogeneity in the count values. The Poisson distribution is nested in the family of negative binomial distributions when $a \to 0$.

The process models on the binary probability $p_{t,i}$ and the mean of the count $\lambda_{t,i}$ are constructed within the framework of generalized linear mixed model as

$$\text{binary part}: \; g(p_{t,i}) = \mathbf{x}_{t,i}' \boldsymbol{\beta}_{t,i} + w_{t,i}, \tag{3}$$

$$\text{count part}: \; \log(\lambda_{t,i}) = \tilde{\mathbf{x}}_{t,i}' \boldsymbol{\alpha}_{t,i} + \tilde{w}_{t,i}, \tag{4}$$

Table 1 Five regression models for count data

Model	Binary part	Count part
Model 1	$g(p_i) = \mathbf{x}_i'\boldsymbol{\beta}$,	$\log(\lambda_i) = \tilde{\mathbf{x}}_i'\boldsymbol{\alpha}$
Model 2	$g(p_{t,i}) = \mathbf{x}_{t,i}'\boldsymbol{\beta} + w_{t,i}$ $w_{t,i} \overset{iid}{\sim} N(0,1)$	$\log(\lambda_{t,i}) = \tilde{\mathbf{x}}_{t,i}'\boldsymbol{\alpha}$
Model 3	$g(p_{t,i}) = \mathbf{x}_{t,i}'\boldsymbol{\beta} + w_{t,i}$, $\mathbf{w}_t \sim MVN_N(0, \Sigma_b(\phi_b))$, for $t = 1, \ldots, T$	$\log(\lambda_{t,i}) = \tilde{\mathbf{x}}_{t,i}'\boldsymbol{\alpha}$
Model 4	$g(p_{t,i}) = \mathbf{x}_{t,i}'\boldsymbol{\beta} + w_{t,i}$, $\mathbf{w}_t \sim MVN_N(0, \Sigma_b(\phi_b))$, for $t = 1, \ldots, T$	$\log(\lambda_{t,i}) = \tilde{\mathbf{x}}_{t,i}'\boldsymbol{\alpha} + \tilde{w}_i$, $\tilde{\mathbf{w}} \sim MVN_N(0, \tau^2\Sigma_c(\phi_c))$
Model 5	$g(p_{t,i}) = \mathbf{x}_{t,i}'\boldsymbol{\beta} + w_{t,i}$, $\mathbf{w}_t \sim MVN_N(0, \Sigma_b(\phi_b))$, for $t = 1, \ldots, T$	$\log(\lambda_{t,i}) = \tilde{\mathbf{x}}_{t,i}'\boldsymbol{\alpha} + \tilde{w}_{t,i}$, $\tilde{\mathbf{w}} \sim MVN_{NT}(0, \tau^2\Sigma_c(\phi_c, \rho_c))$

where g is the link function for the binary regression, $\mathbf{x}_{t,i}$ and $\tilde{\mathbf{x}}_{t,i}$ are the vectors of covariates, which may be spatially and temporally related, $\boldsymbol{\beta}_{t,i}$ and $\boldsymbol{\alpha}_{t,i}$ are the vectors of the corresponding regression coefficients, and $w_{t,i}$ and $\tilde{w}_{t,i}$ are the random components. The link function $g(\cdot)$ is chosen to be Probit link here. Other link functions are also possible but we do not explore further here.

Wang et al. (2015) discussed and compared count data models with different specifications on the random components $w_{t,i}$ and $\tilde{w}_{t,i}$ with the regression coefficients $\boldsymbol{\beta}_{t,i}$ and $\boldsymbol{\alpha}_{t,i}$ constant across space and time. Only ZIP models were considered in Wang et al. (2015). Here we extend the ZIP model to the ZINB model to account for potential extra overdispersion presented in count data. Specifically, the five types of ZIP or ZINB models are constructed and shown in Table 1.

These five models represent a few most commonly used regression models for count data. For example, Model 3 is similar to the one used in Fei and Rathbun (2006), where the spatial random effects are included only in the binary part. Model 5 is similar to those in Ver Hoef and Jansen (2007) and Wang et al. (2015) with correlated spatial and temporal random effects in both the binary part and the count part. These models differ in the specification of the structure of the random effects. Here we describe the model structures and introduce our proposed model (Model 5) by changing the random effects in the systematic component module gradually. In all five models, the regression coefficients $\boldsymbol{\beta}$ and $\boldsymbol{\alpha}$ are constant across space and time. For details, see Wang et al. (2015).

Model 1 is a simple zero-inflated model, without considering any random effects. Model 2 is a zero-inflated model assuming independent random effects in the binary part.

Model 3 is a zero-inflated model assuming spatially correlated random effects in the binary part only. We employ the conditional autoregressive model (CAR) on the spatial random effects $\boldsymbol{\omega}_t = (\omega_{t,1}, \ldots, \omega_{t,N})$ in year t (Cressie 1993). That is, $\boldsymbol{\omega}_t \sim \text{MVN}(\mathbf{0}, \sigma^2(\mathbf{I} - \phi\mathbf{W})^{-1})$, where $\text{MVN}(\boldsymbol{\mu}, \boldsymbol{\Sigma})$ is a multivariate normal distribution with a mean vector $\boldsymbol{\mu}$ and a variance-covariance matrix $\boldsymbol{\Sigma}$, σ^2 is the spatial nugget parameter, ϕ is the spatial range parameter, and $\mathbf{W}$ is the adjacency matrix with $\mathbf{w}_{ii} = 0$, $\mathbf{w}_{i\ell} = 1$ if the areal unit i and ℓ are neighbors, and $\mathbf{w}_{i\ell} = 0$

if they are not ($i \neq \ell$). The neighborhoods of two areal units are defined according to a second-order neighbor definition (Banerjee et al. 2004). To make $(\mathbf{I} - \phi\mathbf{W})^{-1}$ nonsingular, we assume $\phi \in (1/\theta_{(1)}, 1/\theta_{(N)})$, where $\theta_{(1)} < \theta_{(2)} < \ldots < \theta_{(N)}$ are the ordered eigenvalues of $\mathbf{W}$. To ensure identifiability, σ^2 is set to 1 (De Oliveira 2000; Fei and Rathbun 2006). The latent variables $\mathbf{Z}$ are introduced in the model to facilitate the data augmentation method in MCMC computation (Albert and Chib 1993).

Model 4 is a zero-inflated count model incorporating spatial random effects in both binary and count parts. The structure of the spatial random effects in the binary part is the same as in Model 3. For the spatial random effects in the count part, Model 4 assumes a continuous spatial covariance depending on distance, instead of the neighborhood structure as in the CAR model. This is because the spatial correlation in the count part is only estimated using the data from two areal units with the binary part $E_{t,i} = 1$. This may lead to one or a group of isolated areal units, which are assumed spatially independent from the rest of the region if the spatial covariance structure is assumed depending on the neighborhood structure. We find this unsatisfactory and thus propose to use a continuous correlation function (Fernandes et al. 2009; Wang et al. 2015; Wikle and Anderson 2003). Here we use the Matérn correlation function specified as $(\Gamma(\phi_2)2^{(\phi_2-1)})^{-1}\ (2\phi_2^{1/2}d(\mathbf{s},\mathbf{s}')/\phi_1)^{\phi_2}\mathscr{K}_{\phi_2}(2\phi_2^{1/2}d(\mathbf{s},\mathbf{s}')/\phi_1)$, where $\mathscr{K}_{\phi_2}$ is a modified Bessel function of the second kind of order ϕ_2, $d(\mathbf{s},\mathbf{s}')$ is the Euclidean distance between two locations $\mathbf{s}$ and $\mathbf{s}'$, ϕ_1 is the range parameter which measures how fast the correlation decays with distance, and ϕ_2 is the smoothness parameter that measures the degree of smoothness of the spatial process. The higher the value of ϕ_2, the smoother the spatial process would be. We assume the parameter $\phi_2 = 1$ to avoid the weak identification problem (Whittle 1954).

A continuous correlation structure makes it possible to investigate "hot spots" or "cold spots" effects (Wang et al. 2015). A challenge using the continuous covariance function is that it involves the inversion of an $N \times N$ matrix with the dimension increasing with the number of locations N and the computation of the order of N^3. Here, we employ the Gaussian predictive process approach (Banerjee et al. 2008) and specify the spatial random effects $\tilde{w}_i$ as $\tilde{w}_i = \mathbf{D}_i'\boldsymbol{\gamma}$, where the basis function $\mathbf{D}$ is constructed using the predictive process with $\mathbf{D} = [\mathbf{D}(\mathbf{s})]_i = \mathbf{V}(\mathbf{s})'\mathbf{H}^{-1}$, $\mathbf{V}(\mathbf{s}) = \tau^2(\mathbf{v}(\mathbf{s},\mathbf{s}_1^*;\boldsymbol{\phi}), \ldots, \mathbf{v}(\mathbf{s},\mathbf{s}_M^*;\boldsymbol{\phi}))$, and $\mathbf{H}_{lk} = \tau^2\mathbf{v}(s_l^*, s_k^*;\boldsymbol{\phi})$, $s_1^*, \ldots, s_M^*$ are the selected knots in the study area with $M << N$, $\mathbf{v}(\cdot;\cdot)$ is a valid correlation function, and $\boldsymbol{\gamma} \sim N(\mathbf{0},\mathbf{H})$.

Model 5 is recently proposed for the zero-inflated Poisson regression model with spatial-temporal random effects (Wang et al. 2015). The random effects $\tilde{w}_{t,i}$ are specified as $\tilde{w}_{t,i} = \mathbf{D}_i'\boldsymbol{\gamma}_t$, with the same basis function as in Model 4. The temporal evolution of $\boldsymbol{\gamma}_t$ is specified as $\boldsymbol{\gamma}_t = \rho\boldsymbol{\gamma}_{t-1} + \mathbf{v}_t$, where $\mathbf{v}_t \sim N(0,\mathbf{H})$ and $-1 < \rho < 1$. An interesting result was derived based on the spectral decomposition of $\mathbf{H}$ (Salazar et al. 2011): $\mathbf{H} = \tau^2\mathbf{P}\boldsymbol{\Lambda}\mathbf{P}$, where $\mathbf{P}$ is an orthogonal matrix and $\boldsymbol{\Lambda}$ is a diagonal matrix with the eigenvalues of $\mathbf{H}/\tau^2$ as the diagonal elements. Letting $\boldsymbol{\gamma}_t = \mathbf{P}\boldsymbol{\xi}_t$ for all t, we have

$$\mathbf{D}(\mathbf{s})\mathbf{P}\boldsymbol{\xi}_t = \boldsymbol{\Psi}(\mathbf{s})\boldsymbol{\xi}_t, \ \ \boldsymbol{\xi}_t \sim N(\rho\boldsymbol{\xi}_{t-1}, \tau^2\boldsymbol{\Lambda}), \tag{5}$$

where $\boldsymbol{\Psi}(\mathbf{s}) = \mathbf{D}(\mathbf{s})\mathbf{P} = \mathbf{V}(\mathbf{s})'\mathbf{H}^{-1}\mathbf{P}$ and $\boldsymbol{\xi}_t = \rho\boldsymbol{\xi}_{t-1} + \boldsymbol{v}_t$ with $\boldsymbol{v}_t \sim N(0, \tau^2\boldsymbol{\Lambda})$ and $\boldsymbol{\xi}_0 \sim N(\mathbf{m}_0, \mathbf{C}_0)$. As a result, the temporal changes in spatial patterns can be modeled as M independent processes $\tilde{\boldsymbol{\xi}}_i = \{\xi_{1,i}, \xi_{2,i}, \ldots, \xi_{t,i}, \ldots, \xi_{T,i}\}$, $i = 1, \ldots, M$.

The model complexity increases from Model 1 to 5 in the random effects structure. We also include both the Poisson distribution and the negative binomial distribution in the random component in the count part. Thus, we fit both the ZIP and ZINB models with various types of spatial-temporal random effects. With this model development trajectory, we hope to address the following potential complications which are common in modeling count data: (1) overdispersion; (2) excess zeros; (3) spatial-temporal correlations; and (4) computational challenges when the data are large.

2.2 *Prior Specification, Posterior Computation and Model Assessment*

We discuss the prior specification under Model 5, which has the largest set of parameters to be estimated. The prior specifications under other models are similar. The parameters under Model 5 include $\boldsymbol{\beta}, \boldsymbol{\alpha}, \phi_b, \tau^2, \phi_c, \rho$, and a. The priors for these parameters are specified as follows: $\boldsymbol{\beta} \sim N(0, g_{\beta}(\mathbf{X}'\mathbf{X})^{-1})$, where $g_{\beta} = 1000$; $\boldsymbol{\alpha} \sim N(0, g_{\alpha}I)$, where $g_{\alpha} = 1000$; $\phi_b \sim U(\phi_{\min}, \phi_{\max})$, which ensures the positive definiteness of the dispersion matrix $(\mathbf{I} - \phi\mathbf{W})^{-1}$; $\tau^2 \sim IG(c, d)$, where $c = 2$ and $d = 1$; $\rho \sim U(-1, 1)$, and $a \sim Gamma(1/\epsilon, \epsilon)$, where $\epsilon = 3$. The prior for the range parameter ϕ_c in the Matérn correlation function is set as $\phi_c \sim IG(2, h)$, where $h = \max(d(\mathbf{s}, \mathbf{s}'))/(-2\log(0.05))$. With this prior specification, ϕ_c has a large variance and mean based on a crude estimated range, $-\log(0.05) \cdot \phi_c$, taken to be the half of the maximum interlocation distance $\max(d(\mathbf{s}, \mathbf{s}'))$. Details on this prior specification can be found in Banerjee et al. (2004), Banerjee (2005), Lopes et al. (2008), and Salazar et al. (2011). The hyper-parameters in priors for all the other parameters are also chosen to ensure that relatively weak informative priors are used in Bayesian estimation.

Since there is no prior information available on $\boldsymbol{\xi}_0$ in our application, we specify a normal prior for the first state vector $\boldsymbol{\xi}_1 \sim N(\mathbf{m}_1, \mathbf{C}_1)$ (West and Harrison 1997). The hyperparameters $\mathbf{m}_1$ and $\mathbf{C}_1$ are specified as an $M \times 1$ vector $\mathbf{0}$ and an $M \times M$ diagonal covariance matrix $10^6 \cdot \mathbf{I}$.

The posterior estimates of the parameters are computed via MCMC sampling. The detailed development of the MCMC sampling algorithm for the ZIP model is given in Section S1 in Supplementary Material of Wang et al. (2015). The computation for the extension of Bayesian ZIP model to ZINB model is carried out by considering the negative binomial distribution as a mixture of Poisson-

Gamma distribution. Assuming $Y_{t,i}|E_{t,i} = 1, \gamma_{t,i} \sim Poisson(\gamma_{t,i}\lambda_{t,i})$ and $\gamma_{t,i} \sim$ Gamma$(1/a, a)$, the marginal distribution of $Y_{t,i}$ is $NB(\lambda_{t,i}, a)$. The conditional posterior distribution for the gamma random variable $\gamma_{t,i}$ is Gamma$(1/a, a)$ if $E_{t,i} = 0$ and Gamma$(y_{t,i} + 1/a, [1/a + \exp(\tilde{\mathbf{x}}'_{t,i}\boldsymbol{\alpha} + \boldsymbol{\Psi}(s_i)'\boldsymbol{\xi}_t)]^{-1})$ if $E_{t,i} = 1$. The conditional posterior distribution of the dispersion parameter a does not have a closed form. It is sampled using the Metropolis-Hastings algorithm. The `R boa` package (Smith 2007) is used for convergence diagnostics of MCMC chains.

We use two Bayesian model selection criteria; namely, the deviance information criterion (DIC) (Spiegelhalter et al. 2002) and the conditional predictive ordinates (CPO) (Gelfand et al. 1992).

The DIC can be calculated in different ways depending on what is in 'focus' (Spiegelhalter et al. 2002). Here we use the method in Hadfield (2010) and calculate the likelihood for the lowest level of the hierarchy. Therefore, the likelihood function of a data point $y_{t,i}$ depends on the Bernoulli probabilities and the means $(p_{t,i}, \lambda_{t,i})$ for the ZIP model, and $(p_{t,i}, \lambda_{t,i})$ as well as the overdispersion parameter a for the ZINB model. That is, for $i = 1, \ldots, N$ and $t = 1, \ldots, T$, the logarithm of the likelihood function of the observation in the areal unit i in year t is

$$l(y_{t,i}|\boldsymbol{\theta}_{t,i}) = \log\{(1 - p_{t,i})I(y_{t,i} = 0) + p_{t,i}P_{\text{Count}}(y_{t,i}|\boldsymbol{\theta}_{t,i})\},$$

where $P_{\text{Count}}(y_{t,i}|\boldsymbol{\theta}_{t,i})$ is as specified as in Eq. (1) (ZIP) or (2) (ZINB), and $\boldsymbol{\theta}_{t,i} = \{p_{t,i}, \lambda_{t,i}\}$ in the ZIP model or $\{p_{t,i}, \lambda_{t,i}, a\}$ in the ZINB model. Based on the GLMM model specified in Eqs. (3) and (4), $p_{t,i} = g^{-1}(\mathbf{x}'_{t,i}\boldsymbol{\beta}_{t,i} + w_{t,i})$ and $\lambda_{t,i} = \exp(\tilde{\mathbf{x}}'_{t,i}\boldsymbol{\alpha}_{t,i} + \tilde{w}_{t,i})$, where $\boldsymbol{\alpha}, \boldsymbol{\beta}, \{w_{t,i}\}, \{\tilde{w}_{t,i}\}$ as well as the overdispersion parameter a are obtained using MCMC sampling.

The DIC measure is then calculated as $DIC = \hat{D}_{avg}(\mathbf{y}) + p_D$, where p_D is the effective number of parameters of a Bayesian model. The average deviance function $\hat{D}_{avg}(\mathbf{y})$ is calculated as $\hat{D}_{avg}(\mathbf{y}) = \{\sum_{l=1}^{L} D(\mathbf{y}, \boldsymbol{\theta}_l)\}/L$ using L sampling points, where $\boldsymbol{\theta}_l$ is the lth sampling value for the parameter $\boldsymbol{\theta} = \{\boldsymbol{\theta}_{t,i}\}$. The deviance function $D(\mathbf{y}, \boldsymbol{\theta})$ is negative two times the logarithm of the likelihood, $-2\sum_{t=1}^{T}\sum_{i=1}^{N} l(y_{t,i}|\boldsymbol{\theta}_{t,i})$. We calculated p_D as $\hat{p} = \hat{D}_{avg}(\mathbf{y}) - D_{\hat{\theta}}(\mathbf{y})$, where $D_{\hat{\theta}}(\mathbf{y}) = D(\mathbf{y}, \hat{\boldsymbol{\theta}}(\mathbf{y}))$ and $\hat{\boldsymbol{\theta}}$ is the posterior mean of the MCMC samples. The smaller the DIC value, the better the model fits the data.

CPO is a Bayesian cross-validation statistic by computing the conditional predictive distribution after deleting a single observation. Let $\mathbf{D}_{obs}^{-(t,i)}$ denote the data with the observation in the areal unit i in year t deleted, $i = 1, \ldots, N$ and $t = 1, \ldots, T$. For the deleted observation $y_{t,i}$, CPO$_{t,i}$ is the marginal posterior predictive density of $y_{t,i}$ given $\mathbf{D}_{obs}^{-(t,i)}$, which can be expressed as (Dey et al. 1997)

$$\text{CPO}_{t,i} = \left\{\int_{\boldsymbol{\theta}} \frac{\pi(\boldsymbol{\theta}|\mathbf{D}_{obs})}{l(y_{t,i}|\mathbf{D}_{obs}^{-(t,i)}, \boldsymbol{\theta})} d\boldsymbol{\theta}\right\}^{-1}.$$

A Monte Carlo approximation of $\mathrm{CPO}_{t,i}$ is given by

$$\widehat{\mathrm{CPO}}_{t,i} = \left\{ \frac{1}{M} \sum_{m=1}^{M} \frac{1}{l(y_{t,i}|\mathbf{D}_{obs}^{-(t,i)}, \boldsymbol{\theta}^{(m)})} \right\}^{-1}.$$

By assuming conditional independence of $y_{t,i}$, where $i = 1, \ldots, N$ and $t = 1, \ldots, T$, $l(y_{t,i}|D_{obs}^{-(t,i)}, \boldsymbol{\theta}^{(m)})$ is simplified to $l(y_{t,i}|\boldsymbol{\theta}^{(m)})$. We compute the log-pseudo marginal likelihood (LPML) by summarizing all $\mathrm{CPO}_{t,i}$'s, which is

$$\mathrm{LPML} = \sum_{t=1}^{T} \sum_{i=1}^{N} \log(\widehat{\mathrm{CPO}}_{t,i}).$$

The larger the value of LPML is, the better the fit of the model is.

3 Application: Analysis of the Presence and Abundance of Atlantic Cod in the Gulf of Maine-Georges Bank Region

The Northeast Fisheries Sciences Center (NEFSC) has been collecting data on ocean fishery through a standardized research survey since Fall, 1963. The survey is carried out on a regular basis in each of the four seasons each year. Geographically, the survey area covers the area from the Gulf of Maine to Cape Hatteras, NC. Approximately 350–400 stations are surveyed during each survey season, with locations selected by a stratified random sampling design to assure that the number of stations allocated to strata are roughly in proportion to area. Samples are collected in depths of 27–350 m with 4 depth zones. Data recorded on site include the species caught, weight, counts of fish, surface and bottom water temperature, and bottom depth of the tow along with many other variables.

Wang et al. (2015) are the first to apply a Bayesian spatial-temporal model in understanding the presence and abundance of Atlantic cods stocks. The study area is divided into 1325 ($N = 1325$) 10 km by 10 km grids. The survey data used here were collected during the period of fall 1970 to fall 2008 ($T = 39$). The ocean geographical characteristics included in the model are the average depth of the ocean and the depth standard deviation (see Figure S1 in Wang et al. 2015) that show a wide variation in the area. The latitude and the sampling year are considered in the model. All of the covariates are standardized by their corresponding means and standard deviations to improve MCMC convergence.

The study conducted by Wang et al. (2015) was based on the Poisson assumption in the count data part. As discussed in the Introduction section, the data exhibits evidence of overdispersion in a simple ZIP fit. A negative binomial model may improve the fit of these count data, with or without the spatial and spatial-temporal random effects. We fit both the ZIP and ZINB distributions in Model 1–5. Table 2

Table 2 Model comparison among ZIP and ZINB Model 1–5

	Model 1	Model 2	Model 3	Model 4	Model 5
DIC					
ZIP	42110.66	41891.21	40954.10	34918.73	25086.17
ZINB	17370.98	17268.20	16807.35	16388.40	16254.58
LPML					
ZIP	−21040.56	−20929.13	−19604.22	−16629.97	−11263.29
ZINB	−8674.22	−8621.38	−8100.34	−7956.95	−7654.31

DIC is the deviance information criterion and LPML is the log-pseudo marginal likelihood

shows the DIC and LPML for all models. Model 5 with ZINB distribution is the best model, which accounts for spatial-temporal correlation, excess zeros, and the overdispersion in the count data. Comparison between models under the same column with either Poisson or NB distributions assumption confirms the importance of modeling overdispersion in the data.

We proceed with detailed discussion on ZINB Model 1–5. Tables 3 and 4 show detailed results on these models as well as those of ZIP Model 4 and 5 for comparison. For the details regarding the fit of all ZIP models, see Wang et al. (2015).

ZINB Model 1, which is a simple negative binomial zero-inflated model, is clearly not sufficient to fit the data. It has the largest DIC as 17370.98. ZINB Model 2 includes independent random effects in the binary part and adds the time as a covariate in the count part. It shows improvement over Model 1 with a smaller DIC. The spatial random effects are included in the binary part in Model 3 and in both binary and count parts in Model 4, which leads to a lower DIC value. While the direction and significance of most covariates effects do not change a lot from Models 2–4, the latitude becomes an insignificant factor in abundance variation when the spatial random effects are included in the count part (Model 4). All these 4 models assume the same pattern across years, independent or spatially correlated random effects, with the only change in the overall probability or abundance.

ZINB Model 5 does not require this assumption and it models the inseparable spatial-temporal random effects. The estimates based on Model 5, then, do not assume the same spatial correlation patterns across the years. Figure 3 shows the posterior means of the mean count estimates $(p_{t,i}\lambda_{t,i})$ under ZIP Model 4, ZIP Model 5, ZINB Model 4, and ZINB Model 5 for the four snap-shot years in Fig. 1. As shown in Fig. 3, the estimates from ZIP Model 5 and ZINB Model 5 exhibit an overall decreasing trend in the mean estimates of the Atlantic cod abundance, however, the spatial patterns are different from year to year and more importantly, the abundance increases relatively to 10 years ago in the west in 2007. Thus, the proposed spatial-temporal model captures the dynamic changes in the spatial patterns and the nonlinear trend in some regions. As to Table 4, ZIP Models 4 and 5 have higher DIC values compared to the ZINB models. Thus, the ZINB model is more appropriate for the motivating count data. The covariate "time" is significantly

Table 3 Posterior estimates under Models 1–3

	ZINB Model 1		ZINB Model 2		ZINB Model 3	
Variables	Est.	SD	Est.	SD	Est.	SD
Binary part						
Intercept	2.00	0.13	2.32	0.14	3.01	0.21
Mean depth	0.29	0.10	0.43	0.11	0.43	0.15
(meandepth)^2	−0.15	0.07	−0.14	0.08	−0.20	0.09
sd.of depth	−0.07	0.05	−0.13	0.05	−0.11	0.07
Latitude	1.90	0.09	2.06	0.10	2.68	0.14
ϕ					0.1255	0.00006
Count part						
Intercept	1.12	0.03	1.02	0.04	1.07	0.03
Mean depth	−1.29	0.04	−1.29	0.04	−1.31	0.04
(meandepth)^2	−0.16	0.05	−0.17	0.06	−0.14	0.05
sd.of depth	0.48	0.04	0.50	0.04	0.48	0.04
Latitude	−0.09	0.04	−0.06	0.04	−0.10	0.04
Time			−0.31	0.03	−0.28	0.03
a	2.52	0.09	2.49	0.09	2.29	0.08
ϕ_1	–	–				
τ^2	–	–				
ρ	–	–				
DIC	17370.98		17268.20		16807.35	
−2llike	17352.27		17247.20		16521.59	
p_D	9.36		10.50		142.88	

DIC is the deviance information criterion; −2llike is the deviance evaluated at the posterior means of parameters; p_D is the effective number of model parameters in DIC. Model 1: the ZINB model on data combined across years and locations. Model 2: the ZINB model on the data combined across locations with year as a covariate (time) in the count part. Model 3: the ZINB model with the spatial correlation on the binary part and with time as a covariate in the count part

negative and this effect is consistent across ZINB Model 1–5. The effect is only slightly weaker in Model 5 when the temporal random effects are included. This reflects the overall decreasing trend in the fish's abundance. The overdispersion parameter a in the ZINB distribution decreases from ZINB Model 1 to ZINB Model 5, as part of the overdispersion is modeled by spatial random effects or spatial-temporal random effects.

4 Discussion

The significant dynamic spatial patterns may imply that there are some important factors to be considered in estimation and prediction of the Atlantic cod abundance. For example, our preliminary study showed that the abundance has a similar

Table 4 Posterior estimates under Models 4–5 for ZIP and ZINB

	ZINB Model 4		ZINB Model 5		ZIP Model 4		ZIP Model5	
Variables	Est.	SD	est.	SD	Est.	SD	Est.	SD
Binary part								
Intercept	2.99	0.34	3.12	0.14	0.09	0.05	0.27	0.05
Mean depth	0.61	0.21	0.47	0.14	−0.26	0.04	−0.25	0.05
(meandepth)^2	−0.08	0.15	−0.16	0.09	−0.28	0.05	−0.23	0.06
sd.of depth	−0.19	0.13	−0.12	0.07	0.22	0.03	0.20	0.03
Latitude	1.90	0.27	2.68	0.11	0.29	0.04	0.36	0.05
ϕ	0.1255	0.0001	0.1255	0.00007	0.1250	0.0002	0.1251	0.0002
Count part								
Intercept	0.19	0.29	0.81	0.10	−0.78	0.22	0.36	0.17
Mean depth	−1.21	0.05	−1.21	0.05	−0.92	0.02	−1.02	0.02
(meandepth)^2	−0.26	0.06	−0.27	0.06	−0.09	0.02	−0.13	0.03
sd.of depth	0.44	0.04	0.43	0.04	0.25	0.01	0.22	0.01
Latitude	0.13	0.20	−0.08	0.08	−0.68	0.11	−0.49	0.08
Time	−0.37	0.03	−0.30	0.08	−0.17	0.01	−0.64	0.13
a	2.13	0.08	1.73	0.07				
ϕ_1	74.87	1.54	61.53	0.25	92.33	5.58	66.35	1.45
τ^2	2.65	0.98	1.37	0.21	6.19	2.22	8.06	0.75
ρ			0.13	0.05			0.42	0.03
DIC	16388.40		16254.58		34918.73		25086.17	
−2llike	16197.54		15651.32		33961.71		23431.25	
p_D	95.43		301.63		478.51		827.46	

DIC is the deviance information criterion; −2llike is the deviance evaluated at the posterior means of parameters; p_D is the effective number of model parameters in DIC. ZINB Model 4: the ZINB model with spatial correlation on the binary part and the count part and with time as a covariate in the count part. For the predictive process, 16 knots were selected as shown in the left panel of Figure S5 in Wang et al. (2015). ZINB Model 5: the ZINB model with spatial correlation on the binary part and with spatial-temporal correlation in the count part and with time as a covariate in the count part. Knots were selected as in ZINB Model 4. ZIP model 4 and ZIP model 5 are the corresponding models with the ZIP distribution

temporal pattern with the index of the North Atlantic Oscillation (NAO), which can be used as an indicator for the strength and direction of westerly winds and storm tracks across the North Atlantic. Our empirical results then suggest a further investigation of potential important factors on studying the Atlantic cod, which can be explored to see if it can explain the spatial, temporal, or spatial-temporal patterns in the random effects and thus reduce the overdispersion in the count data.

While such information is not readily available, a statistical model that considers these complications is important. There are different methods to deal with these types of count data. Our contribution here is to extend the newly developed spatial-temporal model for zero-inflated count data to the count data with overdispersion, under different structures of the spatial-temporal random effects. Another possibility is to use spatially varying regression coefficients as in Wikle and Anderson

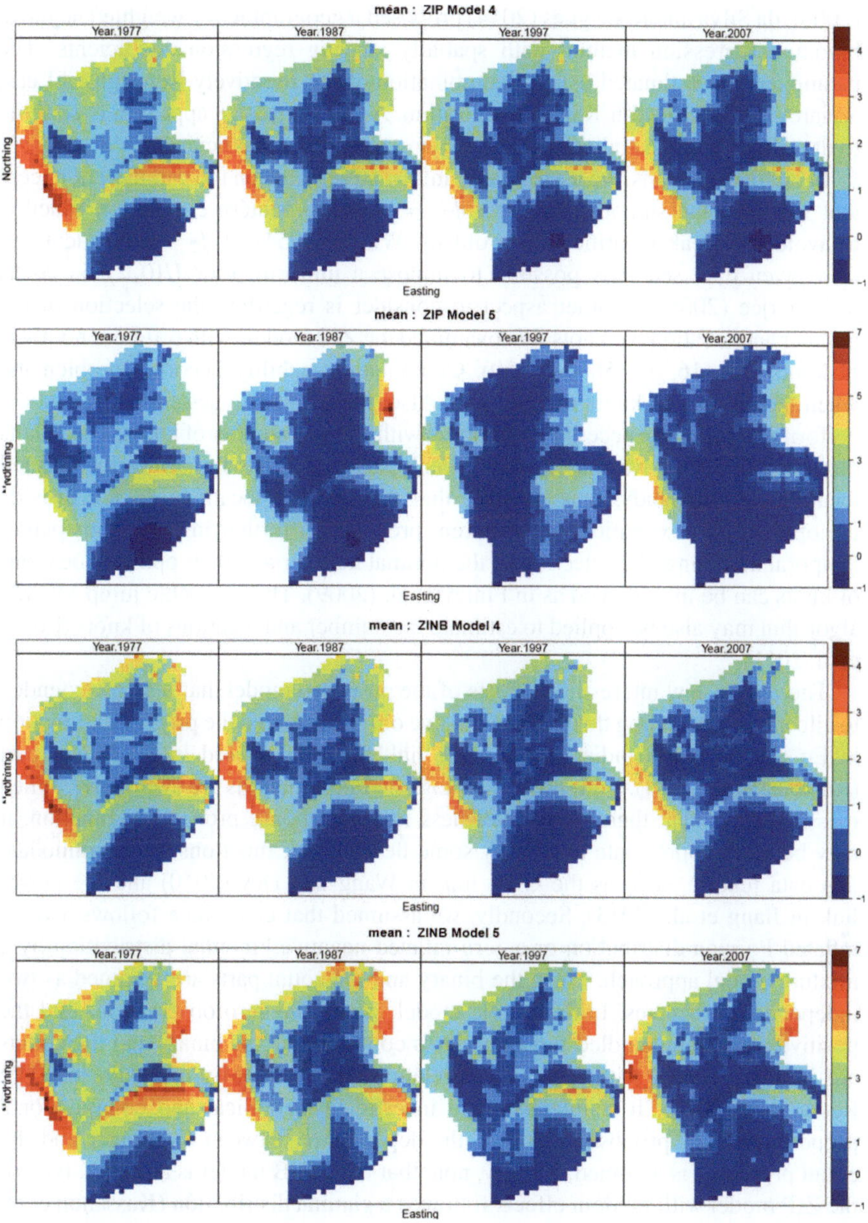

Fig. 3 The logarithm of posterior mean count at each grid from Model 4 and 5 for ZIP and ZINB models

(2003). da Silva and Rodrigues (2014) proposed a geographically weighted negative binomial regression method with spatially varying regression coefficients. The parameters are estimated using a combination of the Iteratively Reweighted Least Squares and the Newton-Raphson algorithm. A fully Bayesian approach is possible to fit a ZINB with spatial-temporally varying regression coefficients.

In our data analysis, we used weakly informative priors on the parameters, except that we fixed the smooth parameter $\phi_2 = 1$ in the Matérn correlation function to avoid the weak identification problem (Whittle 1954). If ϕ_2 can be identified in a given data set, it is possible to impose a uniform prior $U(0, 2)$ on ϕ_2 as in Banerjee (2005). Another aspect to consider is regarding the selection of the number and locations of knots. We examined the ZIP models with different numbers of knots (i.e., 16, 32, 56, 64, 150). Computation stability becomes problematic when the number of knots reached 150. Also, the results suggested that the model performance does not necessarily improve with a larger number of knots. The results discussed in Sect. 3 was based on 16 evenly spaced knots with arbitrarily selected locations in this study. It is possible that the selected locations do not provide the optimal approximation of the parent process. To further improve the spatial-temporal modeling, the selection of the optimal number and their optimal locations of knots can be investigated as in Finley et al. (2009). The reversible jump MCMC algorithm may also be applied to estimate the number and locations of knots (Lopes et al. 2011).

There are a few interesting aspects of the proposed model that may be extended to allow more modeling flexibility. First, we only considered the probit link function in Eq. (3). In some studies, the logistic link function is used in the binary part (Rumisha et al. 2014). Both probit and logistic link functions are symmetric. When it is suspected that there exists skewness in the response probability function, it may be more appropriate to employ some flexible link functions to accommodate this data feature, such as the GEV link in Wang and Dey (2010) and the power link in Jiang et al. (2013). Secondly, we assumed that count data follows a zero-inflated Poisson distribution or a zero-inflated negative binomial distribution by a mixture model approach. Thus, the binary and the count parts are assumed as two independent processes. In the hurdle model, where the zero observations and the positive counts are handled separately, it is common that the binary and the counts are jointly modeled with potential correlation structures (Min and Agresti 2005; Recta et al. 2012). It is interesting to investigate theoretical and computational properties of our proposed model if the dependence between the binary and the count processes is assumed. Thirdly, note that the ZINB model is a special type of the ZIP model with random effects followed a gamma distribution (Kassahun et al. 2015). It is possible to construct a ZIP model with more general assumptions on the random effects to accommodate overdispersion. We thank an anonymous referee for the above comments.

Acknowledgements We thank two referees for their constructive comments and suggestions. Dr. Wang thanks the domestic and international conference travel support provided by the Charles Phelps Taft Center at the University of Cincinnati. Dr. Chen's research was partially supported by NIH grants #GM 70335 and #P01 CA142538.

References

Agarwal, D. K., Gelfand, A. E., & Citron-Pousty, S. (2002). Zero-inflated models with application to spatial count data. *Environmental and Ecological Statistics, 9*, 341–355.

Albert, J. H., & Chib, S. (1993). Bayesian analysis of binary and polychotomous response data. *Journal of the American Statistical Association, 88*, 669–679.

Alexander, N., Moyeed, R., & Stander, J. (2000). Spatial modelling of individual-level parasite counts using the negative binomial distribution. *Biostatistics, 1*(4), 453–463.

Banerjee, S. (2005). On geodetic distance computations in spatial modeling. *Biometrics, 61*(2), 617–625.

Banerjee, S., Carlin, B. P., & Gelfand, A. E. (2004). *Hierarchical modeling and analysis for spatial data*. Boca Raton, London, New York, Washington, DC: Chapman & Hall/CRC.

Banerjee, S., Gelfand, A., Finley, A., & Sang, H. (2008). Gaussian predictive process models for large spatial datasets. *Journal of the Royal Statistical Society Series B, 70*, 825–848.

Breslow, N. E., & Clayton, D. G. (1993). Approximate inference in generalized linear mixed models. *Journal of the American Statistical Association, 88*, 9–25.

Cressie, N. (1993). *Statistics for spatial data* (revised edn.) New York: Wiley.

da Silva, A. R., & Rodrigues, T. C. V. (2014). Geographically weighted negative binomial regression – incorporating overdispersion. *Statistics and Computing, 24*(5), 769–783.

De Oliveira, V. (2000). Bayesian prediction of clipped Gaussian random fields. *Computational Statistics & Data Analysis, 34*, 299–314.

Dey, D. K., Chen, M. H., & Chang, H. (1997). Bayesian approach for nonlinear random effects models. *Biometrics, 53*(4), 1239–1252.

Diggle, P. J., Tawn, J. A., & Moyeed, R. A. (1998). Model-based geostatistics (with discussion). *Applied Statistics, 47*, 299–350.

Fei, S., & Rathbun, S. L. (2006). A spatial zero-inflated Poisson model for oak regeneration. *Environmental and Ecological Statistics, 13*, 406–426.

Fernandes, M. V., Schmidt, A. M., & Migon, H. S. (2009). Modelling zero-inflated spatio-temporal processes. *Statistical Modelling, 9*(1), 3–25.

Finley, A. O., Sang, H., Banerjee, S., & Gelfand, A. E. (2009). Improving the performance of predictive process modeling for large datasets. *Computational Statistics & Data Analysis, 53*(8), 2873–2884.

Fu, Y. Z., Chu, P. X., & Lu, L. Y. (2015). A Baysian approach of joint models for clustered zero-inflated count data with skewness and measurement errors. *Journal of Applied Statistics, 42*(4), 745–761.

Gelfand, A. E., Dey, D. K., & Chang, H. (1992). Model determination using predictive distributions with implementation via sampling-based methods. In J. M. Bernardo, J. O. Berger, A. P. Dawid, & A. F. M. Smith (Eds.), *Bayesian statistics* (Vol. 4, pp. 147–167). Oxford: Oxford University Press.

Ghosh, S. K., Mukhopadhyay, P., & Lu, J. C. (2006). Bayesian analysis of zero-inflated regression models. *Journal of Statistical Planning and Inference, 136*, 1360–1375.

Hadfield, J. D. (2010). MCMC methods for multi-response generalized linear mixed models: The MCMCglmm R package. *Journal of Statistical Software, 33*(2), 1–22.

Jiang, X., Dey, D. K., Prunier, R., Wilson, A. M., & Holsinger, K. E. (2013). A new class of flexible link functions with application to species co-occurrence in Cape floristic region. *The Annals of Applied Statistics, 7*(4), 2180–2204.

Kassahun, W., Neyens, T., Molenberghs, G., Faes, C., & Verbeke, G. (2015). A joint model for hierarchical continuous and zero-inflated overdispersed count data. *Journal of Statistical Computation and Simulation, 85*(3), 552–571.

Lee, K. L., & Bell, D. R. (2009). A spatial negative binomial regression of individual-level count data with regional and person-specific covariates. Working Paper Series, The Wharton School, University of Philadelphia.

Li, H. (2008). Bayesian hierarchical models for spatial count data with application to fire frequency in British Columbia. Master's thesis, Department of Mathmatics and Statistics, University of Victoria, Victoria, Canada.

Lopes, H. F., Gamerman, D., & Salazar, E. (2011). Generalized spatial dynamic factor models. *Computational Statistics & Data Analysis, 55*, 1319–1330.

Lopes, H. F., Salazar, E., & Gamerman, D. (2008). Spatial dynamic factor analysis. *Bayesian Analysis, 3*(4), 759–792.

Min, Y., & Agresti, A. (2005). Random effect models for repeated measures of zero-inflated count data. *Statistical Modelling, 5*, 1–19.

Mohebbi, M., Wolfe, R., & Forbes, A. (2014). Disease mapping and regression with count data in the presence of overdispersion and spatial autocorrelation: A Bayesian model averaging approach. *International Journal of Environmental Research and Public Health, 11*, 883–902.

Nelder, J. A., & Wedderburn, R. M. (1972). Generalized linear models. *Journal of the Royal Statistical Society, Series A, 135*, 370–384.

Recta, V., Haran, M., & Rosenberger, J. L. (2012). A two-stage model for incidence and prevalence in point-level spatial count data. *Environmetrics, 23*, 162–174.

Rumisha, S. F., Smith, T., Abdulla, S., Masanja, H., & Vounatsou, P. (2014). Modelling heterogeneity in malaria transmission using large sparse spatial-temporal entomological data. *Global Health Action, 7*, 22682. http://dx.doi.org/10.3402/gha.v7.22,682.

Salazar, E., Sansó, B., Finley, A., Hammerling, D., Steinsland, I., Wang, X. (2011). Comparing and blending regional climate model prediction for the American southwest. *Journal of Agricultural, Biological, and Environmental Statistics, 16*, 586–605.

Smith, B. J. (2007). boa: An R package for MCMC output convergence assessment and posterior inference. *Journal of Statistical Software, 21*(11), 1–37.

Spiegelhalter, D. J., Best, N. G., Carlin, B. P., & Van Der Linde, A. (2002). Bayesian measures of model complexity and fit (with discussion). *Journal of the Royal Statistical Society, Series B, 64*, 583–639.

Ver Hoef, J. M., & Jansen, J. K. (2007). Space-time zero-inflated count models of harbor seals. *Environmetrics, 18*, 697–712.

Wang, X., Chen, M. H., Kuo, R. C., & Dey, D. K. (2015). Bayesian spatial-temporal modeling of ecological zero-inflated count data. *Statistica Sinica, 25*, 189–204.

Wang, X., & Dey, D. K. (2010). Generalized extreme value regression for binary response data: An application to B2B electronic payments system adoption. *Annals of Applied Statistics, 4*(4), 2000–2023.

West, M., & Harrison, J. (1997). *Bayesian forecasting and dynamic models* (2nd ed.). Berlin: Springer.

Whittle, P. (1954). On stationary processes in the plane. *Biometrika, 41(3/4)*, 434–449.

Wikle, C. K., & Anderson, C. J. (2003). Climatological analysis of tornado report counts using a hierarchical Bayesian spatiotemporal model. *Journal of Geophysical Research (Atmospheres), 108*, 9005–9019.

Bias-Corrected Estimators of Scalar Skew Normal

Guoyi Zhang and Rong Liu

Abstract One problem of a skew normal model is the difficulty in estimating the shape parameter, for which the maximum likelihood estimate may be infinite when sample size is moderate. The existing estimators suffer from large bias even for moderate size samples. In this paper, we proposed five estimators of the shape parameter for a scalar skew normal model, either by bias correction method or by solving a modified score equation. Simulation studies show that except bootstrap estimator, the proposed estimators have smaller bias compared to those estimators in literature for small and moderate samples.

1 Introduction

The skew normal $Y \sim SN(\mu, \sigma, \lambda)$ is a class of distributions that includes the normal distribution ($\lambda = 0$) as a special case. Its density function is as follows

$$f(y; \lambda, \mu, \sigma) = \frac{2}{\sigma}\phi\left(\frac{y-\mu}{\sigma}\right)\Phi\left(\lambda \cdot \frac{y-\mu}{\sigma}\right),$$

where ϕ and Φ are the $N(0, 1)$ density and distribution function, parameters μ, σ and λ regulate location, scale and shape respectively. The distribution is positively or negatively asymmetric, in agreement with the sign of λ.

Azzalini (1985, 1986) introduced scalar skew normal problem and derived properties of the scalar skew normal density function. Generalization to the multivariate case is given by Azzalini and Dalla Valle (1996), Azzalini and Capitanio (1999), and Azzalini (2005, 2011). The skew t family has been investigated by Branco and Dey (2001), Azzalini and Capitanio (2003), Gupta (2003) and Lagos-Álvarez and

G. Zhang (✉)
Department of Mathematics and Statistics, University of New Mexico, Albuquerque, NM 87131-0001, USA
e-mail: gzhang123@gmail.com

R. Liu
Department of Mathematics and Statistics, University of Toledo, Toledo, OH 43606, USA
e-mail: rong.liu@utoledo.edu

Z. Jin et al. (eds.), *New Developments in Statistical Modeling, Inference and Application*, ICSA Book Series in Statistics, DOI 10.1007/978-3-319-42571-9_11

Jiménez-Gamero (2012). Based on the method introduced by Firth (1993), Sartori (2006) investigated bias prevention of the maximum likelihood estimate (MLE) for scalar skew normal and t distribution. If the MLE is subject to a positive bias $b(\lambda)$ (true for skew normal), Firth (1993) suggested shifting the score function $U(\lambda)$ downward by an amount of $U'(\lambda)b(\lambda)$ at each point of λ (illustrated in Fig. 1) to derive a modified score function $U(\lambda) + U'(\lambda)b(\lambda)$. It is proved by Firth (1993) that bias of the MLE could be reduced by modifying the score function. Bayes and Branco (2007) developed a simple closed form for the bias correction factor suggested by Sartori (2006) through a rescaled logistic distribution. Azzalini and Arellano-Valle (2013) formulated a general frame work for penalization of the log-likelihood function and proposed maximum penalized likelihood estimate (MPLE) to correct some undesirable behavior of the MLE. Genton (2004) gives a general overview of the skew distributions and their applications.

The existing work of skew normal and t distribution mainly include the bias prevention estimators: Sartori (2006)'s estimator (call $\tilde{\lambda}_1$), Bayes and Branco (2007)'s estimator (call $\tilde{\lambda}_2$) and Azzalini and Arellano-Valle (2013)'s estimator (call $\tilde{\lambda}_3$). With a moderate sample $n = 20$, and shape parameter $\lambda = 10$, the probability that all observations are nonnegative reaches 52.5 %, for which MLE $= \infty$ and bias is ∞ as well. For such situations, $\tilde{\lambda}_1$, $\tilde{\lambda}_2$ and $\tilde{\lambda}_3$ provided finite solutions for the shape parameter λ, but with large bias. For example, simulations from Sartori (2006) show that under the setting with $\lambda = 10, n = 20$, bias of $\tilde{\lambda}_1$ reached -5.897. Similar results can be found from $\tilde{\lambda}_2$ and $\tilde{\lambda}_3$. The bias prevention estimators work well only for large samples.

In this paper, we proposed five estimators for the shape parameter λ from different perspectives: bias correction approach and score function modification approach. This paper is organized as follows. In Sect. 2, we give a background review of Sartori (2006)'s bias prevention estimator, Bayes and Branco (2007)'s approximation estimator and Azzalini and Arellano-Valle (2013)'s MPLE. In Sect. 3, we propose five estimators. In Sect. 4, we perform simulation studies and compare the proposed estimators with those reviewed in Sect. 2. Section 5 gives conclusions.

2 Background

Let $Z_1, Z_2, \cdots, Z_n$ be a random sample from $SN(0, 1, \lambda)$ and let $l(\lambda)$ be the log-likelihood function denoted as

$$l(\lambda) = \text{constant} + \sum_{i=1}^{n} \log\{2\Phi(\lambda Z_i)\}.$$

Let $U(\lambda)$ be the score function of $l(\lambda)$,

$$U(\lambda) = \sum_{i=1}^{n} \frac{\phi(\lambda Z_i)}{\Phi(\lambda Z_i)} Z_i.$$

$U'(\lambda)$ can be derived as follows,

$$U'(\lambda) = -\lambda \sum_{i=1}^{n} \frac{\phi(\lambda Z_i)}{\Phi(\lambda Z_i)} Z_i^3 - \sum_{i=1}^{n} \left(\frac{\phi(\lambda Z_i)}{\Phi(\lambda Z_i)} \right)^2 Z_i^2.$$

Based on Firth (1993), Sartori (2006) modified the usual score equation $U(\lambda) = 0$ by adding an order O(1) term $M(\lambda) = E\{U'(\lambda)b(\lambda)\}$ (the expected value is used to remove the first-order bias of $\hat{\lambda}$), so that the modified score equation is

$$U(\lambda) + M(\lambda) = 0. \tag{1}$$

Sartori's estimator $\tilde{\lambda}_1$ is the solution of Eq. (1) after replacing $M(\lambda)$ by $M_1(\lambda)$ as follows,

$$M_1(\lambda) = -\frac{\lambda}{2} \cdot \frac{a_{42}(\lambda)}{a_{22}(\lambda)},$$

where $a_{kh}(\lambda) = E\left\{ Z^k \left(\frac{\phi(\lambda Z)}{\Phi(\lambda Z)} \right)^h \right\}$, and the expected values need to be numerically computed.

Bayes and Branco (2007)'s estimator is the solution of Eq. (1) after replacing $M(\lambda)$ by

$$M_2(\lambda) = -\frac{3\lambda}{2} \left(1 + \frac{8\lambda^2}{\pi^2} \right)^{-1},$$

where $M_2(\lambda)$ is a simple closed form approximation of $M_1(\lambda)$ using a rescaled logistic distribution.

Azzalini and Arellano-Valle (2013) proposed MPLE $\tilde{\lambda}_3$. They replace $M(\lambda)$ in Eq. (1) by

$$M_3(\lambda) = -2C_1C_2 \frac{\lambda}{1 + C_2\lambda^2}, \tag{2}$$

where $C_1 = 0.875913, C_2 = 0.856250$. It is easy to see that $M_1(\lambda) \approx M_2(\lambda) \approx M_3(\lambda) = O(\lambda^{-1})$. Hence, the finite solution of λ exists for all of the three methods. It can be shown that for $\tilde{\lambda}_1, \tilde{\lambda}_2$ and $\tilde{\lambda}_3$, $E(\tilde{\lambda}_i - \lambda) = O(n^{-2})$.

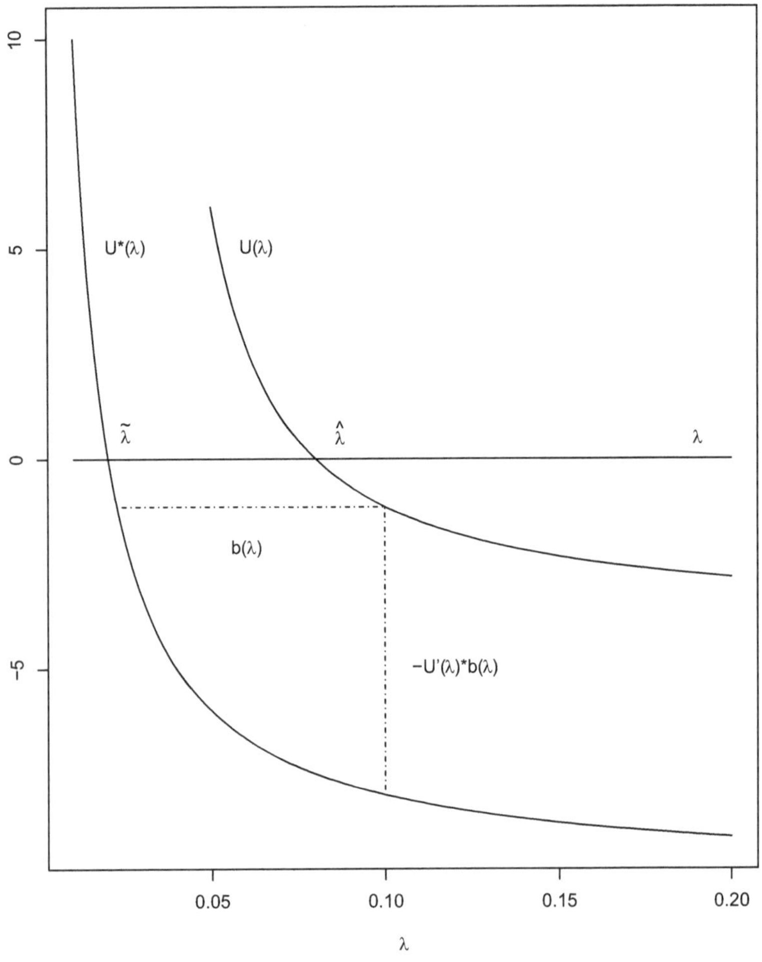

Fig. 1 Modifications of the unbiased score function

3 Bias Reduction Techniques for Scalar Skew Normal

All the three estimators $\tilde{\lambda}_1, \tilde{\lambda}_2$ and $\tilde{\lambda}_3$ suffer from large bias when the sample size is small or moderate. One intuitive way is to estimate the bias and subtract the bias from the estimator. Also notice the systematic negative bias of the three estimators from simulation studies, we propose adjusting the score function to offset the systematic trend. We also examined jackknife and bootstrap bias correction methods for comparison purpose.

3.1 Bias Correction for MLE and $\tilde{\lambda}_3$

For a general MLE $\hat{\lambda}$, it is well known that $\hat{\lambda}$ is consistent with asymptotic distribution

$$\sqrt{n}(\hat{\lambda} - \lambda) \xrightarrow{d} N(0, i(\lambda)^{-1}), n \to \infty,$$

where $i(\lambda)$ is the expected Fisher information for a single observation. Consider the second order expression for the mean of the limiting distribution of $\hat{\lambda}$,

$$0 = U(\hat{\lambda}) = U(\lambda) + (\hat{\lambda} - \lambda)U'(\lambda) + \frac{1}{2}(\hat{\lambda} - \lambda)^2 U''(\lambda) + O_p(n^{-\frac{1}{2}}). \tag{3}$$

Taking expectations through (3), we obtain

$$\begin{aligned} &E(\hat{\lambda} - \lambda)E\left\{U'(\lambda)\right\} + \text{cov}(\hat{\lambda}, U'(\lambda)) \\ &\quad + \frac{1}{2}E(\hat{\lambda} - \lambda)^2 E\{U''(\lambda)\} + \frac{1}{2}\text{cov}\{(\hat{\lambda} - \lambda)^2, U''(\lambda)\} \\ &= O(n^{-\frac{1}{2}}). \end{aligned}$$

Let l_2 be the log-likelihood for one single observation. For convenience, define

$$K_{rs}(\lambda) = E[\{l_2'(\lambda)\}^r \{l_2''(\lambda) + i(\lambda)\}^s].$$

We can show that

$$E\{l_2'''(\lambda)\} = -3K_{11}(\lambda) - K_{30}(\lambda),$$

$$\text{cov}\{\hat{\lambda}, U'(\lambda)\} = o(n^{-1}),$$

and

$$\text{cov}\{(\hat{\lambda} - \lambda)^2, U''(\lambda)\} = o(n^{-1}).$$

For detailed derivation of the above equations in this section, please refer to Cox and Hinkley (1974, p. 309) and Cox and Snell (1968). Some manipulation then gives

$$\begin{aligned} b(\lambda) = E(\hat{\lambda} - \lambda) &= -\frac{K_{11}(\lambda) + K_{30}(\lambda)}{2ni^2(\lambda)} + o(n^{-1}) \\ &= \frac{1}{2} \cdot \frac{\lambda a_{42}(\lambda)}{na_{22}^2(\lambda)} + o(n^{-1}). \end{aligned}$$

The proposed bias-corrected MLE takes the form of

$$\hat{\lambda}_{\text{bc}} = \hat{\lambda} - b(\hat{\lambda}), \tag{4}$$

with $b(\lambda) = \lambda a_{42}(\lambda)/2na_{22}^2(\lambda)$. If the MLE does not exist, the bias prevention estimator $\tilde{\lambda}_1$ will be used instead.

Now, we consider bias correction of the estimator $\tilde{\lambda}_3$. Recall that $\tilde{\lambda}_3$ is the MPLE proposed by Azzalini and Arellano-Valle (2013). Let

$$U^*(\lambda) = U(\lambda) + M_3(\lambda), \tag{5}$$

where $M_3(\lambda)$ is defined as in Eq. (2). Take derivative of $U^*(\lambda)$, we have

$$U^{*'}(\lambda) = U'(\lambda) + M_3'(\lambda),$$

where $M_3'(\lambda) = -2C_1C_2(1 - C_2\lambda^2)/(1 + C_2\lambda^2)^2$. It is easy to show that $M_3(\lambda) = O(\lambda^{-1})$ and $M_3'(\lambda) = O(\lambda^{-2})$. Applying Taylor theorem for $U^*(\tilde{\lambda}_3)$ at the neighborhood of λ, we have

$$0 = U^*(\tilde{\lambda}_3) = U^*(\lambda) + U^{*'}(\lambda)(\tilde{\lambda}_3 - \lambda). \tag{6}$$

Replacing $U^{*'}(\lambda)$ by $E\{U^{*'}(\lambda)\}$ and use the fact that $ni(\lambda) = -E\{U'(\lambda)\}$, $\tilde{\lambda}_3 - \lambda$ can be expressed as the following,

$$\begin{aligned} \tilde{\lambda}_3 - \lambda &= -\frac{U^*(\lambda)}{E\{U^{*'}(\lambda)\}} \\ &= \frac{U(\lambda) + M_3(\lambda)}{ni(\lambda) - M_3'(\lambda)}. \end{aligned} \tag{7}$$

Using the result in Eq. (7) and take expectation through Eq. (6), we have

$$\begin{aligned} 0 &= E\{U^*(\lambda)\} + E\{U^{*'}(\lambda)\}E(\tilde{\lambda}_3 - \lambda) + \operatorname{cov}\{U^{*'}(\lambda), \tilde{\lambda}_3 - \lambda\} \\ &= M_3(\lambda) + \{M_3'(\lambda) - na_{22}(\lambda)\}E(\tilde{\lambda}_3 - \lambda) \\ &+ \frac{1}{na_{22}(\lambda) - M_3'(\lambda)}\{-n(\lambda a_{42}(\lambda) + a_{33}(\lambda))\}. \end{aligned}$$

Therefore, the bias of $\tilde{\lambda}_3$ is

$$\begin{aligned} E(\tilde{\lambda}_3 - \lambda) &= \frac{\dfrac{\lambda na_{42}(\lambda) + na_{33}(\lambda)}{na_{22}(\lambda) - M_3'} - M_3}{M_3' - na_{22}(\lambda)} \\ &= -\frac{\lambda na_{42}(\lambda) + na_{33}(\lambda) + M_3'M_3 - na_{22}(\lambda)M_3}{(M_3' - na_{22}(\lambda))^2}. \end{aligned}$$

The proposed bias-corrected $\tilde{\lambda}_3$ takes the form of

$$\tilde{\lambda}_{\text{SC}} = \tilde{\lambda}_3 - b(\tilde{\lambda}_3), \tag{8}$$

with $b(\tilde{\lambda}_3) = -\left\{\lambda n a_{42}(\lambda) + n a_{33}(\lambda) + M_3' M_3 - n a_{22}(\lambda) M_3\right\} / (M_3' - n a_{22}(\lambda))^2$.

3.2 *Adjusted Estimator*

Considering Fig. 1, $U(\lambda)$ cross the x-axis when Z_is are with opposite sign numbers ($\hat{\lambda}$ exists); and $U(\lambda)$ approaches x-axis without crossing it when Z_is are all positive or all negative ($\hat{\lambda} = \pm\infty$). For $\hat{\lambda} = \pm\infty$ cases, the bias prevention idea is to shift the score function by an amount of $\{-U'(\lambda)b(\lambda)\}$ to force it cross the x-axis to obtain a finite MLE. From simulation studies, we have noticed systematic negative biases of the three estimators $\tilde{\lambda}_1, \tilde{\lambda}_2$ and $\tilde{\lambda}_3$. This means that the amount of shift $\{-U'(\lambda)b(\lambda)\}$ is too large for the three estimators. Therefore it should be reduced by a certain amount to allow the score function $U(\lambda)$ cross the x-axis but produce less bias. We propose adding $M_4(\lambda)$ to the score function $U(\lambda)$, so that

$$U(\lambda) + M_4(\lambda) = 0, \tag{9}$$

where

$$M_4(\lambda) = -\frac{n}{n + d\lambda} \cdot \frac{\lambda a_{42}(\lambda)}{2a_{22}(\lambda)}.$$

Define a constant c such as

$$c = \sup\{d | U(\lambda^*) + M_4(\lambda^*) = 0, \text{where} \quad \lambda^* \quad \text{has negative bias}\}. \tag{10}$$

We can see that for any fixed d and λ, $|M_4(\lambda)| < |M_1(\lambda)|$, i.e. the shifted amount $M_4(\lambda)$ of the score function is smaller than that of $\tilde{\lambda}_1$. As $n \to \infty, n/(n + d\lambda) \to 1$, hence $M_4(\lambda) \longrightarrow M_1(\lambda)$. Equation (10) indicates that $d \in [0, c]$, and that we are looking for a constant c such that λ^* has the smallest negative bias (close to the true value). The proposed adjusted estimator $\tilde{\lambda}_{ad}$ naturally follows as the solution of Eq. (11),

$$U(\lambda) + M_5(\lambda) = 0, \tag{11}$$

with $M_5(\lambda) = -\frac{n}{n + c\lambda} \cdot \frac{\lambda a_{42}(\lambda)}{2a_{22}(\lambda)}$. The following theorem can be derived.

Theorem 1. *The adjusted estimator $\tilde{\lambda}_{ad}$ has the following properties: (1) $\tilde{\lambda}_{ad}$ has finite solution; (2) $Bias(\tilde{\lambda}_{ad}) = O(n^{-2})$; and (3) $\tilde{\lambda}_{ad}$ converges in probability to Sartori (2006)'s estimator $\tilde{\lambda}_1$ as $n \to \infty$, i.e., $\tilde{\lambda}_{ad} \xrightarrow{p} \tilde{\lambda}_1$.*

Proof. Proof follows from Sartori (2006).

3.3 Jackknife and Bootstrap Bias Correction

Following Lagos-Álvarez et al. (2011) for bias correction in the Type I generalized logistic distribution, we consider jackknife and bootstrap bias correction. The jackknife was introduced by Quenouille (1949, 1956) to reduce bias of estimators. Shao and Tu (1995) discussed several forms of the jackknife. The bootstrap was introduced by Efron (1990) for estimating the sampling distribution of a statistic and its characteristics. Both jackknife and bootstrap are popularly used since then. In the following, we will consider delete-1 jackknife and bootstrap bias correction of the estimator $\tilde{\lambda}_3$.

Recall that $Z_1, Z_2, \cdots, Z_n$ is a random sample from $SN(0, 1, \lambda)$. Let $\tilde{\lambda}_{3(i)}$ be the solution of the equation

$$U(\lambda) + M_3(\lambda) = 0, \tag{12}$$

with observation Z_i deleted. Define $\bar{\tilde{\lambda}}_3 = \sum_{i=1}^{n} \tilde{\lambda}_{3(i)}/n$. The jackknife bias is defined as $\widehat{bias}_{jack} = (n-1)(\bar{\tilde{\lambda}}_3 - \tilde{\lambda}_3)$ and the jackknife bias-corrected estimator of λ is

$$\tilde{\lambda}_{jack} = \tilde{\lambda}_3 - \widehat{bias}_{jack} = n\tilde{\lambda}_3 - (n-1)\bar{\tilde{\lambda}}_3. \tag{13}$$

For bootstrap bias correction, we use nonparametric bootstrap to approximate the bias of $\tilde{\lambda}_3$. First, we draw B independent bootstrap samples from $Z_1, Z_2, \cdots, Z_n$ with replacement. Let $Z_1^{(i)}, Z_2^{(i)}, \cdots, Z_n^{(i)}, i = 1, \cdots, B$, be the ith bootstrap sample, and $\tilde{\lambda}_3^{(i)}$ be the solution of Eq. (12) with the ith bootstrap samples. The bias can be estimated as follows

$$\widehat{bias}_{boot} = \frac{\sum_{b=1}^{B} \tilde{\lambda}_3^{(i)}}{B} - \tilde{\lambda}_3.$$

The bootstrap bias-corrected estimator of λ is

$$\tilde{\lambda}_{boot} = \tilde{\lambda}_3 - \widehat{bias}_{boot} = 2\tilde{\lambda}_3 - \sum_{b=1}^{B} \tilde{\lambda}_3^{(i)}/B. \tag{14}$$

4 Simulation Studies

In this section, a small simulation study was conducted to evaluate the five proposed estimators. We consider the shape parameter $\lambda = 5$ and $\lambda = 10$, and generate 2000 skew normal $SN(\lambda)$ samples with sizes $n = 5, 10, 20, 50$ and 100. For each generated sample, the following estimators and their bias were computed: $\tilde{\lambda}_1$ Sartori (2006), $\tilde{\lambda}_2$ Bayes and Branco (2007), $\tilde{\lambda}_3$ Azzalini and Arellano-Valle (2013), $\hat{\lambda}_{\mathrm{bc}}$ (bias-corrected MLE), $\tilde{\lambda}_{\mathrm{SC}}$ (bias-corrected $\tilde{\lambda}_3$), $\tilde{\lambda}_{\mathrm{ad}}$ (adjusted estimator), $\tilde{\lambda}_{jack}$ (jackknife bias-corrected estimator) and $\tilde{\lambda}_{boot}$ (bootstrap bias-corrected estimator). The adjusted estimator $\tilde{\lambda}_{\mathrm{ad}}$ is calculated as the solution of (9) with $d = 2$, which is found by a comparison of several numbers of d in reducing the bias and was used to approximate the constant c in (10). Empirical mean bias, mean variance and mean MSE (mean square error) are reported by Tables 1, 2 and 3 respectively. Notice that the three estimators $\tilde{\lambda}_1$, $\tilde{\lambda}_2$ and $\tilde{\lambda}_3$ perform similarly without any noticeable difference in bias and variance.

Tables 1, 2 and 3 show that except bootstrap method, all the four proposals work very well for small and medium samples ($n \leq 20$) in bias reduction. For large samples, the existing methods work better. We also notice that bias correction is more needed for samples with large shape parameter. From MSE perspective, only $\tilde{\lambda}_{sc}$ is admissible for small and moderate samples. We think that there is still room to improve $\tilde{\lambda}_{\mathrm{ad}}$. In simulation study, we used $d = 2$ to approximate the constant c defined in (10). Future research may consider looking for a better approximation of the constant c.

5 Conclusions

The difficulty of the shape parameter estimation in a scalar skew normal model lies in the fact that there is a considerable percentage of samples in which MLE goes to infinity. The bias prevention estimators in literature are based on large sample properties. They do not work well for small and moderate samples. In this research, we have studied this problem from different perspectives, such as bias correction approach and score function modification approach. Simulation studies show that $\hat{\lambda}_{\mathrm{bc}}$ (bias-corrected MLE), $\tilde{\lambda}_{\mathrm{SC}}$ (bias-corrected $\tilde{\lambda}_3$),$\tilde{\lambda}_{\mathrm{ad}}$ (adjusted estimator) and $\tilde{\lambda}_{jack}$ (jackknife bias-corrected estimator) are all effective in reducing bias for small and moderate samples. However, the price paid for reduced bias is the relatively large variance. For scalar skew normal shape parameter estimation, if sample size is large, the existing estimators $\tilde{\lambda}_1$, $\tilde{\lambda}_2$, $\tilde{\lambda}_3$ all work well, there is no need to perform bias correction; if sample size is small or moderate, we suggest using the proposed estimators $\tilde{\lambda}_{\mathrm{SC}}$ since it has smaller bias and MSE.

Acknowledgements The authors thank the referees for their constructive and insightful comments and suggestions to improve the manuscript.

Table 1 Bias comparison among eight estimators: $\tilde{\lambda}_1$ (Sartori 2006), $\tilde{\lambda}_2$ (Bayes and Branco 2007), $\tilde{\lambda}_3$ (Azzalini and Arellano-Valle 2013), $\hat{\lambda}_{\text{bc}}$ (bias-corrected MLE), $\tilde{\lambda}_{\text{sc}}$ (bias-corrected $\tilde{\lambda}_3$), $\tilde{\lambda}_{\text{ad}}$ (adjusted estimator), $\tilde{\lambda}_{jack}$ (jackknife estimator) and $\tilde{\lambda}_{boot}$ (bootstrap estimator)

λ	n	Bias comparison								$(\hat{\lambda} < +\infty)$ %	Theoretical %
		$\tilde{\lambda}_1$	$\tilde{\lambda}_2$	$\tilde{\lambda}_3$	$\hat{\lambda}_{\text{bc}}$	$\tilde{\lambda}_{\text{sc}}$	$\tilde{\lambda}_{\text{ad}}$	$\tilde{\lambda}_{jack}$	$\tilde{\lambda}_{boot}$		
5	5	−3.8367	−3.8378	−3.8169	1.5487	−2.8557	−0.6169	−3.0074	−3.8370	29.45	27.70
	10	−2.9321	−2.9799	−2.9317	2.2052	−1.9755	0.1329	−1.4557	−3.0246	49.30	47.73
	20	−1.7206	−1.7886	−1.6813	1.5455	−0.5224	−0.0725	0.2866	−1.9125	74.45	72.68
	50	−0.2506	−0.4367	−0.3167	0.8166	0.7034	0.3035	0.6606	−0.8950	95.20	96.10
	100	0.0130	−0.0455	−0.0139	0.2286	0.6055	0.1164	0.1411	−0.5138	99.85	99.84
10	5	−8.7893	−8.8078	−8.7728	−2.0213	−7.7877	−4.2517	−7.8898	−8.7821	14.70	14.88
	10	−7.7206	−7.8064	−7.6863	−0.4815	−6.6637	−3.4285	−5.8375	−7.8352	27.85	27.55
	20	−5.9499	−6.0674	−5.8859	0.7907	−4.3533	−2.6139	−2.8286	−6.1351	47.65	47.52
	50	−2.5310	−2.8728	−2.5830	0.6848	−0.3144	−0.5205	1.3768	−3.0968	81.40	80.05
	100	−0.5412	−0.7596	−0.5230	0.7716	1.3282	0.2560	0.6022	−1.3407	95.90	96.02

The last two columns are the estimated percentage of $\hat{\lambda} < \infty$ samples and the theoretical percentage respectively

Table 2 Variance comparison among eight estimators: $\tilde{\lambda}_1$ (Sartori 2006), $\tilde{\lambda}_2$ (Bayes and Branco 2007), $\tilde{\lambda}_3$ (Azzalini and Arellano-Valle 2013), $\hat{\lambda}_{bc}$ (bias-corrected MLE), $\tilde{\lambda}_{sc}$ (bias-corrected $\tilde{\lambda}_3$), $\tilde{\lambda}_{ad}$ (adjusted estimator), $\tilde{\lambda}_{jack}$ (jackknife estimator) and $\tilde{\lambda}_{boot}$ (bootstrap estimator)

		Variance comparison							
λ	n	$\tilde{\lambda}_1$	$\tilde{\lambda}_2$	$\tilde{\lambda}_3$	$\hat{\lambda}_{bc}$	$\tilde{\lambda}_{sc}$	$\tilde{\lambda}_{ad}$	$\tilde{\lambda}_{jack}$	$\tilde{\lambda}_{boot}$
5	5	0.0733	0.0675	0.0781	49.9059	0.1746	32.115	0.4369	0.0778
	10	0.3078	0.2815	0.3002	52.8567	0.7884	39.1468	2.5469	0.3582
	20	1.1035	0.9790	1.1616	42.6702	2.7217	16.1576	8.3396	1.2477
	50	3.3111	2.4887	2.7447	15.4587	5.6216	8.5271	16.6452	2.7521
	100	2.5556	2.2694	2.5770	3.9826	3.7198	3.0563	8.9424	2.4476
10	5	0.0567	0.0569	0.0570	60.5340	0.1472	45.0309	0.3815	0.0625
	10	0.3970	0.2752	0.3695	69.2983	0.9511	47.9203	2.9509	0.4101
	20	1.3551	1.2935	1.5519	65.8202	4.2194	34.7103	10.7657	1.7632
	50	6.6020	5.0796	6.1174	41.4082	14.0655	27.7209	40.6141	7.2765
	100	11.4856	10.5395	10.8033	27.2896	23.5940	20.3222	37.6914	13.2780

Table 3 MSE comparison among eight estimators: $\tilde{\lambda}_1$ (Sartori 2006), $\tilde{\lambda}_2$ (Bayes and Branco 2007), $\tilde{\lambda}_3$ (Azzalini and Arellano-Valle 2013), $\hat{\lambda}_{bc}$ (bias-corrected MLE), $\tilde{\lambda}_{sc}$ (bias-corrected $\tilde{\lambda}_3$),$\tilde{\lambda}_{ad}$ (adjusted estimator), $\tilde{\lambda}_{jack}$ (jackknife estimator) and $\tilde{\lambda}_{boot}$ (bootstrap estimator)

		Mean square errors comparison							
λ	n	$\tilde{\lambda}_1$	$\tilde{\lambda}_2$	$\tilde{\lambda}_3$	$\hat{\lambda}_{bc}$	$\tilde{\lambda}_{sc}$	$\tilde{\lambda}_{ad}$	$\tilde{\lambda}_{jack}$	$\tilde{\lambda}_{boot}$
5	5	14.7938	14.7969	14.6470	52.2797	8.3296	32.4795	9.4817	14.801
	10	8.9050	9.1615	8.8955	57.6934	4.6910	39.1449	4.6647	9.5066
	20	4.0637	4.1777	3.9881	46.4340	2.9933	16.1548	8.4176	4.9049
	50	3.3722	2.6783	2.8437	16.1178	6.1136	8.6150	17.0733	3.5518
	100	2.5545	2.2703	2.5759	4.0328	4.0847	3.0684	8.9534	2.7092
10	5	77.3094	77.6356	77.0203	64.5895	60.7964	63.0859	62.6313	77.1880
	10	60.0059	61.2160	59.4488	69.4955	45.3560	59.6515	37.0267	61.8014
	20	36.7557	38.1067	36.1955	66.4125	23.1692	41.5257	18.7614	39.4021
	50	13.0050	13.3305	12.7865	41.8565	14.1574	27.9780	42.4897	16.8631
	100	11.7729	11.1113	11.0714	27.8714	25.3464	20.3776	38.0165	15.0624

References

Azzalini, A. (1985). A class of distributions which includes the normal ones. *Scandinavian Journal of Statistics, 12*, 171–178.

Azzalini, A. (1986). Further results on a class of distributions which includes the normal ones. *Statistica, 46*, 199–208.

Azzalini, A. (2005). The skew-normal distribution and related multivariate families (with discussion). *Scandinavian Journal of Statistics, 32*, 159–188.

Azzalini, A. (2011). Skew-normal distribution. *International Encyclopedia of Statistical Sciences, 19*, 1342–1344.

Azzalini, A., & Arellano-Valle, R. B. (2013). Maximum penalized likelihood estimation for skew-normal and skew-t distributions. *Journal of Statistical Planning and Inference, 143*, 419–433.
Azzalini, A., & Capitanio, A. (1999). Statistical applications of the multivariate skew normal distribution. *Journal of the Royal Statistical Society: Series B, 61*, 579–602.
Azzalini, A., & Capitanio, A. (2003). Distributions generated by perturbation of symmetry with emphasis on a multivariate skew t distribution. *Journal of the Royal Statistical Society: Series B, 65*, 367–389.
Azzalini, A., & Dalla Valle, A. (1996). The multivariate skew normal distribution. *Biometrika, 83*, 715–726.
Bayes, C. L., & Branco, M. D. (2007). Bayesian inference for the skewness parameter of the scalar skew-normal distribution. *Brazilian Journal of Probability and Statistics, 21*, 141–163.
Branco, M. D., & Dey, D. K. (2001). A general class of multivariate skew-elliptical distributions. *Journal of Multivariate Analysis, 79*, 99–113.
Cox, D. R., & Hinkley, D. V. (1974). *Theoretical statistics.* Boca Raton, FL: Chapman & Hall/CRC.
Cox, D. R., & Snell, E. J. (1968). A general definition of residuals. *Journal of the Royal Statistical Society: Series B, 30*, 248–275
Efron, B. (1990). More efficient bootstrap computations. *Journal of the American Statistical Association, 85*, 79–89.
Firth, D. (1993). Bias reduction of maximum likelihood estimates. *Biometrika, 80*, 27–38.
Genton, M. G. (2004). *Skew-elliptical distributions and their applications: A journey beyond normality*. Boca Raton, FL: Chapman & Hall/CRC.
Gupta, A. K. (2003). Multivariate skew t-distribution. *Statistics, 37*, 359–363.
Lagos-Álvarez, B., & Jiménez-Gamero, M. D. (2012). A note on bias reduction of maximum likelihood estimates for the scalar skew t distribution. *Journal of Statistical Planning and Inference, 142*, 608–612.
Lagos-Álvarez, B., Jiménez-Gamero, M. D., & Alba Fernández, M. (2011). Bias correction in the type I generalized logistic distribution. *Communication in Statistics-Simulation and Computation, 40*, 511–531.
Quenouille, M. H. (1949). Problems in plane sampling. *Annals of Mathematical Statistics, 20*, 355–375.
Quenouille, M. H. (1956). Notes on bias in estimation. *Biometrika, 43*, 353–360.
Sartori, N. (2006). Bias prevention of maximum likelihood estimates for scalar skew normal and skew t distributions. *Journal of Statistical Planning and Inference, 136*, 4259–4275.
Shao, J., & Tu, D. (1995). *The jackknife and bootstrap.* New York: Springer.

MIX
Papier aus verantwortungsvollen Quellen
Paper from responsible sources
FSC® C105338

If you have any concerns about our products,
you can contact us on
ProductSafety@springernature.com

In case Publisher is established outside the EU,
the EU authorized representative is:
Springer Nature Customer Service Center GmbH
Europaplatz 3, 69115 Heidelberg, Germany

Printed by Libri Plureos GmbH
in Hamburg, Germany